Xenotransplantation

Xenotransplantation

Edited by
Jeffrey L. Platt

Professor of Surgery, Immunology and Pediatrics
Head of Transplantation Biology
Mayo Clinic, Rochester, Minnesota 55905

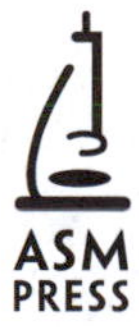

Washington, D.C.

Cover: Histology of porcine kidneys after xenotransplantation into baboons. Inset: rejected control non-transgenic kidney 30 min after transplantation. Background: transgenic porcine kidney expressing human complement regulatory proteins CD59 and decay-accelerating factor (DAF) 24 h after transplantation.

American Society for Microbiology
1752 N Street, N.W.
Washington, DC 20036-2804

Library of Congress Cataloging-in-Publication Data

Xenotransplantation / edited by Jeffrey L. Platt.
p. ; cm.
Includes bibliographical references and index.
ISBN 1-55581-167-1
1. Xenografts. 2. Transplantation immunology. I. Platt, Jeffrey L.
[DNLM: 1. Transplantation, Heterologous. WO 660 X494 2001]
QR188.8 .X45 2001
617.9′5—dc21

00-061838

Printed in the United States of America

Address editorial correspondence to: ASM Press, 1752 N St., N.W., Washington, DC 20036-2804, U.S.A.

Send orders to: ASM Press, P.O. Box 605, Herndon, VA 20172, U.S.A.
Phone: 800-546-2416; 703-661-1593
Fax: 703-661-1501
Email: books@asmusa.org
Online: www.asmpress.org

CONTENTS

CONTRIBUTORS

Rima Abu-Nader • Division of Infectious Diseases, Mayo Clinic, 200 First St., SW, Rochester, MN 55905

I. P. J. Alwayn • Transplantation Biology Research Center, Massachusetts General Hospital/Harvard Medical School, MGH-East, Bldg. 149-9019, 13th St., Boston, MA 02129

M. R. Basker • Transplantation Biology Research Center, Massachusetts General Hospital/Harvard Medical School, MGH-East, Bldg. 149-9019, 13th St., Boston, MA 02129

Thierry Berney • Diabetes Research Institute, University of Miami School of Medicine, 1450 NW 10th Ave., Miami, FL 33136

L. Bühler • Transplantation Biology Research Center, Massachusetts General Hospital/Harvard Medical School, MGH-East, Bldg. 149-9019, 13th St., Boston, MA 02129

Louisa E. Chapman • Retrovirus Diseases Branch, Division of AIDS, STD, and TB Laboratory Research, National Center for Infectious Diseases, Centers for Disease Control and Prevention, Mailstop G-19, 1600 Clifton Rd., NE, Atlanta, GA 30333

Rodica Ciubotariu • Department of Pathology, College of Physicians and Surgeons of Columbia University, 630 West 168th St., P&S 14-401, New York, NY 10032

Adriana Colovai • Department of Pathology, College of Physicians and Surgeons of Columbia University, 630 West 168th St., P&S 14-401, New York, NY 10032

D. K. C. Cooper • Transplantation Biology Research Center, Massachusetts General Hospital/Harvard Medical School, MGH-East, Bldg. 149-9019, 13th St., Boston, MA 02129

Raffaello Cortesini • Department of Surgery, Servizio Trapianti d'Organo, Istituto di II Clinica Chirurgia, Università Degli Studi di Roma "La Sapienza," Rome, Italy

Agustin P. Dalmasso • Department of Surgery and Department of Laboratory Medicine and Pathology, University of Minnesota Medical School, Minneapolis, MN 55455

Roger W. Evans • 2251 Baihly Hills Dr., S.W., Rochester, MN 55902

Jay A. Fishman • Infectious Disease Division and Transplantation Unit, Massachusetts General Hospital and Harvard Medical School, 55 Fruit St., Boston, MA 02114

Michael M. Frank • Department of Pediatrics and Department of Immunology, Duke University Medical Center, Durham, NC 27710

Ronald G. Gill • Barbara Davis Center for Childhood Diabetes, University of Colorado Health Sciences Center, 4200 East 9th Ave., Box B-140, Denver, CO 80262

Luca Inverardi • Diabetes Research Institute, University of Miami School of Medicine, 1450 NW 10th Ave., Miami, FL 33136

Peter J. Matthews • 10046 161st St., Chippewa Falls, WI 54729

Marian G. Michaels • Division of Allergy, Immunology, and Infectious Diseases, University of Pittsburgh School of Medicine, and The Children's Hospital of Pittsburgh, Pittsburgh, PA 15213

B. Paul Morgan • Complement Biology Group, University of Wales College of Medicine, Heath Park, Cardiff CF14 4XN, Wales, U.K.

Carlos V. Paya • Division of Infectious Diseases, Mayo Clinic, 200 First St., SW, Rochester, MN 55905

Antonello Pileggi • Diabetes Research Institute, University of Miami School of Medicine, 1450 NW 10th Ave., Miami, FL 33136

Jeffrey L. Platt • Department of Surgery, Department of Immunology, and Department of Pediatrics, Mayo Clinic, 2-66 Medical Sciences Building, Rochester, MN 55905

D. H. Sachs • Transplantation Biology Research Center, Massachusetts General Hospital/Harvard Medical School, MGH-East, Bldg. 149-9019, 13th St., Boston, MA 02129

Nicole Suciu-Foca • Department of Pathology, College of Physicians and Surgeons of Columbia University, 630 West 168th St., P&S 14-401, New York, NY 10032

Eric Wagner • Department of Pediatrics and Department of Surgery, Duke University Medical Center, Durham, NC 27710; *present address*, Division of Hematology-Oncology, Ste. Justine Hospital, Montreal Quebec H3T 1C5, Canada

Robin A. Weiss • Windeyer Institute of Medical Sciences, University College London, 46 Cleveland St., London W1P 6DB, United Kingdom

PREFACE

The diversity of species in animals, plants, and microbial organisms reflects, in part, the ways in which species use each other to thrive. The coevolution of mitochondria and the eukaryotic cell host, the mutual survival of gut microorganisms and coelomates, and the interactions of an ancient retrovirus with a primordial host species that gave rise to the recombinase activity needed for the evolution of lymphocyte diversity—these all speak to the evolutionary mechanisms by which interactions between species allow individuals to adapt. It may be thought that humans, having complex cultures and technologies, are less dependent on interspecies interactions to allow them to inhabit forbidding environments. However, the development of agriculture, animal husbandry, and, more recently, medical science speaks to the way in which culture uses interactions between species. In this context, xenotransplantation might be viewed as one of many experiments, some of nature and some of culture, in which our species gains a survival advantage by heterologous interactions.

Experiments of nature do not always work and usually fail. Most experiments in xenotransplantation have, to this point, failed. The main reason for failure has been the immunological reaction of the host against the graft—a subject considered extensively in this volume. Recent work in laboratories around the world has provided keen insights into the basis for this immunological reaction and has sparked new hope that the reaction can be suppressed or prevented.

If the immunological response of the transplant recipient can be overcome as a hurdle to xenotransplantation, then the next hurdle of importance would be the physiologic properties of the graft: will the graft function appropriately in the foreign environment? Indeed, there is much concern that xenografts of certain types may not function appropriately and may be exceedingly difficult to justify on a physiologic basis. However, given the widespread application of transplantation of nearly every organ system and the cleverness of those engaged in the field, it seems reasonable to think that some types of xenografts will be found that can provide physiologic function of advantage to the patient.

If xenografts, then, survive and function in the foreign host, then the next challenge will be the possibility that xenografts would transfer infectious agents from the donor species to the recipient. This question has taken a preeminent position in the field of xenotransplantation in recent years and is a subject considered in detail in this volume. In the end, though, the risk of infection in xenotransplantation may prove as much an advantage as an obstacle, for cross-species infections are significant mechanisms by which new organisms infect a species. Xenotransplantation may provide an arena that monitors, for the first time, the potential for such infections to occur. Viewed in this context, xenotransplantation may provide a further means by which our species can adapt to hostile elements in the environment.

The genesis of this book reflects, in large part, the conviction of the editor that obstacles to xenotransplantation can be turned to advantages. Gaining the most from efforts to surmount the obstacles to xenotransplantation seems to require the application of novel technologies and novel ideas. This, in turn, will spring from the recruiting of new scientists, clinicians, and others to the field. Few of the authors of this volume began their careers in the field of xenotransplantation, and, on consideration, it can be seen that the most prodigious contributions of these authors came from applying insights and skills originating outside of the field. The editor is thus grateful to this outstanding group of contributors, not only for their efforts in helping to produce this volume, but also for their many efforts to make xenotransplantation a feasible endeavor. Likewise, the editor thanks his colleagues in Minnesota and North Carolina and in so many places around the world for their energy, encouragement, and spirited support.

Jeffrey L. Platt
Transplantation Biology
Mayo Clinic
200 First Street SW
Rochester, MN 55905

Section I

INTRODUCTION

Xenotransplantation
Edited by Jeffrey L. Platt

Chapter 1

A Primer on Xenotransplantation

Jeffrey L. Platt

No area of medicine stimulates as much excitement or as much controversy as transplantation. The excitement of transplantation stems, in part, from its dramatic medical effects; transplanting kidneys, hearts, livers, and lungs potentially transforms a patient from being desperately ill to being physiologically normal. The excitement of transplantation also stems from the circumstances in which transplants are performed; in most cases transplantation brings together, by surgical means, the untimely and tragic death of one person, the transplant donor, and the near resurrection of another, the transplant recipient. The controversy over transplantation derives mainly from the shortage of donors, which limits the number of procedures to as few as 5% of those needed (30), and this requires that difficult decisions—who will receive a transplant and who will be left to suffer or to die—be made. Also controversial is the fact that transplantation is an imperfect cure, potentially leading to the transfer of infectious disease from the donor to the recipient and always requiring treatment of the recipient with pharmaceutical agents that compromise immunity.

If transplantation is exciting and controversial now, it was equally so at its inception at the turn of the 20th century. The development of the vascular anastomosis by Jaboulay, Ullman, Carrel, and Guthrie, among others, stimulated the imagination of experimental surgeons to believe that they could, at last, replace failing organs with healthy ones. In the first several years of the 20th century, vascular anastomosis led to a number of experimental transplants of organs, limbs, and even the head and neck, as well as to early clinical trials (40). In some instances, successful transplantation of organs between different individuals was claimed; however, in no case, except for autografts, was the success enduring (18). Still, Alexis Carrel was awarded the Nobel Prize in 1912 for his work on vascular suture and the transplantation of blood vessels and organs.

The first attempts to use the vascular anastomosis for the treatment of organ failure in humans was made by Ullman and Jaboulay in 1906 (47). While it was obvious then that the best source of organs for human patients would be another human, it was not clear how a human organ could be obtained. Some opined that since cells of the body survive for a period after the heart ceases to beat, the deceased should not be surgically violated. Therefore, the organs to be used for transplantation to a human subject might

Jeffrey L. Platt • Departments of Surgery, Immunology, and Pediatrics, Mayo Clinic, Rochester, MN 55905.

have to be obtained from a non-human source. Accordingly, the first efforts at clinical transplantation were conducted by connecting pig and sheep kidneys to the blood vessels of human subjects with renal failure (47, 106). These first efforts at xenotransplantation were successful from the standpoint of the vascular connection, but the kidneys failed to emit more than a few drops of urine and the procedure failed to correct the medical condition of the patients.

Most accounts of the history of transplantation credit Voronoy with the first attempt to transplant a kidney from a human donor in 1929 (12). However, the *New York Times* reported a human kidney allograft in 1911 in Philadelphia (4). The physician who performed the transplant in Philadelphia was Dr. L. J. Hammond. The transplant recipient was a patient dying of renal tuberculosis, and the donor was the victim of an automobile accident. The physicians attending to the dying patient brought the deceased donor into the hospital, harvested the kidneys, and transplanted them into the patient with kidney disease. The outcome of this first kidney allotransplant was not recorded, but it might be surmised that the transplant rapidly failed as there was no further report in the *New York Times*. Perhaps the most significant outcome of the transplant, aside from its historical interest, was a prescient comment by the reporter: "The percentage of fatalities of healthy human beings to the number of diseased organs in living persons has never been computed. It can not be large. If the organs and tissues of animals can be utilized there will be enough to go around; and lives that might in former time have been despaired of may be considerably prolonged" (5).

A RATIONALE FOR XENOTRANSPLANTATION

Today, there is much interest in xenotransplantation. Ironically, this interest stems, in large part, from the successful application of allotransplantation in humans. The development of increasingly better agents and regimens for suppressing immune-mediated rejection and treating infectious complications has allowed transplantation to become the preferred treatment for chronic failure of the heart, kidneys, liver, lungs, and, some would add, the pancreas for treatment for diabetes. The 21st century will, no doubt, bring further advances in the application of transplantation such as augmentation or replacement of the small bowel, musculoskeletal cells, and neuronal tissue, increasing the shortage of human tissues even further. Not only may transplantation be used for the replacement of failing tissues and organs, it may be used to impart new therapeutic functions. For instance, hematopoietic stem cells may be used to modify immune responses or to bring about immunological tolerance for the treatment of autoimmune disease or the prevention of transplant rejection. Still, the application of transplantation remains limited today, as it was at the turn of the 20th century, by the shortage of human tissues and organs. Thus, some in the field of transplantation are turning, once again, to the possibility of using animals in lieu of humans as a source of organs and tissues.

The rationale for xenotransplantation given most attention is the shortage of human organs and tissues. As severe as the shortage may be in the United States, it is worse by orders of magnitude in countries where culture or religion precludes the donation of organs or tissues after death. It is worse, too, in some countries of the developing world, where only limited means exist to sustain patients with chronic organ failure until a human organ donor can be found. As important as the shortage of organs is as a rationale for xenotransplantation, it may be eclipsed by other potential uses.

Another important prospect for xenotransplantation is as an approach to preventing the occurrence of disease. As one example, transplantation might someday be used to prevent the occurrence of a genetic or metabolic disease such as severe hypercholesterolemia or hereditary predisposition to cardiac arrhythmia; however, such applications of human transplants in advance of the onset of symptoms would hardly be ethical when thousands await transplants for treatment of the complications of organ failure or to prevent early death. Such a use could be undertaken, however, if organs and tissues were not limited. As another example, the transplantation of animal tissues might be undertaken to avoid reinfection by an infectious agent. Thus, xenotransplantation might be used to treat organ failure caused by viruses such as hepatitis B or hepatitis C that would be likely to recur in an allotransplant but not in the xenotransplant. Reinfection of the transplant not only causes persistent disease, but also leads to the use of additional human organs, which might be provided to other patients. Preliminary attempts at such therapies for the treatment of hepatitis B and human immunodeficiency virus (HIV) infection have been made (31, 103). It is not difficult to imagine the broad application of preemptive therapy. Prevention of reinfection might be undertaken someday if animal organs and xenotransplantation were to become an effective modality, and a widespread epidemic of hepatitis, myocarditis, etc., were to occur.

A third rationale for interest in xenotransplantation relates to the use of transplants as a vehicle for gene delivery. Among the more reliable approaches to gene therapy is to house the transferred genetic material inside a cell, which could then be transplanted into the patient. For example, Blau has proposed the use of myoblasts as a cellular vehicle for delivery of genes related to muscle diseases, or potentially, unrelated to muscle diseases (10). While current methods of gene transfer are realizing increasing success, the use of animals instead of humans as a source of cells allows the application of transgenic techniques that deliver and integrate a gene into the fertilized egg, thus giving rise to a line of animals with the exogenous gene. Accompanied by suitable regulatory elements, that gene might potentially be expressed at a high level or under conditions of regulation in selected tissues of the transgenic animals (23, 61, 84, 85). Expression of genetic material in this way potentially allows the delivery of genetic material in a predictable manner, without repeated transduction of a target cell or the use of transformed, clonally expanded cells as a vehicle for gene delivery. It also assures delivery, and potentially expression, of the gene to stem cells, currently a significant hurdle in gene therapy.

Species Used as a Source of Xenografts

The advent of immunosuppressive drugs in the 1950s made it finally possible to transplant organs and tissues between individuals. Still, the question raised in 1911, what would be the source of organs and tissues for transplantation, remained to be addressed. Before the enactment of laws defining brain death, the availability of donors was somewhat limited. The shortage of transplant donors in turn spurred interest in the potential use of animals as a source of organs.

It was intuitive then as it would be now that the best source of xenogeneic organs and tissues for transplantation into humans would be primate species closely related to humans. Accordingly, Reemtsma, Starzl, and others (90, 104) transplanted kidneys from chimpanzees and baboons into humans. Some of the chimpanzee kidneys functioned for many months, although the recipients died from complications unrelated to the function of the transplant. Given this experience and the revolutionary advances in immunosuppressive and antimicrobial therapies, xenotransplants from primates might be expected to function for prolonged periods today. For several reasons, however, most in the field of xenotransplantation have abandoned the use of nonhuman primates. One reason for abandoning the use of non-human primates as a source of xenotransplants is that the number of primates potentially available as a source of organs and tissues does not approach the enormous number needed. Another reason relates to the risk of transmitting zoonotic agents from the primate to the human. Nor is it presently possible (and some would add that it is not ethical) to introduce genetic material into the germ cells of primates. Therefore, instead of using primates, most in the field of transplantation focus on the use of pigs or other non-primate species.

The reasons for using pigs number at least four. First, the supply of pigs, unlike the supply of primates, is unlimited. Second, porcine organs, especially the heart, are of an appropriate size for use in humans. Third, pigs can be genetically engineered whereas primates presently cannot. Fourth, the risk of zoonotic infection from pigs might be limited and more easily controlled. The hurdles to the use of pigs, however, are significant.

The Hurdles to Xenotransplantation

If opportunities offered by xenotransplantation are great, the hurdles, at present, appear equally so. These hurdles include (i) the immune response of the host against the graft leading to rejection of the graft, (ii) the inherent physiologic limitations of the animal tissue or organ in a human system or induced disruption of the normal functions of the recipient, and (iii) the possibility of transferring infectious agents from the transplant to the recipient and, potentially, more broadly to the general population. The sections that follow will focus on the hurdles to transplanting porcine organs and cells into humans. The hurdles to xenotransplantation involving the immune response and the physiological limitations depend very much on the type of tissue transplanted (Table 1 and Fig. 1). The type of transplant is in turn usefully categorized as being isolated cells, free tissue, or a vascularized organ.

Isolated cells, such as dispersed hepatocytes, muscle cells, or bone marrow cells, receive their vascular supply from the recipient. This vascular supply consists of blood vessels that have grown from recipient cells into the transplant and provide a vascular network

Table 1. Xenograft classification[a]

Type of xenograft	Examples	Type of vascular supply	Microenvironment
Isolated cells	Hepatocytes Bone marrow	Neovascularization	Recipient
Free tissue	Pancreatic islets Skin	Neovascularization + anastomosis of donor and recipient vessels	Donor and recipient
Organs	Kidney Heart	Primary anastomosis of donor and recipient vessels	Donor

[a] Adapted from Takahashi et al. (105)

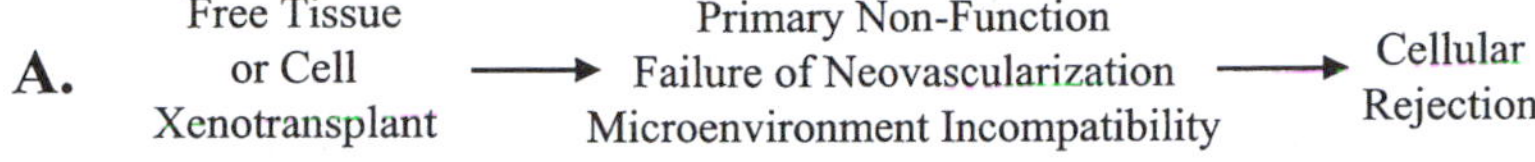

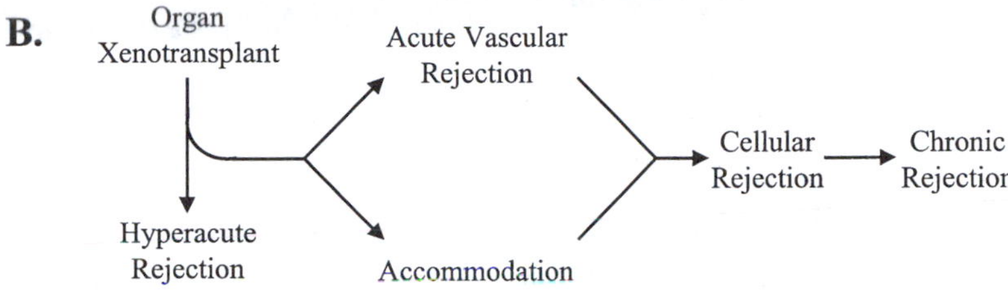

Figure 1. The immunological responses to xenotransplantation of various tissue types. **A**. Xenografts of free tissues such as pancreatic islets or isolated cells such as bone marrow cells are subject to early failure due to primary non-function, failure to neovascularize, or molecular incompatibilities and subsequent cell-mediated rejection. **B**. A porcine organ transplanted into a human would be subject to one or more of the immunological reactions shown here. Transplantation into an untreated recipient would give rise to hyperacute rejection. If hyperacute rejection is avoided, for example, by the inhibition of complement, the graft is subjected to acute vascular rejection. If anti-donor antibodies are depleted from the recipient, the graft may undergo accommodation, a condition in which acute vascular rejection does not occur despite the presence of anti-donor antibodies in the circulation of the recipient. If acute vascular rejection is avoided, the graft will undergo cell-mediated rejection or chronic rejection.

of recipient origin. One potential hurdle to xenotransplantation, then, is the ability of the transplant to stimulate the formation of a vascular network. Although the failure of vascularization owing to incompatibility between species may occur, it has yet to be established as an important problem. However, it seems not unlikely that cells transplanted between disparate species may fail to induce the full differentiation of ingrowing blood vessels, and this problem could in turn impair the function of the graft. Another related hurdle is the potential for incompatibility of the transplant with growth factors and hormones of the recipient. Bone marrow transplanted between disparate species may fail to engraft because the growth factors of the recipient fail to optimally stimulate donor cells (38, 71). One growth factor known to be incompatible between species is GM-CSF. Whether the incompatibility is absolute, leaving the transplanted cells unstimulated, or whether the incompatibility is relative, giving rise to a competitive advantage for bone marrow cells of the recipient, is a question of importance for systems such as bone marrow in which the growth of one cell can eclipse the growth of another.

Although the need to induce vascularization of the cellular transplant is portrayed as a hurdle, the formation of a vascular network by the recipient is also an advantage. The blood vessels of the host present a barrier to antibodies, components of the complement system, and in some cases, lymphocytes that readily destroy organ transplants. As a result of this barrier, some of the types of rejection (hyperacute and acute vascular rejection), which will be seen to be major impediments to the xenotransplantation of organs, do not apparently occur in cellular and free tissue grafts. Furthermore, cellular transplants might be kept alive and functioning by current immunosuppressive regimens, which would be woefully inadequate if applied to organ transplants.

Free tissues, such as skin and pancreatic islets, are organized aggregates of cells. Transplanted free tissues derive a vascular supply in part through the ingrowth of blood vessels of the recipient and in part through the spontaneous anastomosis of capillaries of the transplant with capillaries of the recipient. The significance of these two types of blood supply has not been established; it is conceivable that the survival or failure of the graft could depend on how this interaction is achieved. Free tissue grafts derive some growth factors and elements of the microenvironment from the donor and some from the recipient. Thus, these grafts, like cellular grafts, may suffer from incompatibilities between donor and recipient. Free tissue grafts are generally not subject to the types of vascular injury found in organ transplants; however, owing to the spontaneous anastomosis of donor and recipient blood vessels, the grafts can under some circumstances be attacked by antibodies directed against the donor (48).

Cellular and free tissue transplants are subject to "primary non-function" (51). Primary non-function is the apparent failure of grafted tissues to establish complete function. It may reflect failure of engraftment due to biological factors, the effects of inflammatory mediators on the survival and function of the transplant, or it may be mediated by immune elements, especially T lymphocytes and natural killer cells. In some systems, primary non-function can be overcome by providing a graft of larger size.

Organ transplants provide their own vascular network and microenvironment. As a result, organ transplants are not subject to such problems as "failure to engraft" or failure to vascularize. On the other hand, the vascular system of the organ transplant can be directly attacked by the immune system of the recipient. This direct interaction of the immune system of the recipient with the blood vessels of the donor gives rise to severe forms of "vascular rejection" as summarized in Fig. 1B. The problem of vascular rejection appears to be the most daunting hurdle to the clinical application of organ xenotransplantation.

IMMUNOLOGICAL HURDLES TO XENOTRANSPLANTATION

Hyperacute Rejection

A pig organ transplanted into an unmodified non-human primate or human is subject to hyperacute rejection (78). Hyperacute rejection is characterized pathologically by interstitial hemorrhage and formation of platelet thrombi. The changes occur almost immediately upon perfusion of the organ by recipient blood, and they cause the very rapid loss of graft function. In pig-to-human transplantation, hyperacute rejection is initiated by the binding of human xenoreactive IgM to the endothelium of the porcine organ (80). Antibody binding triggers activation of the complement system of the recipient, and it is the activation of complement on donor blood vessels that causes the dramatic manifestations of hyperacute rejection.

Xenoreactive Natural Antibodies and the Antigens They Recognize

Greater than 90% of xenoreactive antibodies that bind to porcine organs are specific for Galα1-3Gal (21, 37, 98). This antigen is synthesized by the enzyme α1,3-galactosyltransferase (α1,3GT), which exists in lower mammals and New World monkeys but is absent in Old World monkeys, apes, and humans (32). Xenoreactive antibodies specific for Galα1-3Gal are members of a family of antibodies that includes isohemagglutinins (76) and comprise 1 to 4% of circulating IgM (73). Upon binding to glycoproteins and/or glycolipids bearing Galα1-3Gal on the endothelial surface, these antibodies activate complement, setting into motion a series of events leading to the destruction of the newly transplanted organ.

Most abundant of the natural antibodies are "polyreactive" antibodies, a term denoting the remarkable ability of these antibodies to bind to diverse structures. Although polyreactive antibodies clearly recognize xenogeneic cells (36), it is uncertain whether these antibodies play any role in the rejection of xenotransplants.

Complement Activation and Complement Regulatory Proteins

Binding of xenoreactive antibodies to the endothelium of a porcine organ activates the complement system through the classical pathway (80), and the activation of complement in the xenograft is an essential step in the pathogenesis of hyperacute rejection. Studies in rodents suggest that terminal complement complexes may be needed for the development of hyperacute rejection, as this process does not occur in recipients deficient in C6 (11). Although the membrane attack complex of complement is probably the most potent effector of hyperacute rejection, the susceptibility of CD59 transgenic organs, in which assembly of the membrane attack complex is inhibited, to hyperacute rejection (28) and the finding that C5b67 complexes can disrupt endothelial integrity (94) suggest that the entire complement cascade may not be necessary to bring about hyperacute rejection and that C5b67 or C5b678 may be sufficient. In sum, it is likely that hyperacute rejection depends on the rapid assembly of terminal complement on endothelium of the newly transplanted organ.

Consisting of more than 20 proteins in the blood, the complement system includes a pivotal protein, C3, which can form amide or ester bonds with foreign surfaces or even with autologous cell surfaces. Attachment of C3b to foreign surfaces allows association of that protein with factor B and, thus, the formation of a C3 convertase, which cleaves C3 and C5, inducing the complement cascade through the alternative pathway. Activation of complement on autologous cells by the alternative pathway is inhibited by factor H, a plasma protein that recognizes C3b and disrupts C3 convertase by several mechanisms. The function of factor H is highly specific for the surface on which complement is affixed, and, thus, it does not inhibit C3b on the surface of many foreign cells or infectious organisms, this constituting perhaps the most important mechanism of non–self-discrimination for the complement system.

Table 2 shows quantitative measures for alternative pathway activation of complement from various species on the cells of disparate species. It will be noted that the alternative pathway of human complement does not become activated on porcine cells, thus making pigs compatible xenotransplant sources from this perspective. The human alternative pathway is activated on the cells of many other species. This is an important distinction because the alternative pathway of complement provides a major defense against extracellular microorganisms, and interfering with that system to promote the survival of xenografts would potentially subject the recipient to severe infectious complications. Because the human alternative pathway of complement is not activated directly on porcine cells, hyperacute rejection of porcine organs can be prevented by depleting xenoreactive antibodies, possibly without inhibition of the complement system.

The susceptibility of porcine organs to complement-mediated damage is not entirely a function of the binding of xenoreactive natural antibodies. The very rapid activation of complement in xenografts reflects in part the failure of complement regulatory proteins

Table 2. Activation of complement via the alternative pathway on xenogeneic cells[a]

Cells	Serum									
	Cow	Rabbit	Horse	Pigeon	Pig	Human	Dog	Rat	Guinea pig	Sheep
Cow		<0.28	<0.28	<0.28	<0.28	<0.28	<0.28	<0.28	<0.28	<0.28
Rabbit	2.6		<0.28	1.14	0.58	1.08	1.27	0.35	0.45	0.41
Horse	0.59	<0.28		0.67	0.41	0.49	2.34	0.74	<0.28	<0.28
Pigeon	2.34	0.48	<0.28		1.14	0.37	1.78	<0.28	<0.28	<0.28
Pig	<0.28	<0.28	<0.28	1.23		<0.28	2.46	0.29	<0.28	<0.28
Human	>4.4	<0.28	<0.28	0.35	**0.40**		<0.28	<0.28	<0.28	0.73
Dog	<0.28	1.43	3.4	1.85	0.56	4.4		4.4	4.4	>4.4
Rat	0.36	0.28	<0.28	0.37	0.39	0.41	2.2		0.41	0.38
Guinea pig	>4.4	0.41	<0.28	0.55	2.3	0.55	2.46	0.61		>4.4
Sheep	<0.28	<0.28	<0.28	<0.28	<0.28	<0.28	0.70	<0.28	<0.28	

[a]The number of units of complement per milliliter of serum of 10 different species capable of lysing 50% of 5×10^8 RBCs of other species by alternative pathway. Adapted from Edwards (29).

expressed in the endothelium of porcine organs to effectively control the human complement cascade (26, 86). Thus, decay accelerating factor (DAF) and membrane cofactor protein (MCP), which regulate complement activation by dissociating and degrading C3 convertase, and CD59, which prevents formation of the C8 and C9 components, function much better against homologous complement than against heterologous complement (6). The failure of these donor complement regulatory proteins to control activation of the complement system of the recipient might make the xenograft more susceptible to hyperacute rejection (86). The importance of aberrant complement control was recently demonstrated by studies in which expression of low levels of human DAF and CD59 in transgenic pigs was sufficient to prevent the hyperacute rejection of porcine organs transplanted into primates (15, 66).

It is widely believed that nearly all porcine organ xenografts are subject to hyperacute rejection by primates. However, some reports suggest that the lung (50) and the liver (16) might resist antibody-mediated hyperacute rejection. Another recent report suggests that hyperacute rejection of porcine kidneys and hearts does not always occur in unmodified primates (110). In considering what now appear to be exceptions to the dogma of species susceptibility to hyperacute rejection, it will be important to ensure that the exception does not reflect simply a low level of xenoreactive antibodies found in young animals and humans (49) or the use of treatments that inhibit complement or prevent endothelial damage.

Prevention of Hyperacute Rejection

Hyperacute rejection, once viewed as the most daunting hurdle to xenotransplantation, can now be circumvented by various therapeutic means. One specific approach to the prevention of hyperacute rejection is the inhibition of antibody binding to Galα1-3Gal. The first effort toward this end involved the infusion of soluble saccharides to block antibody binding (109). Unfortunately, this approach was not successful because the large amounts of sugar needed were toxic and because the sugar used (Galα1-6Gal) would probably fail to block 30% of the xenoreactive antibodies (74). An alternative approach is to deplete anti–Galα1-3Gal antibodies from the recipient. Sablinski et al. (95) and Lin et al. (58) used columns bearing Galα1-3Gal to immunodeplete xenoreactive natural antibodies from baboons, observing that this procedure alone without depleting complement would prevent hyperacute rejection.

An approach commonly advanced for preventing the binding of xenoreactive natural antibodies involves the development of lines of pigs expressing low levels of Galα1-3Gal (35). Various approaches to decreasing expression of Galα1-3Gal have been considered (79). One approach to decreasing antigen expression is to overexpress another glycosyltransferase that can compete with α1,3galactosyltransferase in catalyzing the termination of saccharide chains. This approach, pursued by Sandrin et al. (97) and Sharma et al. (101), consists of expression of α1,2fucosyltransferase that causes synthesis of H antigen, to which humans are tolerant, in transgenic animals. Other potential approaches are illustrated in Fig. 2. No approach to decreasing antigen expression, yet tested, prevents the rejection of xenografts, and given the effectiveness of antibody removal combined with inhibition of complement, it seems difficult to justify modification of antigen expression solely for the prevention of hyperacute rejection.

Another therapeutic approach to hyperacute rejection involves inhibition of complement. Infusion of complement inhibitors such as cobra venom factor (CVF) (56), soluble complement receptor type I (SCR1) (89), or IVIg (62) reliably prevents hyperacute rejection. Unfortunately, CVF and SCR1 impair host defense by inhibiting complement early in the cascade. More enduring inhibition of complement mediated injury might be achieved through the use of organs from transgenic pigs expressing human complement regulatory proteins. This goal has now been achieved through the expression of human DAF and human CD59 in transgenic pigs (15, 24), as discussed above.

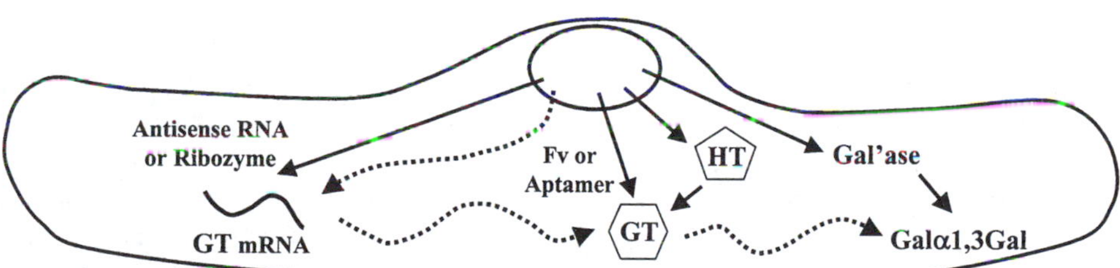

Figure 2. Possible ways in which Galα1-3Gal expression could be decreased by genetic engineering. Synthesis of Galα1-3Gal is catalyzed by α1,3-galactosyltransferase (GT); the biosynthetic pathway is shown by dashed arrows. This enzyme adds galactose residues at the termini of oligosaccharide chains. Four possible approaches to preventing the synthesis of the sugar are shown by normal arrows. First, the expression of antisense RNA or a ribozyme might disrupt the structure or function of the GT mRNA. Second, introduction of a gene for an inhibitory ligand for GT, such as an appropriate Fv (an antibody-like molecule) or an aptamer (a small oligonucleotide inhibitor), might inhibit the function of the enzyme. Third, overexpression of another glycosyl transferase, such as H transferase, which adds fucose residues, might compete for the subterminal residues on oligosaccharide chains. This has been achieved in rats by the overexpression of a human H transferase, resulting in the addition of fucose rather than Galα1-3Gal to oligosaccharide side chains (101). Fourth, expression of a glycosidase, such as α-galactosidase, might lead to cleavage of the antigenic saccharide chains. Reprinted by permission from *Nature* 392(Suppl.):11–17, 1998, Macmillan Magazines Ltd.

Acute Vascular Rejection

When hyperacute rejection is averted, a xenograft is confronted with another rejection process, which we have called "acute vascular rejection" (55) and some have referred to as "delayed xenograft rejection." Acute vascular rejection may begin within 24 h of reperfusion and leads to failure of the xenograft within days to weeks following transplantation. The pathologic features of acute vascular rejection of xenografts, like those of acute vascular rejection of allografts, include endothelial swelling, ischemia, and thrombosis. In light of recent success in preventing hyperacute rejection, acute vascular rejection looms as the next major hurdle to the enduring survival of xenografts, and accordingly, the pathogenesis of acute vascular rejection has become a critical subject of investigation.

Pathogenesis

Acute vascular rejection initially appears as a patchy discoloration on the graft, reflecting small areas of focal ischemia. These changes occur relatively early, and in the case of cardiac xenografts, the intensity of contractions is still vigorous and the consistency of the xenograft is still soft. Discoloration of the graft is typically observed in all regions of the heart. Areas of congestion are also noted. The next clinical change characteristic of acute vascular rejection is arrhythmia, in the form of ectopies such as premature ventricular contractions or bigeminy. Arrhythmias are generally observed in the days following the appearance of discoloration. The walls of the ventricles also begin to thicken and the consistency of myocardium gradually hardens as fibrosis develops. Over the ensuing hours to days, the cardiac contractions become perceptibly weaker and the frequency of ectopies increases until the ventricles finally cease contracting. Although cessation of atrial contraction seems to portend a poor prognostic outcome, the timing of atrial asystole in relationship to the cessation of ventricular contraction is variable, possibly depending on such factors as the approach to the atria during the organ harvest. Finally, perhaps peculiar to the heterotopic cardiac transplant model is the development of a thickened layer of inflammatory fibrosis outside the epicardium; this change, however, does not usually affect the viability of the xenograft not undergoing acute vascular rejection.

Clinical laboratory findings characteristic of acute vascular rejection vary with the type and size of the organ transplant. Acute vascular rejection may be marked by thrombocytopenia and coagulopathy, owing presumably to consumption in the graft. Progressive anemia may also be seen, presumably due to hemolysis in damaged blood vessels.

The histopathological manifestations of acute vascular rejection are quite dramatic. The earliest changes seen in acute vascular rejection include deposits of fibrin and fibrin microthrombi, noted as early as 24 h after reperfusion (60). In conjunction with fibrin deposition there occurs a thickening of endothelium due in part to endothelial cell swelling and in part to vasoconstriction. Next, the intralumenal space of small blood vessels becomes widened, owing to partial occlusion by fibrin thrombi, and areas of focal ischemia appear. The ischemia is often associated with the adhesion of inflammatory cells to vascular walls and the influx of these same cells into the interstitium. During the next period of days, the ischemia progresses to frank necrosis accompanied by prominent inflammatory changes.

The immunopathology of acute vascular rejection includes several typical features. Consistent with the potential involvement of antibodies in the pathogenesis of the lesions, there is typically a diffuse deposition of recipient IgM and sometimes IgG along endothelial surfaces early in the course of acute vascular rejection. Immunoglobulin deposits may become less pronounced or even vanish in more advanced lesions, perhaps owing to degradation or endocytosis of cell-bound proteins. Terminal complement components are generally not seen, as in most cases the assembly of these components is inhibited by the therapies that prevent hyperacute rejection. An exception can be found in xenografts in recipients from which anti-donor antibodies, but not complement, were depleted. Furthermore, as immunopathology is not sufficiently sensitive to detect low levels of terminal complex assembly, the absence of these components should not be taken as evidence that the components do not contribute to the pathogenesis of rejection. The presence of fibrin is also detected at an early time.

Listed in Table 3 are various immune and nonimmune factors that have been postulated to initiate or predispose xenografts to acute vascular rejection. While it is not unlikely that several of these factors are brought to bear in the initiation of rejection, certain priorities of importance can be deduced from experimental models.

Work in my laboratory and studies from other laboratories suggest that anti-donor antibodies are of preeminent importance in the initiation of acute vascular rejection; indeed, five lines of evidence support this view. First, the immunopathology of xenogeneic organs undergoing acute vascular rejection almost invariably reveals Ig of recipient origin bound to the endothelial lining of graft blood vessels (55, 62, 80). Second, the synthesis of anti-donor antibodies increases following exposure to a xenogeneic organ (22, 67), and this increase coincides with the most prominent manifestations of acute vascular rejection. Third, administration of immunosuppressive regimens calculated to inhibit synthesis of antibodies may prevent acute vascular rejection (24). Fourth, depletion of antibodies from xenograft recipients prevents the occurrence of acute vascular rejection (60). Fifth, administration of anti-donor antibodies to recipients of allografts or xenografts induces tissue lesions typical of acute vascular rejection.

If anti-donor antibodies seem to play an important role in the pathogenesis of acute vascular rejection, the importance of other mechanisms can be postulated as well. Blakely et al. (9) suggested that monocytes, which are known to express tissue factor, a cofactor for the formation of prothrombinase complexes, might cause the fibrin deposition and thus the tissue manifestations of acute vascular rejection. This view was supported by the observation that acute vascular rejection in rodents is associated with the influx of macrophages expressing tissue factor. On the other hand, lesions early in the course of acute vascular rejection, especially in pig-to-primate transplants, do not reveal significant numbers of macrophages (60, 62). Nor is the onset or the pathology of acute vascular rejection

Table 3. Factors implicated in the initiation of acute vascular rejection[a]

Initiating factor	Mechanism	Reference
Xenoreactive antibodies	Activation of EC by binding to signaling molecules	44
Complement	Activation of EC by MAC	62
	Activation of EC by C5a	87
Macrophages	Elaboration of tissue factor	9
Natural killer cells	Cytotoxicity and activation of EC	64
Neutrophils	Oxidant mediated injury	112
	Activation of EC	13
Platelets	Secretion of vasoactive factors	14
Molecular incompatibility	Thrombomodulin incompatibility with recipient proteins	53

[a]EC, endothelial cell; MAC, membrane attack complex. Adapted from Platt et al. (82).

more than modestly inhibited by the administration of agents that inhibit the interaction of inflammatory cells with xenogeneic endothelium (112), in contrast to the results achieved by antibody depletion that significantly prolongs the survival of the transplants (60). Nor, conversely, do allotransplants with cellular rejection, which are often found to have large numbers of invading macrophages, necessarily exhibit lesions typical of acute vascular rejection (81). Thus, while a role for macrophages cannot be excluded at this juncture, it seems more likely that these cells are a marker for tissue injury rather than the cause in acute vascular rejection of xenotransplants.

Another mechanism thought to be of import in the pathogenesis of acute vascular rejection is an intrinsic incompatibility between the plasma coagulation proteins of the recipient and the cell surface regulators of coagulation in the donor organ. Recently it was found that porcine thrombomodulin functions poorly or not at all in combination with human thrombin and human protein C in the generation of activated protein C (54). A similar mechanism was postulated by Bach et al. (8). One argument against the importance of these intrinsic incompatibilities between the donor and the recipient of xenotransplants as the main pathogenic mechanism is that in pig-to-primate xenografts, with control of complement and the inhibition or depletion of xenoreactive antibodies or administration of cyclophosphamide, the diffuse intravascular coagulation characteristic of acute vascular rejection does not occur (24). Moreover, the finding of acute vascular rejection in concordant xenografts and in allografts in which molecular incompatibilities are less significant or nonexistent suggests that acute vascular rejection of discordant xenotransplants would probably occur anyway, even if the incompatibilities were corrected.

Yet another mechanism that might contribute to the pathogenesis of acute vascular rejection is the action of lymphocytes or natural killer cells on graft endothelium. The potential involvement of natural killer cells has been of special interest because the cells might be expected to be activated in xenograft recipients through stimulation of carbohydrate receptors, Fc receptors, and failure to stimulate MHC class I receptors (45, 46). Consistent with this concept, human natural killer cells have been found to exert cytotoxic and noncytotoxic effects, such as induction of procoagulant activity, on porcine endothelial cells in vitro (63, 64). Although natural killer cells and other lymphocytes have been found in some rodent xenografts (8), this finding is not always observed (55), as they are not major components of pig-to-primate xenografts (60, 62). Therefore, while lymphoid cells may well contribute to tissue injury in acute vascular rejection, they may not be essential for the manifestation of tissue lesions. If inflammatory cells are sometimes absent from tissues undergoing acute vascular rejection, platelet aggregates are nearly always present. These aggregates may form in response to thrombin generation or endothelial injury. However, Bustos et al. recently showed that platelets can mediate endothelial cell activation (14), raising the prospect that they might be involved in the initiation of acute vascular rejection.

Activation of Endothelial Cells in Acute Vascular Rejection

It was originally postulated that regardless of which factors may be involved in the initiation of xenograft rejection, the pathogenesis of rejection might be linked to the activation of endothelial cells in the graft (75, 86). This conception has proved a useful paradigm for studying vascular responses to immune injury (92, 93); however, it is clearly too simplistic to explain the principal manifestations of hyperacute rejection and may fail to account for certain important aspects of pathogenesis for acute vascular rejection.

This pathogenic link was postulated because of the association of acute vascular rejection with severe and diffuse intravascular coagulation and inflammation, pathological changes that might be expected to be induced by endothelium expressing increased procoagulant and proinflammatory activity, as would be manifest by activated endothelium. Consistent with the concept regarding the importance of endothelial cell activation, investigators including the author have found changes in the endothelium of organs undergoing acute vascular rejection consistent with activation (9). Among these changes is the de novo expression of tissue factor and PAI-1, which would give rise to a thrombotic diathesis (92). Likewise, E-selectin, MCP-1, and IL1β might promote the influx and activation of inflammatory cells (9, 100). Whether in fact acute vascular rejection depends on endothelial cell activation in the strictest sense is not certain, however. It is not inconceivable that inflammatory changes or ischemia could in turn cause endothelial cell activation as a secondary event. This distinction is important because some have proposed that acute vascular rejection might be prevented if the activation of endothelium could be suppressed. Apart from the validity of the concept, however, there is also the question of what biological price might be paid for suppressing the ability of endothelial cells to be activated.

Strategies for the Prevention and Treatment of Acute Vascular Rejection

At least five approaches might have potential application to the prevention and treatment of acute vascular rejection. These approaches address acute vascular rejection from the perspectives of the interaction of antibodies with the donor organ and the pathophysiologic changes in endothelium that give rise to the tissue lesions and the induction of "accommodation," a condition described in 1990 (86) as acquired resistance to humoral injury.

To the extent that interaction of anti-donor antibodies with the transplant triggers acute vascular rejection, strategies that would deplete those antibodies, such as immunoabsorption with affinity columns, or that would inhibit antibody synthesis, such as splenectomy and treatment with cyclophosphamide, may benefit the graft. Clearly, one important question is the specificity of the antibodies that cause vascular damage. The studies listed above suggest that in the presence of immunosuppression the major specificity of xenoreactive antibodies remains Galα1-3Gal (22, 67). However, other antibodies can be detected (67). If the specificity of the offending antibodies is predominantly Galα1-3Gal, as the work suggests, then strategies that would specifically lower the levels of those antibodies, or lower the expression of the antigen they recognize, would be a rational approach to prevention and therapy of acute vascular rejection. Specific depletion of these antibodies can be achieved using immunoabsorbent columns. For logistic reasons, repeated depletion procedures or suppression of synthesis by administration of high doses of immunosuppressive agents is not particularly desirable. Fortunately, temporary depletion of these anti-donor antibodies may be sufficient to allow the occurrence of accommodation as described below. Suppressing the synthesis of antibodies via specific immunological tolerance would be a useful alternative. Sykes and coworkers have reported exciting progress in this area (108). Another approach is to manipulate the donor to decrease expression of Galα1-3Gal. Various other approaches to antigen manipulation were reviewed (59, 79). One approach exploits natural variation in antigen expression and the genetic basis for this variation to develop lines of animals with "low" levels of antigen expression (3, 35). Another approach, mentioned above, involves the expression of H transferase in transgenic animals that leads to the synthesis of increased amounts of the H antigen to which humans are tolerant and decreased synthesis of Galα1-3Gal (97, 101). Expression of other transferases might also be practical depending on the biological effect of the sugars expressed in increased amounts. It was recently determined that antigen expression needs to be decreased by greater than 95% to avert acute vascular rejection. In light of this, multiple approaches or specific targeting of the α1,3galactosyltransferase gene will be necessary.

Accommodation

Another approach to preventing acute vascular rejection is the establishment of accommodation, a state in which the graft appears inured to the presence of anti-donor antibodies in the circulation (86). Accommodation was first observed in the transplantation of kidneys across ABO-blood group barriers where temporary depletion of anti–blood group antibodies proved sufficient to allow enduring survival of kidney allografts (20). The mechanisms of accommodation are uncertain, although they may involve a change in the antibody repertoire, change in the antigen, or the acquired resistance of endothelium to humoral injury. An acquired resistance of endothelium to humoral injury has been described in rodent models (7); however, the relevance of this observation for primates has not been ascertained. Accommodation is typically seen when anti-donor antibodies are removed from the circulation of an organ graft recipient and then allowed to return to the circulation. In some instances, the returning antibodies do not mediate destruction of the transplant; rather, the transplant continues to function as if inured to the presence of these antibodies. Regardless of the mechanisms responsible for accommodation, there is little doubt that establishment in a porcine-to-primate xenograft setting would be an important step toward the clinical application of xenotransplantation.

Cellular Rejection

The cellular immune response to a xenograft has been the subject of increasing attention in recent years. Cellular rejection may be seen in vascularized xenografts if hyperacute rejection and acute vascular rejection are averted. Cellular rejection is the first type of rejection seen in cell and tissue xenografts.

Still uncertain is the extent to which the cell-mediated immune response to a xenograft differs from the response to an allograft and the extent to which this response can be controlled by conventional immunosuppressive therapy. There is a general sense that the cell-mediated immune response to a xenograft may be more severe than the cell-mediated response to an allograft (96). This vigor may reflect various factors, two in particular being the very large variety of foreign antigens available for indirect presentation and the amplifying effects of humoral immunity.

One important question has been the mechanism of T-cell recognition of xenogeneic cells. The intensity of the cellular response may also reflect failure of some of the normal immunoregulatory mechanisms to work across species. Yet another factor that may tend to promote a vigorous cellular immune reaction is humoral immunity. The extent to which the direct versus the indirect pathways of T-cell recognition might be utilized in the cellular immune response to xenotransplantation has been one topic of interest because potential defects in corecognition by CD4 and CD8 and in costimulation (69) distinguish the xeno-response from the allo-response. The human anti-porcine T-cell response is similar to the allogeneic response in that human T cells can recognize porcine MHC class II antigens through the direct pathway (70, 107). Still, given the diversity of foreign antigenic peptides in a xenograft, there is concern that antigen presentation by recipient antigen-presenting cells, i.e., through the indirect pathway, will be especially potent. The mechanism by which T cells recognize xenogeneic cells is important for at least three reasons. First, as suggested above, the mechanism(s) may dictate the intensity of the immune response or the extent to which an elicited humoral response will ensue. Second, to the extent that the direct pathway predominates, genetic engineering of donors might be used to impair T-cell activation. Third, the mechanism(s) of recognition may dictate the types of immunomodulatory therapies that can be directed at the recipient.

Given the potential strength of the T-cell response to xenotransplantation and the potential importance of elicited antibodies, some have suggested that the success of xenotransplantation may depend on the generation of immunological tolerance (96). Although there are a growing number of approaches to inducing tolerance to allografts, there is a limited amount of information about inducing tolerance to xenografts. One approach may involve the generation of mixed chimerism leading to deletion of "xenoreactive" cells (96). A related strategy may well involve the transplantation of donor thymus to allow the maturation of a mature T-cell repertoire that will not be reactive with the donor (113). Another approach involves the manipulation of the mature T-cell repertoire through the generation of microchimerism or other means so that xenoreactive cells are depleted or inhibited (57, 102).

Another aspect of cellular rejection is the potential importance of natural killer cells, the function of which might contribute to acute vascular rejection or cellular rejection (46). There is some evidence that natural killer cells accumulate in xenografts, recognize Galα1-3Gal, and may fail to be controlled by inhibitory receptors specific for MHC class I. Recent studies have revealed noncytotoxic mechanisms by which natural killer cells may injure xenogeneic endothelial cells—a change in morphology and endothelial cell activation (63). Yet to be determined, however, is the relative importance of natural killer cell–mediated injury and which therapeutic strategy might best deal with this problem.

Prevention of Xenograft Rejection: Implications for the Defense Against Infectious Disease

Among the most challenging problems in the field of transplantation is the set of complications caused by immunosuppressive therapy. These complications include heightened risk of infection and tumor formation caused by abrogation of elements of host defense. Since the immune response to xenotransplantation involves nearly all elements of host defense, the challenge of developing safe and effective approaches to preventing immune destruction of xenografts is greater than the corresponding challenge for allografts.

Clearly the various components of the immune response to xenotransplants contribute to host defense. In particular, complement and natural antibodies provide a critical defense against invasive extracellular microorganisms and some viruses. Abridging the function of complement, natural antibodies, macrophages, T cells, etc., would overly compromise the well-being of the graft recipient. Therefore, one critical question in research in xenotransplantation is which of the many components of the immune system implicated in responses to xenotransplantation are in fact not involved or are critical to such responses; that is to say, which elements of immunity can be left intact in the recipient of a xenotransplant.

The components of the immune system that provide a defense against pyogenic microorganisms are the complement system and phagocytes. System interference with the ability to opsonize bacteria, particularly by inhibition of the alternative pathway of complement or interference with phagocytosis, would be expected to increase profoundly the risk of life-threatening infection. The advent of transgenic animals expressing human complement regulatory proteins has addressed this problem, at least in part, since the control of complement does not require systemic inhibition of the complement cascade. On the other hand, the utilization of complement regulatory proteins as viral receptors may make transgenic organs more susceptible to infection.

Still uncertain is the extent to which natural antibodies, particularly anti–Galα1-3Gal antibodies, contribute to host defense and surveillance. Anti–Galα1-3Gal have been postulated to clear senescent cells from the circulation, contribute to a primary barrier against infection of humans by animal viruses (33), and prevent translocation and infection by enteric pathogens (34, 91). Depletion of anti–Galα1-3Gal antibodies thus seems to impose a risk of various severe infections. However, some individuals have very low levels of these antibodies and yet do not have a demonstrably increased risk of serious infection (83).

PHYSIOLOGIC HURDLES TO XENOTRANSPLANTATION

Clearly the most salient question, from a clinical perspective, is whether and to which extent a xenotransplant can mediate the physiologic functions needed to replace the function of a failing organ or tissue. Currently there is only limited information to address this question. Recent studies have suggested that the pig kidney can maintain relatively normal fluid and electrolyte levels in non-human primates (2, 95, 111). Porcine hearts transplanted orthotopically in baboons can keep baboons alive, but the level of cardiac function achieved in pig-to-baboon cardiac xenografts has yet to be quantitated (99). The pig lung can maintain normal gas exchange in baboons for periods of hours (25), but long-term studies are needed to substantiate the conclusion that porcine pulmonary xenografts could be satisfactory from a physiologic perspective. The porcine liver has been used with some success as a temporary extracorporeal device to treat patients with fulminant hepatic failure (19), and there are a few reports in which baboons have survived for days with porcine liver transplants (17). However, critical analysis of the function of porcine livers in primates has not been reported, and there are reasons to think that the porcine liver might not suffice as an organ xenograft (88). One limitation of the porcine liver is that proteins of the coagulation and complement cascades seem incompatible with human proteins and control mechanisms. Other possible problems could stem from differences in the detoxifying enzymes between species. It should be considered, however, that where physiologic limitations are found, there is the possibility that function can be corrected by genetic engineering of the donor.

There is the possibility that a xenograft, particularly a liver transplant, might secrete products that would impair various systems of the recipient. For example, the complement secreted by the pig liver may be spontaneously activated on primate cells (Table 2). Likewise, the coagulation proteins of the pig may not be compatible with thrombomodulin and other control elements of the primate system. These or other incompatibilities may induce systemic physiologic disturbances. This concern is greatest for the liver, as the heart, kidney, and lungs do not secrete substantial amounts of proteins. One potential difficulty is the possibility that the antigenic material, secreted by the porcine organ, may lead to the formation of immune complexes that may be pathogenic. This problem seems particularly likely in the case of the lung, where substantial amounts of von Willebrand factor can be shown to be emitted in immune complexes formed in the systemic circulation (42).

Where xenotransplantation is used as a bridge to allotransplantation, or where xenotransplants might be followed by another type of allotransplant (e.g., transplantation of porcine islets followed by a human kidney transplant for diabetic nephropathy), the possibility must be considered that the xenotransplant will sensitize the recipient to cross-reactive alloantigens. For example, it is possible that antibodies developed against porcine histocompatibility antigens (SLA) will cross-react with some human histocompatibility antigens (HLA). The development of such antibodies and cross-reactivity might then preclude the carrying out of certain allotransplants. Evidence of such cross-reactivity has not been reported, but neither has it been extensively sought.

Preliminary studies suggest that the kidney of a pig can provide a physiologic replacement for a human kidney, save perhaps for the maintenance of red blood cell mass. Preliminary studies over a short period indicate that the porcine heart may be capable of providing hemodynamic support and the porcine lung pulmonary support for primates. Yet uncertain is whether subtle defects in physiology, intrinsic to porcine organs or arising as a result of inadequately controlled immune-mediated processes described above, may limit clinical application of cardiac xenotransplantation. Were physiologic limitations to be found, there is the possibility that function could be amplified by the introduction of genes that would enhance organ function or protect the transplanted organ from deleterious effects of the host's immune response. Some have thought that the function of allografts or of the failing heart might be improved by gene therapy. Because in a xenograft, extrinsic genes (transgenes) can be expressed in all cells and without the typical limitations of gene therapy, this possibility is perhaps greater in a xenograft. As one example, such efforts have been undertaken by Koch et al. (1, 52).

XENOTRANSPLANTATION AND INFECTIOUS DISEASE

There is concern about the possible transmission of "new" infectious agents from the graft into the recipient, especially if such agents might then be transmitted to the population as a whole. This issue was highlighted by the discovery that an endogenous porcine retrovirus might be able to infect human cells in culture (65, 77). Furthermore, a new porcine virus related to human hepatitis virus E was recently reported (68). However, it still remains to be proven that these viruses or other "new" agents could actually infect humans and whether such infection could lead to transmission to other individuals or to disease. Thus far, no evidence has emerged that these agents can infect humans (41, 72). Nevertheless, the subject of zoonosis will remain of importance because genetic modifications of xenografts that lower expression of Galα1-3Gal or increase resistance to complement could allow zoonotic agents from these animals to evade immune surveillance.

LIVER-ASSIST DEVICES AND LIVER PERFUSION

Among the more daunting challenges in clinical medicine is the treatment of severe liver failure. One potential approach to this problem is the use of a liver-assist device. Such a device might consist of isolated hepatocytes housed in an apparatus that brings together the blood of the patient and cultured hepatocytes, separated by a semipermeable membrane, that would temporarily address the life-threatening complications of liver failure. In contrast to most other types of xenotransplantation, liver-assist devices can presently be used in human subjects. Another approach involves the ex vivo perfusion of livers unsuitable for transplantation. While it is intuitive that the optimal liver-assist device or the intact perfused liver would consist of human cells or tissues, the availability of human livers is limited, and accordingly, in recent years efforts have been made to use animal, especially porcine, livers as a source of cells or liver tissue. Use of animal organs or cells outside the body, for example, liver-assist devices, is not strictly speaking transplantation. However, this type of use for organs and cells raises some issues pertaining to xenotransplantation. This section will consider some of these issues.

Immunological Hurdles to Application of Hepatic-Assist Devices

Discussions of the immunology of xenotransplantation generally focus on the fate of the transplanted organ—the fate of the patient being, in general, inextricably linked with the fate of the organ. In contrast to this perspective, however, the issues of greatest import for use of xenogeneic devices are not so much related to the fate of the devices as they are to the function of the device and complications experienced by the patient. The immune response of the patient to the cells in a hepatic-assist device might lead, in principle, to three categories of complications, referred to as (i) rejection, (ii) immune complexes, and (iii) sensitization. These terms do not fully describe the range of issues to be considered but are intended, rather, to represent various problems that can be explained from the perspective of the immune system. In the category of rejection, I shall consider the range of functional impairments of livers or hepatocytes brought about by exposure to xenogeneic blood. In the category of immune complexes, I shall consider the range of toxic effects caused by the products of the xenogeneic liver or cells. In the category of sensitization, I shall consider the implications of the immune responses engendered by the use of xenogeneic livers or hepatocytes.

Rejection

The permeable membrane associated with hepatic-assist devices isolates the hepatocytes, to a certain extent, from the immune system of the recipient. Accordingly, the major immune reactions that one encounters in a perfused or transplanted foreign organ would not occur within the protected barrier of the hepatic-assist device. Still, some types of injury to those cells may occur; this injury is referred to as "rejection." Although most elements of humoral immunity and, clearly, the elements of cellular immunity would be prevented from contacting the foreign cells, anaphylatoxins, the molecular mass of which is less than 10,000 Da, generated in the vicinity of the device, might well pass toward the hepatocytes and alter their function. Depending on the size of the membrane used, it might be anticipated that some immunoglobulins could also permeate. Some immune reactions may occur outside the device, owing to the binding of antibodies to proteins secreted from xenogeneic hepatocytes, leading to engagement of the complement system. These reactions, although potentially not fatal or even severe, might add to ischemic injury caused by the limited accessibility of the foreign cells to the treated patients' blood.

Formation of Immune Complexes

The second immunological hurdle to the use of hepatic-assist devices is a range of disorders caused by the interaction of pig and human proteins, one example of which is the formation of immune complexes. Immune complexes may form when material secreted by the perfused organ or device becomes bound by antibodies in the blood of the treated patient. These responses may generate inflammatory mediators that can injure the hepatocytes, as discussed above. In addition to this effect, the immune complexes may incite systemic injury to the treated patient. It was recently reported that immune complexes can form following organ xenotransplantation (43), and it is highly likely that such complexes will form from the products secreted by the foreign hepatocytes. In the case of lung xenotransplants, the major immune reaction involves recognition of Galα1-3Gal by foreign antibodies. Combination of natural antibodies with Galα1-3Gal is also likely to be the dominant reaction when liver perfusion is first applied in a given patient. Because the individuals treated by hepatic-assist devices or liver perfusion may not be immunosuppressed, it is likely that sensitization to foreign proteins will also occur, allowing the formation of other types of immune complexes with repeated treatments. Other protein–protein interactions, such as the reaction of porcine von Willebrand factor with human platelet Ib receptors, could lead to medical complications, in this case thrombocytopenia, and need to be considered as potential hazards.

Sensitization

The third category of immune response to the transplant that serves as a hurdle to the application of hepatic-assist devices or liver perfusion is sensitization of the patient. Such sensitization may give rise to the formation of immune complexes with systemic or focal peripheral complications, as discussed above. In addition, there is concern that the patient will be sensitized to porcine histocompatibility antigens and that antibodies generated against such antigens might cross-react with HLA antigens. Should sensitization to porcine histocompatibility (SLA) occur, and should this sensitization be cross-reacted with some HLA antigens, the use of hepatic-assist devices or liver perfusion could erect a hurdle to subsequent allotransplantation.

Physiologic Hurdles to Application of Hepatic-Assist Devices

It is intuitive that the hepatic-assist device or perfused liver, whether it is xenogeneic or allogeneic, will likely fail to perform all of the synthetic and detoxifying functions of a native liver. Not only will the function of the device or perfused organ likely be deficient, but the patient's clinical condition would be expected to deteriorate during periods when treatment is not conducted. Still, it is clear that the most urgent physiologic needs, particularly the maintenance of normal intracranial pressure, can be provided by a perfused liver (19) and, probably, by liver hepatic-assist devices. Further information regarding the physiologic limitations of these devices and procedures will be forthcoming as clinical application is expanded, and this information might be usefully applied to improving the functional performance of the procedures. One aspect of physiology that also warrants comment is the impact of "rejection," as defined above, on the performance of the device or perfused organ. There is little doubt from studies of organ xenotransplants that the major barrier to physiologic functioning is not intrinsic differences between species, but, rather, the effects of the host immune system on the functioning of the organ transplant. It is likely, too, that rejection, as broadly construed above, will be an important limiting factor on performance. Thus, efforts to understand these immune reactions will likely be rewarded by improvements in efficacy. Further, in contrast to the setting of animal husbandry, slaughtering, etc., the animals used as a source of livers for xenoperfusion can be screened for all infectious agents known to be of relevance to the treated patient.

Infection

The risk of zoonosis, as such, is thought to be heightened for xenotransplants because the recipient of a xenotransplant has animal cells in continuity with the recipient's own cells for protracted periods and, in part, because the recipient is treated with immunosuppressive agents. These risks, however, are effaced in the case of liver perfusion and use of hepatic-assist devices because these procedures do not involve protracted contact between the cells of the animal and the cells of the recipient and because the patient is not generally immunosuppressed. Thus, the condition of exposure to animal tissues in the course of xenoperfusion or use of xeno-assist devices is not substantively different from the contact that occurs between the blood of human and animal cells in the course of animal husbandry, slaughtering, etc. Clearly, there is a finite risk of zoonosis. However, if the source of tissues and organs is suitably screened, this risk may be less than the risk attendant with exposure to pigs under occupational circumstances.

PROSPECTS FOR CLINICAL APPLICATION OF XENOTRANSPLANTATION

The past few years have brought significant progress in defining the hurdles to xenotransplantation and progress in overcoming the immunologic and physiologic hurdles in this field. It is our view that the entry of xenotransplantation into the clinical area may be a step-by-step process. First, there will occur free tissue xenografts and extracorporeal use of xenogeneic organs. Limited clinical trials of this sort are in progress (19, 27, 39), and there is encouraging early evidence that porcine free tissue grafts may endure in a human recipient (27). Next, xenogeneic organs will probably be used as "bridge" transplants while patients wait for more suitable organs. Bridge transplants will not address the critical shortage of organs available for transplantation, but the transplants will allow the gathering of vital information regarding the remaining immune and biological hurdles. Third, there will be the use of porcine organs as permanent replacements, but this use will probably be restricted to patients who cannot receive a human organ allograft. Only with further refinements may there eventually be a fourth and final step in which xenotransplantation is used as an alternative to allotransplantation.

Acknowledgments. Portions of this text have been adapted from Platt, J. L., *Nature* **392**(Suppl.)**:**11–17, 1998; Platt, J. L., S. S. Lin, and C. G. A. McGregor, *Xenotransplantation* **5:**169–175, 1998; Platt, J. L., *Pediatric Transplantation* **3:**193–200, 1999.

Work in the author's laboratory is supported by grants from the National Institutes of Health.

REFERENCES

1. **Akhter, S. A., C. A. Skaer, A. P. Kypson, P. H. McDonald, K. C. Peppel, D. D. Glower, R. J. Lefkowitz, and W. J. Koch.** 1997. Restoration of β-adrenergic signaling in failing cardiac ventricular myocytes via adenoviral-mediated gene transfer. *Proc. Nat. Acad. Sci. USA* **94:**12100–12105.
2. **Alexandre, G. P. J., P. Gianello, D. Latinne, M. Carlier, A. Dewaele, L. Van Obbergh, M. Moriau, E. Marbaix, J. L. Lambotte, L. Lambotte, and J. P. Squifflet.** 1989. Plasmapheresis and splenectomy in

experimental renal xenotransplantation, p. 259–266. *In* M. A. Hardy (ed.), *Xenograft 25*. Elsevier Science Publishers, New York, N.Y.

3. **Alvarado, C. G., A. H. Cotterell, K. R. McCurry, B. H. Collins, J. C. Magee, J. Berthold, J. S. Logan, and J. L. Platt.** 1995. Variation in the level of xenoantigen expression in porcine organs. *Transplantation* **59:**1589–1596.
4. **Anonymous.** November 14, 1911. Dr. Hammond gives patient new kidney. *The New York Times*, New York, N.Y.
5. **Anonymous.** November 15, 1911. A new surgical feat. *The New York Times*, New York, N.Y.
6. **Atkinson, J. P., T. J. Oglesby, D. White, E. A. Adams, and M. K. Liszewski**. 1991. Separation of self from non-self in the complement system: a role for membrane cofactor protein and decay accelerating factor. *Clin. Exp. Immunol.* **86**(Supp. 1)**:**27–30.
7. **Bach, F. H., C. Ferran, P. Hechenleitner, W. Mark, N. Koyamada, T. Miyatake, H. Winkler, A. Badrichani, D. Cardinas, and W. H. Hancock.** 1997. Accommodation of vascularized xenografts: expression of "protective genes" by donor endothelial cells in a host Th2 cytokine environment. *Nature Med.* **3:**196–204.
8. **Bach, F. H., H. Winkler, C. Ferran, W. W. Hancock, and S. C. Robson**. 1996. Delayed xenograft rejection. *Immunol. Today* **17:**379–384.
9. **Blakely, M. L., W. J. Van Der Werf, M. C. Berndt, A. P. Dalmasso, F. H. Bach, and W. W. Hancock.** 1994. Activation of intragraft endothelial and mononuclear cells during discordant xenograft rejection. *Transplantation* **58:**1059–1066.
10. **Blau, H. M., and M. L. Springer.** 1995. Muscle-mediated gene therapy. *N. Engl. J. Med.* **333:**1554–1556.
11. **Brauer, R. B., W. M. Baldwin III, M. R. Daha, S. K. Pruitt, and F. Sanfilippo**. 1993. Use of C6-deficient rats to evaluate the mechanism of hyperacute rejection of discordant cardiac xenografts. *J. Immunol.* **151:**7240–7248.
12. **Brent, L.** 1997. Clinical aspects and immunosuppression, p. 306–343. *In A History of Transplantation Immunology*. Academic Press, San Diego, Calif.
13. **Bustos, M., and J. L. Platt.** 1997. Platelet-endothelial cell interactions in a xenograft model. *Transplant. Proc.* **29:**886.
14. **Bustos, M., S. Saadi, and J. L. Platt.** Platelet-mediated activation of endothelial cells: implications for the pathogenesis of transplant rejection. Submitted.
15. **Byrne, G. W., K. R. McCurry, M. J. Martin, S. M. McClellan, J. L. Platt, and J. S. Logan.** 1997. Transgenic pigs expressing human CD59 and decay-accelerating factor produce an intrinsic barrier to complement-mediated damage. *Transplantation* **63:**149–155.
16. **Calne, R. Y., D. R. Davis, J. R. Pena, H. Balner, M. De Vries, B. M. Herbertson, V. C. Joysey, P. R. Millard, M. J. Seaman, J. R. Samuel, J. Stibbe, and D. L. Westbroek.** 1970. Hepatic allografts and xenografts in primates. *Lancet* **1:**103–106.
17. **Calne, R. Y., H. J. O. White, B. M. Herbertson, P. R. Millard, D. R. Davis, J. R. Salaman, and J. R. Samuel.** 1968. Pig-to-baboon liver xenografts. *Lancet* **1:**1176–1178.
18. **Carrel, A.** 1914. The transplantation of organs. *N.Y. J. Med.* **99:**839–840.
19. **Chari, R. S., B. H. Collins, J. C. Magee, A. D. Kirk, R. C. Harland, R. L. McCann, J. L. Platt, and W. C. Meyers.** 1994. Treatment of hepatic failure with ex vivo pig-liver perfusion followed by liver transplantation. *N. Engl. J. Med.* **331:**234–237.
20. **Chopek, M. W., R. L. Simmons, and J. L. Platt.** 1987. ABO-incompatible renal transplantation: initial immunopathologic evaluation. *Transplant. Proc.* **19:**4553–4557.
21. **Collins, B. H., W. Parker, and J. L. Platt.** 1994. Characterization of porcine endothelial cell determinants recognized by human natural antibodies. *Xenotransplantation* **1:**36–46.
22. **Cotterell, A. H., B. H. Collins, W. Parker, R. C. Harland, and J. L. Platt.** 1995. The humoral immune response in humans following cross-perfusion of porcine organs. *Transplantation* **60:**861–868.
23. **Cozzi, E., and D. J. G. White.** 1995. The generation of transgenic pigs as potential organ donors for humans. *Nature Med.* **1:**964–966.
24. **Cozzi, E., N. Yannoutsos, G. A. Langford, G. Pino-Chavez, J. Wallwork, and D. J. G. White.** 1997. Effect of transgenic expression of human decay-accelerating factor on the inhibition of hyperacute rejection of pig organs, p. 665–682. *In* D. K. C. Cooper, E. Kemp, J. L. Platt, and D. J. G. White (ed.), *Xenotransplantation: The Transplantation of Organs and Tissues Between Species*, 2nd ed. Springer, Berlin, Germany.
25. **Daggett, C. W., M. Yeatman, A. J. Lodge, E. P. Chen, C. Gullotto, M. M. Frank, J. L. Platt, and**

R. D. Davis. 1998. Total respiratory support from swine lungs in primate recipients. *J. Thorac. Cardiovasc. Surg.* **115:**19–27.

26. **Dalmasso, A. P., G. M. Vercellotti, J. L. Platt, and F. H. Bach.** 1991. Inhibition of complement-mediated endothelial cell cytotoxicity by decay accelerating factor: potential for prevention of xenograft hyperacute rejection. *Transplantation* **52:**530–533.
27. **Deacon, T., J. Schumacher, J. Dinsmore, C. Thomas, P. Palmer, S. Kott, A. Edge, D. Penney, S. Kassissieh, P. Dempsey, and O. Isacson.** 1997. Histological evidence of fetal pig neural cell survival after transplantation into a patient with Parkinson's disease. *Nature Med.* **3:**350–353.
28. **Diamond, L. E., K. R. McCurry, E. R. Oldham, S. B. McClellan, M. J. Martin, J. L. Platt, and J. S. Logan.** 1996. Characterization of transgenic pigs expressing functionally active human CD59 on cardiac endothelium. *Transplantation* **61:**1241–1249.
29. **Edwards, J.** 1981. Complement activation by xenogeneic red blood cells. *Transplantation* **31:**226–227.
30. **Evans, R. W., C. E. Orians, and N. L. Ascher.** 1992. The potential supply of organ donors: an assessment of the efficiency of organ procurement efforts in the United States. *J. Am. Med. Assoc.* **267:**239–246.
31. **Exner, B. G., M. Neipp, and S. T. Ildstad.** 1997. Baboon bone marrow transplantation in humans: application of cross-species disease resistance. *World J. Surg.* **21:**962–967.
32. **Galili, U., M. R. Clark, S. B. Shohet, J. Buehler, and B. A. Macher.** 1987. Evolutionary relationship between the natural anti-Gal antibody and the Galα1-3Gal epitope in primates. *Proc. Nat. Acad. Sci. USA* **84:**1369–1373.
33. **Galili, U., I. Flechner, A. Knyszynski, D. Danon, and E. A. Rachmilewitz.** 1986. The natural anti-α-galactosyl IgG on human normal senescent red blood cells. *B. J. Haematol.* **62:**317–324.
34. **Galili, U., R. E. Mandrell, R. A. Hamadeh, S. B. Shohet, and J. M. Griffiss.** 1988. Interaction between human natural anti-α-galactosyl immunoglobulin G and bacteria of the human flora. *Infect. Immun.* **56:**1730–1737.
35. **Geller, R. L., P. Rubinstein, and J. L. Platt.** 1994. Variation in expression of porcine xenogeneic antigens. *Transplantation* **58:**272–277.
36. **Geller, R. L., M. Turman, F. H. Bach, and J. L. Platt.** 1992. Deposition of polyreactive antibodies in xenograft rejection: detection using anti-idiotype monoclonal antibodies. *Transplant. Proc.* **24:**595.
37. **Good, A. H., D. K. C. Cooper, A. J. Malcolm, R. M. Ippolito, E. Koren, F. A. Neethling, Y. Ye, N. Zuhdi, and L. R. Lamontagne.** 1992. Identification of carbohydrate structures that bind human antiporcine antibodies: implications for discordant xenografting in humans. *Transplant. Proc.* **24:**559–562.
38. **Gritsch, H. A., R. M. Glaser, D. W. Emery, L. A. Lee, C. V. Smith, T. Sablinski, J. S. Arn, D. H. Sachs, and M. Sykes.** 1994. The importance of nonimmune factors in reconstitution by discordant xenogeneic hematopoietic cells. *Transplantation* **57:**906–917.
39. **Groth, C. G., O. Korsgren, A. Tibell, J. Tollemar, E. Moller, J. Bolinder, J. Ostman, F. P. Reinholt, C. Hellerstrom, and A. Andersson.** 1994. Transplantation of porcine fetal pancreas to diabetic patients. *Lancet* **344:**1402–1404.
40. **Guthrie, C. C.** 1912. *Blood-Vessel Surgery and Its Applications*. Longmans, Green & Co., New York, N.Y.
41. **Heneine, W., A. Tibell, W. M. Switzer, P. Sandstrom, G. V. Rosales, A. Mathews, O. Korsgren, L. E. Chapman, T. M. Folks, and C. G. Groth.** 1998. No evidence of infection with porcine endogenous retrovirus in recipients of porcine islet-cell xenografts. *Lancet* **352:**695–699.
42. **Holzknecht, Z. E., S. Coombes, B. A. Blocher, T. B. Plummer, M. Bustos, C. L. Lau, R. D. Davis, and J. L. Platt.** Immune complex formation after xenotransplantation. Submitted.
43. **Holzknecht, Z. E., S. Coombes, B. A. Blocher, T. B. Plummer, M. Bustos, C. L. Lau, R. D. Davis, and J. L. Platt.** Evidence of immunocomplex formation in pulmonary xenografts. *Transplant. Proc.* In press.
44. **Holzknecht, Z. E., and J. L. Platt.** 1995. Identification of porcine endothelial cell membrane antigens recognized by human xenoreactive antibodies. *J. Immunol.* **154:**4565–4575.
45. **Inverardi, L., B. Clissi, A. L. Stolzer, J. R. Bender, and R. Pardi.** 1996. Overlapping recognition of xenogeneic carbohydrate ligands by human natural killer lymphocytes and natural antibodies. *Transplant. Proc.* **28:**552.
46. **Inverardi, L., M. Samaja, R. Motterlini, F. Mangili, J. R. Bender, and R. Pardi.** 1992. Early recognition of a discordant xenogeneic organ by human circulating lymphocytes. *J. Immunol.* **149:**1416–1423.
47. **Jaboulay, M.** 1906. De reins au pli du coude par soutures arterielles et veineuses. *Lyon Med.* **107:**575–577.
48. **Jooste, S. V., R. B. Colvin, and H. J. Winn.** 1981. The vascular bed as the primary target in the destruction of skin grafts by antiserum. *J. Exp. Med.* **154:**1332–1341.

49. **Kaplon, R. J., R. E. Michler, H. Xu, P. A. Kwiatkowski, N. M. Edwards, and J. L. Platt.** 1994. Absence of hyperacute rejection in newborn pig-to-baboon cardiac xenografts. *Transplantation* **59:**1–6.
50. **Kaplon, R. J., J. L. Platt, P. A. Kwiatkowski, N. M. Edwards, H. Xu, A. S. Shah, and R. E. Michler.** 1995. Absence of hyperacute rejection in pig-to-primate orthotopic pulmonary xenografts. *Transplantation* **59:**410–416.
51. **Kaufman, D. B., J. L. Platt, F. L. Rabe, P. G. Stock, and D. E. R. Sutherland.** 1990. The immunological basis of islet allograft primary non-function. *J. Exp. Med.* **172:**291–302.
52. **Kypson, A. P., K. Peppel, S. A. Akhter, R. E. Lilly, D. D. Glower, R. J. Lefkowitz, and W. J. Koch.** 1998. Ex vivo adenoviral-mediated gene transfer to the adult rat heart. *J. Thorac. Cardiovasc. Surg.* **115:**623–630.
53. **Lawson, J. H., L. Daniels, and J. L. Platt.** 1997. The evaluation of thrombomodulin activity in porcine to human xenotransplantation. *Transplant. Proc.* **29:**884–885.
54. **Lawson, J. H., and J. L. Platt.** 1996. Molecular barriers to xenotransplantation. *Transplantation* **62:**303–310.
55. **Leventhal, J. R., A. J. Matas, L. H. Sun, S. Reif, R. M. Bolman, A. P. Dalmasso, and J. L. Platt.** 1993. The immunopathology of cardiac xenograft rejection in the guinea pig-to-rat model. *Transplantation* **56:** 1–8.
56. **Leventhal, J. R., P. Sakiyalak, J. Witson, P. Simone, A. J. Matas, R. M. Bolman, and A. P. Dalmasso.** 1994. The synergistic effect of combined antibody and complement depletion on discordant cardiac xenograft survival in nonhuman primates. *Transplantation* **57:**974–978.
57. **Li, H., C. Ricordi, A. J. Demetris, C. L. Kaufman, C. Korbanic, M. L. Hronakes, and S. T. Ildstad.** 1994. Mixed xenogeneic chimerism (mouse+rat∗>mouse) to induce donor-specific tolerance to sequential or simultaneous islet xenografts. *Transplantation* **57:**592–598.
58. **Lin, S. S., D. L. Kooyman, L. J. Daniels, C. W. Daggett, W. Parker, J. H. Lawson, C. W. Hoopes, C. Gullotto, L. Li, P. Birch, R. D. Davis, L. E. Diamond, J. S. Logan, and J. L. Platt.** 1997. The role of natural anti-Galα1-3Gal antibodies in hyperacute rejection of pig-to-baboon cardiac xenotransplants. *Transplant. Immunol.* **5:**212–218.
59. **Lin, S. S., and J. L. Platt.** 1998. Genetic therapies for xenotransplantation. *J. Am. Coll. Surg.* **186:**388–396.
60. **Lin, S. S., B. C. Weidner, G. W. Byrne, L. E. Diamond, J. H. Lawson, C. W. Hoopes, L. J. Daniels, C. W. Daggett, W. Parker, R. C. Harland, R. D. Davis, R. R. Bollinger, J. S. Logan, and J. L. Platt.** 1998. The role of antibodies in acute vascular rejection of pig-to-baboon cardiac transplants. *J. Clin. Invest.* **101:**1745–1756.
61. **Logan, J. S., and M. J. Martin.** 1994. Transgenic swine as a recombinant production system for human hemoglobin. *Meth. Enzymol.* **231:**435–445.
62. **Magee, J. C., B. H. Collins, R. C. Harland, B. J. Lindman, R. R. Bollinger, M. M. Frank, and J. L. Platt.** 1995. Immunoglobulin prevents complement mediated hyperacute rejection in swine-to-primate xenotransplantation. *J. Clin. Invest.* **96:**2404–2412.
63. **Malyguine, A. M., S. Saadi, R. A. Holzknecht, C. R. Patte, N. Sud, J. L. Platt, and J. R. Dawson.** 1997. Induction of procoagulant function in porcine endothelial cells by human NK cells. *J. Immunol.* **159:**4659–4664.
64. **Malyguine, A. M., S. Saadi, J. L. Platt, and J. R. Dawson.** 1996. Human natural killer cells induce morphologic changes in porcine endothelial cell monolayers. *Transplantation* **61:**161–164.
65. **Martin, U., V. Kiessig, J. H. Blusch, A. Haverich, K. von der Helm, T. Herden, and G. Steinhoff.** 1998. Expression of pig endogenous retrovirus by primary porcine endothelial cells and infection of human cells. *Lancet* **352**(9129)**:**692–694.
66. **McCurry, K. R., D. L. Kooyman, C. G. Alvarado, A. H. Cotterell, M. J. Martin, J. S. Logan, and J. L. Platt.** 1995. Human complement regulatory proteins protect swine-to-primate cardiac xenografts from humoral injury. *Nature Med.* **1:**423–427.
67. **McCurry, K. R., W. Parker, A. H. Cotterell, B. C. Weidner, S. S. Lin, L. J. Daniels, Z. E. Holzknecht, G. W. Byrne, L. E. Diamond, J. S. Logan, and J. L. Platt.** 1997. Humoral responses in pig-to-baboon cardiac transplantation: implications for the pathogenesis and treatment of acute vascular rejection and for accommodation. *Hum. Immunol.* **58:**91–105.
68. **Meng, X. J., R. H. Purcell, P. G. Halbur, J. R. Lehman, D. M. Webb, T. S. Tsareva, J. S. Haynes, B. J. Thacker, and S. U. Emerson.** 1997. A novel virus in swine is closely related to the human hepatitis E virus. *Proc. Nat. Acad. Sci. USA* **94:**9860–9865.

69. **Moses, R. D., H. J. Winn, and H. Auchincloss, Jr.** 1992. Multiple defects in cell surface molecule interactions across species differences are responsible for diminished xenogeneic T cell responses. *Transplantation* **53:**203–209.

70. **Murray, A. G., M. M. Khodadoust, J. S. Pober, and A. L. M. Bothwell.** 1994. Porcine aortic endothelial cells activate human T cells: direct presentation of MHC antigens and costimulation by ligands for human CD2 and CD28. *Immunity* **1:**57–63.

71. **Ohdan, H., Y.-G. Yang, A. Shimizu, K. G. Swenson, and M. Sykes.** 1999. Mixed bone marrow chimerism induced without lethal conditioning prevents T cell- and anti-Galα1,3Gal-mediated heart graft rejection. *J. Clin. Invest.* **104:**281–290.

72. **Paradis, K., G. Langford, Z. Long, W. Heneine, P. Sandstrom, W. M. Switzer, L. E. Chapman, C. Lockey, and D. Onions.** 1999. Search for cross-species transmission of porcine endogenous retrovirus in patients treated with living pig tissue. *Science* **285:**1236–1241.

73. **Parker, W., D. Bruno, Z. E. Holzknecht, and J. L. Platt.** 1994. Xenoreactive natural antibodies: isolation and initial characterization. *J. Immunol.* **153:**3791–3803.

74. **Parker, W., K. Lundberg-Swanson, Z. E. Holzknecht, J. Lateef, S. A. Washburn, S. J. Braedehoeft, and J. L. Platt.** 1996. Isohemagglutinins and xenoreactive antibodies are members of a distinct family of natural antibodies. *Hum. Immunol.* **45:**94–104.

75. **Parker, W., S. Saadi, S. S. Lin, Z. E. Holzknecht, M. Bustos, and J. L. Platt.** 1996. Transplantation of discordant xenografts: a challenge revisited. *Immunol. Today* **17:**373–378.

76. **Parker, W., P. B. Yu, Z. E. Holzknecht, K. Lundberg-Swanson, R. H. Buckley, and J. L. Platt.** 1997. Specificity and function of "natural" antibodies in immunodeficient subjects: clues to B-cell lineage and development. *J. Clin. Immunol.* **17:**311–321.

77. **Patience, C., Y. Takeuchi, and R. A. Weiss.** 1997. Infection of human cells by an endogenous retrovirus of pigs. *Nature Med.* **3:**282–286.

78. **Platt, J. L.** 1995. *Hyperacute Xenograft Rejection.* R.G. Landes, Austin, Tex.

79. **Platt, J. L.** 1998. New directions for organ transplantation. *Nature* **392**(Suppl)**:**11–17.

80. **Platt, J. L., R. J. Fischel, A. J. Matas, S. A. Reif, R. M. Bolman, and F. H. Bach.** 1991. Immunopathology of hyperacute xenograft rejection in a swine-to-primate model. *Transplantation* **52:**214–220.

81. **Platt, J. L., T. W. LeBien, and A. F. Michael.** 1982. Interstitial mononuclear cell populations in renal graft rejection: identification by monoclonal antibodies in tissue sections. *J. Exp. Med.* **155:**17–30.

82. **Platt, J. L., S. S. Lin, and C. G. A. McGregor.** 1998. Acute vascular rejection. *Xenotransplantation* **5:**169–175.

83. **Platt, J. L., B. J. Lindman, R. L. Geller, H. J. Noreen, J. L. Swanson, A. P. Dalmasso, and F. H. Bach.** 1991. The role of natural antibodies in the activation of xenogenic endothelial cells. *Transplantation* **52:**1037–1043.

84. **Platt, J. L., and J. S. Logan.** 1997. The generation and use of transgenic animals for xenotransplantation, p. 455–460. *In* L. M. Houdebine (ed.), *Transgenic Animals: Generation and Use*, 1st ed. Harwood Academic Publishers GmbH, Amsterdam, The Netherlands.

85. **Platt, J. L., and J. S. Logan.** 1996. Use of transgenic animals in xenotransplantation. *Transplant. Rev.* **10:**69–77.

86. **Platt, J. L., G. M. Vercellotti, A. P. Dalmasso, A. J. Matas, R. M. Bolman, J. S. Najarian, and F. H. Bach.** 1990. Transplantation of discordant xenografts: a review of progress. *Immunol. Today* **11:**450–456.

87. **Platt, J. L., G. M. Vercellotti, B. J. Lindman, T. R. Oegema, Jr., F. H. Bach, and A. P. Dalmasso.** 1990. Release of heparan sulfate from endothelial cells: implications for the pathogenesis of hyperacute rejection. *J. Exp. Med.* **171:**1363–1368.

88. **Powelson, J., A. B. Cosimi, W. Austen, M. Bailen, Jr., R. Colvin, P. Gianello, T. Sablinski, T. Lorf, T. Kawai, M. Tanaka, and D. Sachs.** 1994. Porcine-to-primate orthotopic liver transplantation. *Transplant. Proc.* **26:**1353–1354.

89. **Pruitt, S. K., A. D. Kirk, R. R. Bollinger, H. C. Marsh, Jr., B. H. Collins, J. L. Levin, J. R. Mault, J. S. Heinle, S. Ibrahim, A. R. Rudolph, W. M. Baldwin III, and F. Sanfilippo.** 1994. The effect of soluble complement receptor type 1 on hyperacute rejection of porcine xenografts. *Transplantation* **57:**363–370.

90. **Reemtsma, K., B. H. McCracken, J. U. Schlegel, M. A. Pearl, C. W. Pearce, C. W. DeWitt, P. E. Smith, R. L. Hewitt, R. L. Flinner, and O. Creech.** 1964. Renal heterotransplantation in man. *Ann. Surg.* **160:**384–410.

91. **Rother, R. P., W. L. Fodor, J. P. Springhorn, C. W. Birks, E. Setter, M. S. Sandrin, S. P. Squinto, and S. A. Rollins.** 1995. A novel mechanism of retrovirus inactivation in human serum mediated by anti-α-galactosyl natural antibody. *J. Exp. Med.* **182:**1345–1355.
92. **Saadi, S., N. S. Ihrcke, and J. L. Platt.** 1996. Pathophysiology of xenograft rejection, p. 31–45. *In* R. Lieberman and R. Morris (ed.), *Principles of Immunomodulatory Drug Development in Transplantation and Autoimmunity*, 1st ed. Raven Press, New York, N.Y.
93. **Saadi, S., and J. L. Platt.** 1998. Endothelial cell responses to complement activation, p. 335–353. *In* J. E. Volanakis and M. M. Frank (ed.), *The Human Complement System in Health and Disease*. Marcel Dekker, Inc., New York, N.Y.
94. **Saadi, S., and J. L. Platt.** 1995. Transient perturbation of endothelial integrity induced by antibodies and complement. *J. Exp. Med.* **181:**21–31.
95. **Sablinski, T., D. Latinne, P. Gianello, M. Bailin, K. Bergen, R. B. Colvin, A. Foley, H. Hong, T. Lorf, S. Meehan, R. Monroy, J. A. Powelson, M. Sykes, M. Tanaka, A. B. Cosimi, and D. H. Sachs.** 1995. Xenotransplantation of pig kidneys to nonhuman primates: I. development of the model. *Xenotransplantation* **2:**264–270.
96. **Sachs, D. H., and T. Sablinski.** 1995. Tolerance across discordant xenogeneic barriers. *Xenotransplantation* **2:**234–239.
97. **Sandrin, M. S., W. L. Fodor, E. Mouhtouris, N. Osman, S. Cohney, S. A. Rollins, E. R. Guilmette, E. Setter, S. P. Squinto, and I. McKenzie.** 1995. Enzymatic remodelling of the carbohydrate surface of a xenogeneic cell substantially reduces human antibody binding and complement-mediated cytolysis. *Nat. Med.* **1:**1261–1267.
98. **Sandrin, M. S., H. A. Vaughan, P. L. Dabkowski, and I. F. C. McKenzie.** 1993. Anti-pig IgM antibodies in human serum react predominantly with Galα(1,3)Gal epitopes. *Proc. Nat. Acad. Sci. USA* **90:**11391–11395.
99. **Schmoeckel, M., F. N. K. Bhatti, A. Zaidi, E. Cozzi, P. D. Waterworth, M. J. Tolan, M. Goddard, R. G. Warner, G. A. Langford, J. J. Dunning, J. Wallwork, and D. J. G. White.** 1998. Orthotopic heart transplantation in a transgenic pig-to-primate model. *Transplantation* **65:**1570–1577.
100. **Selvan, R. S., H. B. Kapadia, and J. L. Platt.** 1998. Complement-induced expression of chemokine genes in endothelium: regulation by IL-1-dependent and -independent mechanisms. *J. Immunol.* **161:**4388–4395.
101. **Sharma, A., J. F. Okabe, P. Birch, J. L. Platt, and J. S. Logan.** 1996. Reduction in the level of Gal (α1,3) Gal in transgenic mice and pigs by the expression of an α(1,2) fucosyltransferase. *Proc. Nat. Acad. Sci. USA* **93:**7190–7195.
102. **Starzl, T. E., A. J. Demetris, N. Murase, S. Ildstad, C. Ricordi, and M. Trucco.** 1992. Cell migration, chimerism, and graft acceptance. *Lancet* **339:**1579–1582.
103. **Starzl, T. E., J. Fung, A. Tzakis, S. Todo, A. J. Demetris, I. R. Marino, H. Doyle, A. Zeevi, V. Warty, M. Michaels, S. Kusne, W. A. Rudert, and M. Trucco.** 1993. Baboon-to-human liver transplantation. *Lancet* **341:**65–71.
104. **Starzl, T. E., T. L. Marchioro, G. N. Peters, C. H. Kirkpatrick, W. E. C. Wilson, K. A. Porter, D. Rifkind, D. A. Ogden, C. R. Hitchcock, and W. R. Waddell.** 1964. Renal heterotransplantation from baboon to man: experience with 6 cases. *Transplantation* **2:**752–776.
105. **Takahashi, T., S. Saadi, and J. Platt.** 1997. Recent advances in the immunology of xenotransplantation. *Immunol. Res.* **16:**273–297.
106. **Ullman, E.** 1914. Tissue and organ transplantation. *Ann. Surg.* **60:**195–219.
107. **Yamada, K., D. H. Sachs, and H. DerSimonian.** 1995. Human anti-porcine xenogeneic T cell response. Evidence for allelic specificity of mixed leukocyte reaction and for both direct and indirect pathways of recognition. *J. Immunol.* **155:**5249–5256.
108. **Yang, Y.-G., E. deGoma, H. Ohdan, J. L. Bracy, Y. Xu, J. Iacomini, A. D. Thall, and M. Sykes.** 1998. Tolerization of anti-Galα1-3Gal natural antibody-forming B cells by induction of mixed chimerism. *J. Exp. Med.* **187:**1335–1342.
109. **Ye, Y., F. A. Neethling, M. Niekrasz, E. Koren, S. V. Richards, M. Martin, S. Kosanke, R. Oriol, and D. K. C. Cooper.** 1994. Evidence that intravenously administered α-galactosyl carbohydrates reduce baboon serum cytotoxicity to pig kidney cells (PK15) and transplanted pig hearts. *Transplantation* **58:**330–337.
110. **Zaidi, A., P. Friend, M. Schmoeckel, F. N. K. Bhatti, M. Tolan, P. Waterworth, E. Cozzi, G. Chavez, J. J. Dunning, J. Wallwork, and D. J. G. White.** 1997. Hyperacute rejection is not consistent after pig to primate renal xenotransplantation (abstract). Presented at the 4th International Congress for Xenotransplantation, Nantes, France.

111. **Zaidi, A., M. Schmoeckel, F. Bhatti, P. Waterworth, M. Tolan, E. Cozzi, G. Chavez, G. Langford, S. Thiru, J. Wallwork, D. White, and P. Friend.** 1998. Life-supporting pig-to-primate renal xenotransplantation using genetically modified donors. *Transplantation* **65:**1584–1590.

112. **Zehr, K. J., A. Herskowitz, P. C. Lee, P. Kumar, A. M. Gillinov, and W. A. Baumgartner.** 1994. Neutrophil adhesion and complement inhibition prolongs survival of cardiac xenografts in discordant species. *Transplantation* **57:**900–906.

113. **Zhao, Y., K. Swenson, J. J. Sergio, J. S. Arn, D. H. Sachs, and M. Sykes.** 1996. Skin graft tolerance across a discordant xenogeneic barrier. *Nature Med.* **2:**1211–1216.

Xenotransplantation
Edited by Jeffrey L. Platt

Chapter 2

Coming to Terms with Reality: Why Xenotransplantation Is a Necessity

Roger W. Evans

Transplantation is considered to be established therapy for a variety of end-stage diseases (44, 48, 92, 96). As a result, the number of persons being considered as transplant candidates has grown markedly since 1980. Unfortunately, both the need and demand for all transplant procedures grossly outstrip the supply of donor organs (17, 29–32, 35, 38, 42, 47, 64, 67, 70, 76, 83).

Many attempts have been made to confront the grim reality that many people who could benefit from transplantation fail to do so. Most significantly, in 1985, the National Task Force on Organ Transplantation was given the rather thankless assignment of trying to sort out and resolve many thorny issues surrounding the provision of transplant services (68). For all intents and purposes, the task force faced the same dilemma health services researchers have tried to address when assessing the need and demand for medical care. However, in the general case, more often than not, economics becomes the primary constraint: there are simply too few dollars available to do all the work that needs to be done (25, 26). Therefore, access soon becomes an ethical issue which health care systems worldwide attempt to address with the goal of being efficient, fair, and equitable.

Despite some obvious parallels, transplantation stands in stark contrast to many other health care services. First, while cost is an extremely critical issue, donor organ supply has always been the foremost concern (33, 34, 36, 40, 41, 49, 50). Second, transplantation technology has evolved to the point where the number of persons who could benefit each year has increased manyfold, with the gap between need and demand narrowing. Third, this situation has, in turn, been the source of highly controversial disputes related to the selection of transplant recipients, the criteria for donor selection, the quality and distribution of transplant services, the relative cost-effectiveness of transplant services, methods of donor organ procurement, and the role of new technology (2, 11, 39, 52, 55, 65, 85). Finally, it is conceivable that if we were to resolve the supply issue, the financial one would become even more significant than it is today.

Against this health policy backdrop, the primary objective of this chapter is modest. If we are to appreciate the options available to address the problems of need, supply, and demand,

Roger W. Evans • 2251 Baihly Hills Drive S.W., Rochester, MN 55902.

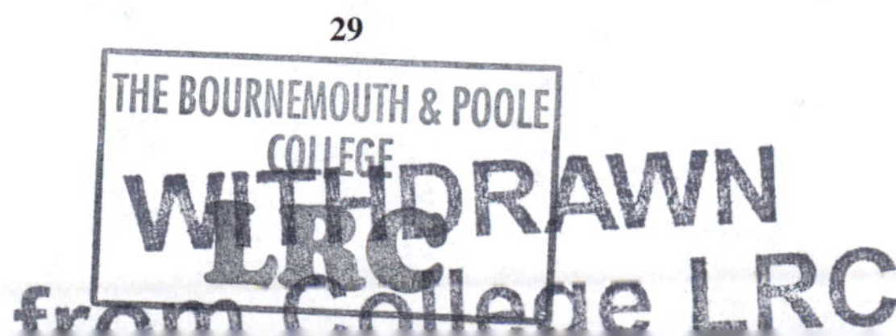

it is critical that we understand, both conceptually and empirically, the situation we are in. Too often, naïve analysts and misleading analyses give us the impression that the future will be unlike the past, since both xenotransplantation and mechanical devices will enable us to overcome the supply constraint (1, 13, 18, 19, 21, 22, 37, 43, 46, 57, 61, 66, 69, 78, 91, 93). In addition, it is hypothesized that new technologies will allow us to eliminate the clinical and immunological hurdles that have made transplantation an excessively expensive therapeutic endeavor. Unfortunately, while optimism may be a source of inspiration, too often, when it is unrealistic, it is a precursor to defeat. Ultimately, hope must be tempered by reality.

THE CONCEPTS OF NEED, DEMAND, AND SUPPLY

Elsewhere I have described a conceptual approach to the analysis of need, demand, and supply in organ transplantation (38). The schematic presented in Fig. 1 captures what I consider to be the essential distinctions between the concepts of need and demand. Too often, the terms need and demand are used interchangeably when, in fact, as I will argue, the concepts are very different from each other. Moreover, even reasonably astute analysts express the demand for transplantation only in terms of the number of persons on the transplant waiting list at the end of a defined period (e.g., year end). This, as shown in Fig. 1, represents, in part, the "unmet demand" for transplantation.

The criteria and process used to select transplant candidates are hardly uniform or, for that matter, consistent. For example, for years kidney transplant surgeons have maintained that only a small fraction of the patients on kidney dialysis who might benefit from a kidney transplant are ever referred for evaluation (31). Economic incentives, critics maintain, have led nephrologists to prefer dialysis over transplantation. Moreover, in the case of extrarenal transplantation, insurance and ability to pay have been considered as demand constraints (27, 28, 84). In other words, people who cannot pay become the victims of a so-called "green screen"—a barrier that precludes their access to services from which they might otherwise benefit. In short, clinical and nonclinical factors may contribute to what I refer to as the "unrecognized need" for transplantation. Individuals in this category are unlikely to be worked up or listed as suitable transplant candidates, even though they may benefit from the surgery they are denied an opportunity to receive.

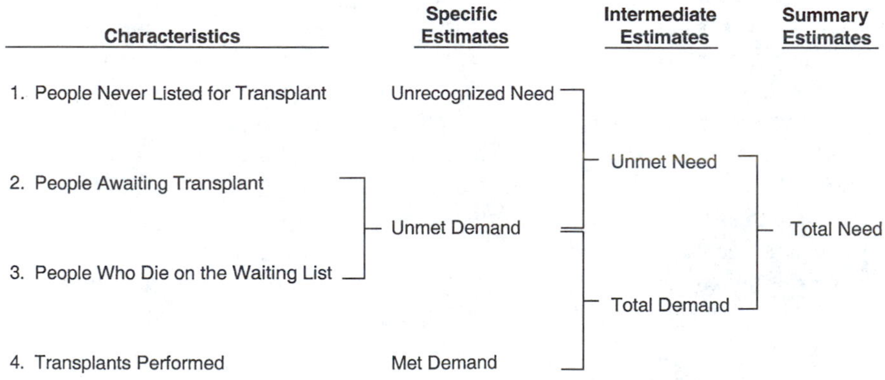

Figure 1. The concepts of need and demand in organ transplantation.

The demand for transplantation, as illustrated in Fig. 1, has three components. First, there are those individuals who are on the list and awaiting the availability of a suitable donor organ. Second, during the course of a year, people on the waiting list die before an organ becomes available to them. Finally, persons who have received a transplant must be included in any attempt to quantify demand. From my perspective, the first two groups of patients constitute "unmet demand," while the third is, perhaps, best described as "met demand." Therefore, as is apparent from Fig. 1, we can talk about three critical concepts—"unrecognized need," "unmet demand," and "met demand"—for which we can derive three "specific estimates."

The next stage in the schematic, labeled as "intermediate estimates," is slightly confusing, since unmet demand factors into both "unmet need" and "total demand." Thus, in decomposing the final "summary estimate" of "total need," we must not double count; unmet demand should enter our calculations only once.

The definitions of the concepts critical to our discussion thus far are summarized in Table 1. However, as noted above, the extent to which demand is met depends on the supply of donor organs, in which case we further distinguish between "actual" and "potential" supply (42, 70). Supply, in turn, can be separately described in terms of donors and organs. The supply of paired organs obviously exceeds the supply of single organs, as in the case of kidneys and lungs. In addition, organ donors may be living-related, living-unrelated, or cadaveric. For purposes of this discussion, we will focus on actual and potential cadaveric donors and donor organs.

Potential donors are individuals from whom organs might have been retrieved or procured for purposes of transplantation. Unfortunately, families do not always consent to organ donation and, even if they do consent, they may be selective in the organs they donate. Thus, the term potential can be applied to both donors and organs.

Data on actual donors are typically compiled by organ procurement organizations and reported to the United Network for Organ Sharing (UNOS) (86–88). In addition, UNOS keeps statistics on the number of donor organs actually procured. As might be expected, although consent may be obtained and organs procured, not every "gift of life" is transplanted. In some cases, a suitable recipient may not be awaiting transplant and, in other cases, logistical considerations may preclude the use of a procured organ. In addition, transplant teams are inconsistent in the criteria they use to define a "suitable" donor organ. In the past, unused

Table 1. Definitions of concepts[a]

Unrecognized need—the number of suitable persons never placed on the transplant waiting list.

Unmet demand—the number of persons awaiting transplant plus the number of persons who die while on the waiting list.

Met demand—the number of transplants performed.

Unmet need—the number of suitable persons never placed on the transplant waiting list plus the number of persons awaiting transplant plus the number of persons who die while on the waiting list.

Total demand—the number of persons awaiting transplant plus the number of persons who die while on the waiting list plus the number of transplants performed.

Total need—the number of persons never listed for transplant plus the number of persons awaiting transplant plus the number of persons who die on the waiting list plus the number of transplants performed.

[a] *Source:* See reference 38, page 14.

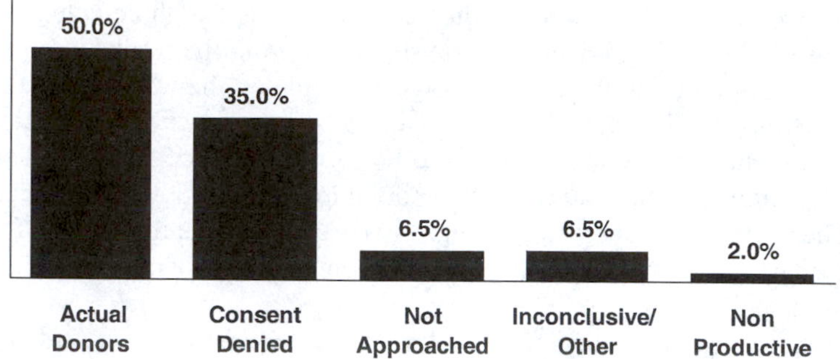

Figure 2. What happened to potential organ donors (January–March 1996)? (Data provided by Susan Gunderson, LifeSource, Inc., Minneapolis, Minn.)

donor organs were described as "wasted," a concept that is now considered to be misleading, offensive, and inappropriate. Every conceivable effort is made to place donor organs, but occasionally they must be discarded or, better yet, used for research purposes.

While the transplant community remains a strong advocate for the technology it offers, most of us now believe that, despite our best efforts, there will always be a significant discrepancy between the number of potential and the number of actual human donors. Many people fail to embrace the concept of organ donation, as is obvious from Fig. 2, wherein LifeSource reports that, in 1996, only 50% of potential donors were actually a source of cadaveric donor organs (60).

At the other end of the foregoing spectrum are those living persons who are willing to donate, either an entire or a part of a vital organ for transplantation to a relative or an "emotionally related" person. Under these circumstances, paired organs are most frequently donated, but today living-related pancreas, liver, and lung donations are feasible and conducted successfully in relatively small numbers (3–5, 10, 20, 51, 54, 56, 59, 62, 79–81, 94, 95). Various proposals have been made in an effort to enhance the opportunities for living-donor organ donation (73).

NEED AND DEMAND ESTIMATES

Data relevant to the demand for transplantation, as well as all aspects of transplant activity, are routinely published by and available from UNOS. Alternatively, need estimation has proven to be a more difficult challenge. Few attempts have been made to develop criteria and guidelines appropriate to the task. Often the indications and contraindications for various transplant procedures are identified in the literature, but little is done to derive estimates of need based on them.

In the past, my colleagues and I have estimated the need for extrarenal transplantation based on mortality data, using both cause of death and age to stratify the data (42, 70). If a person died from a cause that was a recognized indication for transplantation, and was of a suitable age (see Table 2), we assumed he or she could have benefited from a transplantation. This exercise has been relatively straightforward for heart, heart–lung, lung, and liver transplantation although, in the case of lung and heart–lung transplantation, there has been some overlap since some patients might benefit from either procedure.

Table 2. Age criteria for various organ transplants

Transplant procedure	Age (yr)
Kidney	1–64
Liver	0–64
Pancreas	1–49
Heart	0–64
Lung	1–64
Heart–lung	1–54

Estimating the need for kidney and pancreas transplantation is somewhat more complex and potentially more controversial. In both cases, end-stage renal disease (ESRD) is a major consideration. No one can say for sure how many ESRD patients might benefit from a kidney, pancreas, or pancreas–kidney transplant. We know, however, based on several sources, how many ESRD patients of various ages are on dialysis and have diabetes as their primary disease diagnosis (89, 90). From our perspective, this information provides a crude basis for need estimation.

Comorbidity is a major contraindication for most transplant procedures. Patients with multiple coexisting conditions are often unsuitable for transplantation. Even if the transplant surgery proves successful, the patient's postoperative course will, most likely, be eventful with frequent hospitalizations. Unfortunately, even large databases rarely provide the level of clinical detail required to assess the nature and extent of disease comorbidity, as is appropriate for each underlying cause of death or, in the case of ESRD patients, their primary disease diagnosis. Therefore, by definition, need estimation will remain a crude but informative exercise.

In presenting the data that follow, I will focus on overall trends. Depending on the availability of data, the time periods I cover will vary. In addition, some data will obviously be stronger than others. In concluding the chapter, I will summarize all data on an organ-specific basis and then overall.

Need Estimates

Procedure-specific estimates of the total need for transplantation for the period 1979–97 are summarized in Table 3. (For data tables, see p. 36–45. Source for data in Tables 4 through 6, 13, and 14 is the United Network for Organ Sharing, Richmond, Va. [www.UNOS. org], December, 1998.) As indicated, on the one hand, there have been substantial increases in the need for kidney, pancreas, and lung transplantation. On the other hand, there have been significant decreases in the need for liver, heart, and heart–lung transplantation.

Several caveats are relevant to the interpretation of these results. First, due to an anticipated epidemic of hepatitis C, it is conceivable that the need for liver transplantation will increase rather than decrease (23, 74). Second, the need for pancreas transplantation may be understated since the estimates in Table 3 are based on persons with ESRD who have a primary diagnosis of diabetes as the cause of their renal failure. Diabetes remains the single most common cause of ESRD. In 1996, the U.S. Renal Data System reported that 43% of all new ESRD patients are diabetic (90). Third, the decrease in the need for cardiac transplantation undoubtedly reflects the fact that superior methods have become available to treat heart disease as well as heart failure (72). Finally, despite these observations, between 1979 and 1997, the need for all major solid organ transplants has increased by at least 40%.

Demand Estimates

As described previously, three data points, all available from UNOS, are necessary to estimate the demand for transplantation. For the period 1988–97, procedure-specific data are summarized for the following: (i) the year-end waiting list (see Table 4), (ii) reported deaths on the waiting list (see Table 5), and (iii) the number of cadaveric organ transplants by year (see Table 6). Combining these data points yields an estimate of the total demand for transplantation that, in turn, is summarized in Table 7.

Although the procedure-specific data presented in Tables 4 through 7 are of interest, changes in the overall statistics are both salient and noteworthy. First, between 1988 and 1997, the number of persons awaiting transplant at year end has increased by 253%. Second, during this same period, the number of patients who died while awaiting a transplant increased by 199%. Third, all things considered, there has been but a rather modest 56% increase in the number of cadaveric organ transplants. Finally, between 1988 and 1997, we have witnessed a 158% increase in the total demand for transplantation, with organ-specific increases as follows: kidney, 106%; liver, 484%; pancreas, 651%; heart, 118%; lung, 3,276%; and heart–lung, 4%.

Synthesis of Need and Demand Estimates

Figure 1 provides a conceptual basis for synthesizing the data presented here for need and supply. As indicated, we can derive three specific estimates, two intermediate estimates, and one overall summary estimate.

Data on the unrecognized need for transplantation are summarized in Table 8. As shown, overall, 109,900 persons who could have benefited from a transplant procedure in 1997 were never recognized as such. Since 1988, this number of persons has continued to decrease as more patients have been placed on the waiting list. Apparently, despite financial considerations and other barriers, access is becoming a less significant issue than has been the case in the past.

Estimates of the unmet demand for transplantation are presented in Table 9. As indicated, the unmet demand for transplantation has markedly increased since 1988, underscoring the significance of the donor organ supply dilemma. In numerical order, the unmet demand for lung transplantation has been greatest, followed by pancreas, heart, kidney, liver, and heart–lung transplantation. Overall, the unmet demand for transplantation has increased by nearly 250%.

The met demand for transplantation has already been captured in Table 6. Although the number of transplants performed each year has increased, the overall rate of increase, at 56%, has been relatively unimpressive. However, as is apparent from Table 6, since 1988 there have been substantial increases in the number of liver, pancreas, and lung transplants performed each year. There have been more modest gains for heart and kidney transplantation, and a 16% decrease in heart–lung transplantation.

As noted previously, there is some overlap in the calculation of the intermediate estimates, namely unmet need and total demand. In each instance, unmet demand factors into both estimates. Nonetheless, unmet need and total demand are critical to our understanding of the need, demand, and supply dilemma.

Data on unmet need are summarized in Table 10, whereas data on total demand have already been presented in Table 7. Since 1988 we have seen a continued increase in both the overall unmet need for and the overall total demand for transplantation. Interestingly, however, the unmet need for liver and lung transplantation has decreased by 11.1% and 1.9%, respectively. Meanwhile, the unmet need for pancreas transplantation has increased by over 100%. At nearly 56%, the increase in the unmet need for kidney transplantation is also noteworthy.

Finally, the last summary estimate—total need—has already been quantified and, in part, described in relationship to Table 3. While there have been substantial increases in the need for some transplant procedures, there has been a remarkable decline of 7.2% in the need for heart transplantation. Once again, in numerical rank order, the total need for pancreas transplantation has increased by nearly 109%, followed by kidney (50.4%), lung (2.5%), liver (2.0%), and heart–lung (1.7%) transplantation.

SUPPLY ESTIMATES

Since 1975, many attempts have been made to address the problem of donor organ supply (6, 7, 42, 45, 47, 63, 67, 70). In virtually every case, the conclusion has been the same—there are more donor organs available than are procured. However, as shown in Table 11, there has been considerable variation in the projected number of potential donors available per million population (in tables, PMP). When extrapolated to the population of the United States, the most generous estimates suggest that more than 100 donors per million population may be available annually. More conservative estimates put this figure at between 20 and 38 donors per million population.

Upon reviewing the details of each of the studies summarized in Table 11, it is evident that differing assumptions yield varying results. In other words, none of the studies are directly comparable—all use different methods to address the same issue. In some cases death records are reviewed, and in others, summary mortality data are accessed based on electronic files. In nearly all cases, a significant margin of error exists because many clinical considerations are not quantified and meaningfully interpreted.

Data on the actual supply of cadaveric organ donors are more straightforward, with the relevant data for the period 1980–97 summarized in Table 12. As indicated, cadaveric donor supply, when expressed in terms of the number of donors per million population, has essentially doubled, from 9.4 donors per million population in 1980 to 20.5 donors in 1997.

Table 13 provides information on the number of organ-specific cadaveric donors for the period 1988–97. As indicated, there has been a 31% increase in the number of cadaveric kidney donors, a 150% increase in the number of liver donors, a 128% increase in the number of pancreas donors, a 36% increase in the number of heart donors, and a 156% increase in the number of lung donors. Overall, there has been a 34% increase in the number of actual cadaveric donors in the United States.

Data on the actual number of cadaveric donor organs procured each year in the United States since 1988 are summarized in Table 14. Over the period 1988–97 the percentage increases in the number of cadaveric organs procured have been as follows: kidneys, 30%; livers, 144%; pancreases, 125%; hearts, 38%; lungs, 470%; and overall, 62%.

Few attempts have been made to directly address the issue of organ procurement efficiency in the United States. My colleagues and I were among the first to point out with data that, relative to potential, organ procurement organizations (OPOs) were highly variable with respect to the efficiency with which they accomplish this task (42, 70). We came to this conclusion by comparing the potential number of donors available in each OPO service area with the number of donors from whom organs were actually procured. We did this by deriving both a low and a high number of potential donors per million population. Thus, we characterized OPO efficiency in terms of a range.

We concluded that somewhere between 7,000 and 10,800 organ donors were potentially available in 1989. This translated into between 28.5 and 43.7 donors per million population. Using these data, along with census figures for the U.S. population, I have estimated how many potential donors may have been available each year for the period 1990–97. The relevant estimates are provided in Table 15.

In the same study, we derived estimates of organ-specific cadaveric donor availability (see Table 16) and cadaveric donor organ availability (see Table 17) (70). Once again, we expressed these data in terms of numbers, as well as per million population. Because the criteria for organ-specific suitability vary, so do the estimates of availability. Criteria for donor lungs are more stringent than the criteria for donor kidneys. Thus, fewer potential donor lungs than donor kidneys are available.

Table 18 provides organ-specific estimates of the number of potential cadaveric organ donors that may have been available for the period 1988–97. The low figure is based on very stringent criteria, whereas the high estimate reflects slightly more liberal donor selection criteria.

Table 19 characterizes the overall efficiency of donor procurement efforts in the United States. As indicated, in 1988, donor organs were procured from between 38 and 58% of all potential donors. In 1997, the comparable range was between 47 and 72%. Clearly, efficiency varies greatly by organ type. In 1997, between 10 and 15% of potential cadaveric donors contributed lungs, compared with between 43 and 67% for kidneys.

Tables 20 and 21 provide a slightly different take on similar data. In this case, I have depicted the data according to donor organ type. For unpaired organs, such as hearts and livers, the results are the same. However, for paired organs, the situation is quite different. Nonetheless, the efficiency of procuring donors, as opposed to organs, not surprisingly, remains essentially unchanged.

Taken together, the data presented here confirm what we have known all along—more cadaveric donors are available than we currently access. The same is true of cadaveric donor organs. As a result, donor and organ procurement efforts continue to be relatively inefficient at a time when both the need and demand for transplantable cadaveric donor organs are at an all-time high.

ORGAN-SPECIFIC SUMMARY ESTIMATES

The foregoing data are, perhaps, best considered in an organ-specific summary manner. This is accomplished in Tables 22 through 27, with an overall summary provided in Table 28. In addition, Table 29 depicts the percentage change in all estimates for the period 1988–97. As indicated, the potential donor supply estimates have not been varied based on alternative assumptions. I have conservatively assumed that donor selection criteria remained unchanged during the period under scrutiny.

The shortfall in donor organ supply is readily apparent from Table 30. In this table, I am underscoring the size of the discrepancy between the total need for each transplant procedure and the most liberal estimate of donor supply (the high potential column in Tables 22 through 29). This table is slightly confusing since it gives the impression that the supply of donor heart–lungs exceeds need. This is clearly not the case since donor hearts and lungs are required for heart, lung, and heart–lung transplants. Thus, based on the assumption that all potential donor organs were procured in 1997, more than 100,000 persons who could potentially benefit from transplantation would have failed to do so. In effect, even under the best of circumstances, there are far too few human donor organs available to meet the need for them.

DISCUSSION

The data presented here enable us to put xenotransplantation into an appropriate perspective (1, 13, 18, 19, 21, 22, 43, 57, 69, 91, 93). At this time and into the foreseeable future, human donor organ supply is inadequate to meet the demand, let alone the need, for them. Thus, even under the best of circumstances, a viable alternative to human donor organs must become available if we are to meet the patient care needs we now project. In this regard, it is critical that people understand that public policy changes with respect to organ donation will ease but not eliminate the crisis we now experience (58, 71). Moreover, as patient selection criteria become increasingly liberal, the problem will become even more severe.

Of course, critics may argue that living-donor transplantation, split liver transplantation, non-heart beating organ donation, and artificial organs will eliminate the crisis (16, 37, 46, 61, 66, 75, 77, 78). Unfortunately, at this time, these innovations appear to have limited potential. While left ventricular-assist devices are appealing, their long-term use is still limited. Likewise, bioartificial livers have scientific support, but their viability remains unclear (12, 15, 53). And, finally, if living organ donation were to have a major impact, it seems it would have already become a more prevalent means to treat ESRD. Instead, people have chosen to downplay the benefits relative to the risks of living donor transplantation, and of course, these are not inconsequential (1a, 3–5, 10, 20, 51, 54, 56, 79–81, 89, 94, 95). As of this time, at least three living liver donors have died from surgical or postoperative complications. Kidney donors have likewise met the same fate although, proportionately, the number of deaths has been small.

Despite the data reported here, futile health policy efforts will be directed toward eliminating the disparity between the need for solid organ transplantation and the supply of human donor organs. For example, presumed consent has recently been endorsed by the British Medical Association, the Commonwealth of Pennsylvania has implemented financial incentives for organ donation, and the U.S. Department of Health and Human Services continues to make available grant funding for initiatives intended to increase the supply of donor organs (1a, 8, 14, 24). Meanwhile, reports from Spain and elsewhere indicate that the gap between the potential and the actual supply of donors can be narrowed through increasingly aggressive procurement efforts (9). However, as reported here, if all potential human donors became actual donors, the supply of human donor organs in the United States would remain inadequate.

At this time, it is admittedly difficult to predict the long-term outcome of xenotransplantation (13, 18, 19, 21, 22, 43, 57, 69, 82, 91, 93). If it becomes a viable therapeutic option, the donor organ shortage, as we know it, could conceivably be eliminated for most transplants. Nonetheless, the technological, immunological, ethical, and economic hurdles that lie ahead are predictably significant and immensely controversial. The means to the end we all desire is hardly straightforward. Debate is likely to increase as success is achieved. Thus, the pace of progress may be exceedingly slow, as nonclinical issues take center stage as resource constraints become as apparent as they are real.

Table 3. Total need for transplantation, 1979–97[a]

Year	Kidney	Liver	Pancreas[b]	Heart	Lung	Heart–Lung	Total
1979	31,638	23,055	1,458	56,042	14,983	7,886	134,062
1980	34,796	23,280	1,797	57,163	16,118	7,898	141,052
1981	38,353	22,033	2,399	56,453	16,300	7,742	143,280
1982	41,615	20,815	3,128	55,143	16,007	7,560	144,268
1983	44,473	20,641	3,792	55,848	16,919	7,763	149,436
1984	46,271	20,293	4,471	55,181	17,222	7,541	150,979
1985	47,743	19,941	5,106	54,775	17,777	7,515	152,857
1986	48,523	19,258	5,542	54,389	17,754	7,479	152,945
1987	49,991	19,372	6,152	53,009	17,619	7,649	153,792
1988	52,382	19,567	6,786	52,772	17,997	7,620	157,124
1989	55,301	19,518	7,832	50,568	18,382	7,700	159,301
1990	58,122	18,997	8,644	49,423	17,693	7,479	160,358
1991	61,340	18,702	9,709	48,955	17,971	7,611	164,288
1992	65,001	18,850	10,780	48,913	17,540	7,478	168,562
1993	68,159	18,882	11,464	50,169	18,531	7,537	174,742
1994	71,734	19,435	12,531	48,881	18,297	7,502	178,380
1995	75,555	19,575	13,752	48,909	18,358	7,788	183,937
1996	77,992	19,770[c]	14,144	48,950[c]	18,500[c]	7,671[c]	187,027
1997	78,806	19,968[c]	14,175	48,965[c]	18,450[c]	7,688[c]	188,052

[a] Data on kidney and pancreas transplantation provided by Paul Eggers, Ph.D., Health Care Financing Administration, Baltimore, Md.

[b] Based on the number of end-stage renal disease patients with a primary diagnosis of diabetes. While the estimates include kidney–pancreas patients, they must be considered conservative. Idealy, patients in need of a pancreas transplant would receive one before their kidneys fail.

[c] Projected.

Table 4. Year-end waiting list for transplantation, 1988–97

Year	Kidney	Liver	Pancreas[a]	Heart	Lung	Heart–Lung	Total
1988	13,943	616	163	1,030	69	205	16,026
1989	16,294	827	320	1,320	94	240	19,095
1990	17,883	1,237	473	1,788	308	225	21,914
1991	19,352	1,676	600	2,267	670	154	24,719
1992	22,376	2,323	904	2,690	942	180	29,415
1993	24,973	2,997	1,106	2,834	1,240	202	33,352
1994	27,498	4,059	1,289	2,933	1,625	205	37,609
1995	31,149	5,701	1,525	3,468	1,932	208	43,983
1996	34,646	7,480	1,788	3,700	2,318	237	50,169
1997	38,236	9,637	1,952	3,897	2,664	236	56,622

[a] Includes kidney–pancreas patients.

Table 5. Reported deaths on the waiting list, 1988–97

Year	Kidney	Liver	Pancreas[a]	Heart	Lung	Heart–Lung	Total
1988	732	195	5	494	16	62	1,504
1989	749	284	21	518	38	74	1,684
1990	921	318	19	612	50	66	1,986
1991	982	435	36	779	137	41	2,410
1992	1,055	493	48	779	218	43	2,636
1993	1,286	562	61	761	250	51	2,971
1994	1,312	658	77	722	283	47	3,099
1995	1,494	799	86	769	340	28	3,516
1996	1,797	953	94	744	386	48	4,022
1997	2,003	1,131	132	773	409	56	4,504

[a] Includes kidney–pancreas patients.

Table 6. Number of cadaveric organ transplants by year, 1988–97

Year	Kidney	Liver	Pancreas[a]	Heart	Lung	Heart–Lung	Total
1988	7,231	1,713	244	1,669	33	74	10,890
1989	7,087	2,199	431	1,696	93	67	11,555
1990	7,784	2,677	526	2,095	203	52	13,337
1991	7,333	2,931	529	2,122	401	51	13,367
1992	7,696	3,031	554	2,170	535	48	14,034
1993	8,170	3,404	772	2,295	660	60	15,361
1994	8,384	3.592	840	2,338	708	70	15,932
1995	8,603	3,879	1,018	2,361	848	70	16,779
1996	8,571	4,013	1,013	2,342	790	39	16,768
1997	8,607	4,099	1,055	2,292	911	62	17,026

[a] Includes kidney–pancreas patients.

Table 7. The total demand for cadaveric transplantation, 1988–97

Year	Kidney	Liver	Pancreas[a]	Heart	Lung	Heart–Lung	Total
1988	23,718	2,524	417	3,200	118	341	30,318
1989	26,033	3,312	758	3,543	225	381	34,252
1990	28,681	4,245	1,020	4,508	561	343	39,363
1991	30,458	5,064	1,167	5,171	1,212	246	43,330
1992	33,662	5,880	1,509	5,640	1,695	271	48,679
1993	37,279	6,999	1,941	5,892	2,157	313	54,743
1994	40,200	8,370	2,208	5,996	2,631	322	59,750
1995	44,530	10,422	2,638	6,597	3,143	306	67,681
1996	48,482	12,495	2,903	6,787	3,509	324	74,545
1997	48,846	14,867	3,139	6,962	3,984	354	78,152

[a] Includes kidney–pancreas patients.

Table 8. Estimates of the unrecognized need for transplantation, 1988–97

Year	Kidney	Liver	Pancreas[a]	Heart	Lung	Heart–Lung	Total
1988	28,664	17,043	6,369	49,572	17,879	7,279	126,806
1989	29,268	16,206	7,074	47,025	18,157	7,319	125,049
1990	29,441	14,752	7,624	44,915	17,132	7,136	120,995
1991	30,882	13,638	8,542	43,784	16,759	7,365	120,958
1992	31,339	12,970	9,271	43,273	15,845	7,207	119,883
1993	30,880	11,883	9,523	44,277	16,374	7,224	119,999
1994	31,534	11,065	10,323	42,885	15,666	7,180	118,630
1995	31,025	9,153	11,114	42,312	15,215	7,482	116,256
1996	29,510	7,275	11,241	42,163	14,991	7,347	112,482
1997	29,960	5,101	11,036	42,003	14,466	7,334	109,900

[a]Includes kidney–pancreas patients.

Table 9. Estimates of the unmet demand for transplantation, 1988–97

Year	Kidney	Liver	Pancreas[a]	Heart	Lung	Heart–Lung	Total
1988	14,675	811	168	1,524	85	267	17,530
1989	17,043	1,111	341	1,838	132	314	20,779
1990	18,804	1,555	492	2,400	358	291	23,900
1991	20,334	2,111	636	3,046	807	195	27,129
1992	23,431	2,816	952	3,469	1,160	223	32,051
1993	26,259	3,559	1,167	3,595	1,490	253	36,323
1994	28,810	4,717	1,366	3,655	1,908	252	40,708
1995	32,643	6,500	1,611	4,237	2,272	236	47,499
1996	36,433	8,433	1,882	4,444	2,704	285	54,191
1997	40,239	10,768	2,084	4,670	3,073	292	61,126

[a]Includes kidney–pancreas patients.

Table 10. Estimates of the unmet need for transplantation, 1988–97

Year	Kidney	Liver	Pancreas[a]	Heart	Lung	Heart–Lung	Total
1988	43,339	17,854	6,537	51,096	17,964	7,546	144,336
1989	46,311	17,317	7,415	48,863	18,239	7,633	145,828
1990	48,245	16,307	8,116	47,315	17,490	7,427	144,895
1991	51,216	15,749	9,178	46,830	17,566	7,560	148,087
1992	54,770	15,786	10,223	46,742	17,005	7,430	151,934
1993	57,139	15,442	10,690	47,872	17,864	7,477	156,322
1994	60,344	15,782	11,689	46,540	17,574	7,432	159,338
1995	63,668	15,653	12,725	46,549	17,487	7,718	163,755
1996	65,953	15,708	13,123	46,607	17,695	7,632	166,673
1997	70,199	15,869	13,120	46,673	17,539	7,626	171,026

[a]Includes kidney–pancreas patients.

Table 11. Estimates of potential donor supply in the United States

Area studied	Reference(s)	Yr(s)	Donor PMP		No. of donors	
			Low	High	Low	High
Georgia	6	1975–79	43.0	55.0	9,700	12,400
Georgia, Kansas, Missouri	7	1975	55.0	116.0	11,900	25,100
Varied by study	63	1986	68.0	104.0	16,400	25,000
Pennsylvania	67	1987	38.3	55.2	9,300	13,400
Kentucky	45	1989	–	48.0	–	11,900
United States	42, 70	1989	28.5	43.7	6,900	10,700
Rhode Island, Vermont	42	1990	20.0	40.0	5,000	10,000
Selected areas in U.S.	47	1996	47.4	56.9	12,600	15,100

Table 12. Number of cadaveric organ donors, 1980–97

Year	Actual no.	U.S. population (in millions)	Donors PMP
1980	2,138	227.7	9.4
1981	2,142	230.0	9.3
1982	2,300	232.2	9.9
1983	2,705	234.3	11.5
1984	3,290	236.3	13.9
1985	3,637	238.5	15.2
1986	3,990	240.7	16.6
1987	4,000	242.8	16.5
1988	4,084	245.0	16.7
1989	4,019	247.3	16.3
1990	4,512	249.9	18.1
1991	4,528	252.6	17.9
1992	4,521	255.4	17.7
1993	4,861	258.1	18.8
1994	5,100	260.7	19.6
1995	5,357	263.2	20.4
1996	5,417	265.6	20.4
1997	5,475	267.6	20.5

Table 13. Number of cadaveric organ donors by year, 1988–97

Year	Kidney	Liver	Pancreas	Heart	Lung	Total
1988	3,880	1,835	577	1,785	130	4,084
1989	3,817	2,377	799	1,782	191	4,019
1990	4,308	2,871	951	2,168	275	4,512
1991	4,269	3,167	1,066	2,198	395	4,528
1992	4,277	3,335	1,004	2,247	527	4,521
1993	4,609	3,764	1,243	2,442	790	4,861
1994	4,798	4,095	1,360	2,526	918	5,100
1995	4,997	4,324	1,286	2,503	908	5,357
1996	5,069	4,452	1,295	2,459	750	5,417
1997	5,078	4,579	1,316	2,427	836	5,475

Table 14. Number of organs recovered from cadaveric donors, 1988–97

Year	Kidney	Liver	Pancreas	Heart	Lung	Total
1988	7,712	1,843	578	1,785	243	12,161
1989	7,578	2,390	799	1,782	334	12,883
1990	8,553	2,880	951	2,168	461	15,013
1991	8,481	3,173	1,066	2,198	684	15,602
1992	8,503	3,337	1,004	2,247	933	16,024
1993	9,163	3,771	1,244	2,442	1,462	18,082
1994	9,531	4,112	1,360	2,526	1,694	19,223
1995	9,914	4,335	1,288	2,503	1,687	19,727
1996	10,017	4,491	1,300	2,459	1,385	19,652
1997	10,080	4,651	1,312	2,421	1,555	19,960

Table 15. Estimated number of potential cadaveric organ donors by year, 1988–97

Year	U.S. population (in millions)	Low[a] no. (28.5 PMP)	High[a] no. (43.7 PMP)
1988	245.0	6,983	10,707
1989	247.3	7,048	10,807
1990	249.9	7,122	10,921
1991	252.6	7,199	11,039
1992	255.4	7,279	11,161
1993	258.1	7,356	11,279
1994	260.7	7,430	11,393
1995	263.2	7,501	11,502
1996	265.6	7,570	11,607
1997	267.6	7,627	11,694

[a]Based on 1989 data, 247.3 million population.

Table 16. Potential supply of cadaveric organ donors

Estimate	Donor				
	Kidney	Liver	Pancreas	Heart	Lung
Number					
Low	6,900	6,900	6,900	5,200	5,000
High	10,700	9,600	10,700	8,200	8,000
PMP[a]					
Low	28.5	27.9	27.9	21.0	20.2
High	43.7	38.8	43.3	33.2	32.3

[a]Based on 1989 data, 247.3 million population.

Table 17. Potential supply of cadaveric donor organs

Estimate	Donor				
	Kidney	Liver	Pancreas	Heart	Lung
Number					
Low	13,800	6,900	6,900	5,200	10,000
High	21,400	9,600	10,700	8,200	16,000
PMP[a]					
Low	55.8	27.9	27.9	21.0	40.4
High	86.5	38.8	43.3	33.2	64.7

[a]Based on 1989 data, 247.3 million population.

Table 18. Potential supply of cadaveric organ donors by donor type, 1988–97[a]

Year	U.S. population (in millions)	Kidney		Liver		Pancreas		Heart		Lung	
		LO	HI	LO	HI	LO	HI	LO	HI	LO	HI
1988	245.0	6,983	10,707	6,836	9,506	6,836	10,707	5.145	8,134	4,949	7,914
1989	247.3	7,048	10,807	6,900	9,595	6,900	10,807	5,193	8,210	4,995	7,988
1990	249.9	7,122	10,921	6,972	9,696	6,972	10,921	5,248	8,297	5,048	8,072
1991	252.6	7,199	11,039	7,048	9,801	7,048	11,039	5,305	8,386	5,103	8,159
1992	255.4	7,279	11,161	7,126	9,910	7,126	11,161	5,363	8,479	5,159	8,249
1993	258.1	7,356	11,279	7,201	10,014	7,201	11,279	5,420	8,569	5,214	8,337
1994	260.7	7,430	11,393	7,274	10,115	7,274	11,393	5,475	8,655	5,266	8,421
1995	263.2	7,501	11,502	7,343	10,212	7,343	11,502	5,527	8,738	5,317	8,501
1996	265.6	7,570	11,607	7,410	10,305	7,410	11,607	5,578	8,818	5,365	8,579
1997	267.6	7,627	11,694	7,466	10,383	7,466	11,694	5,620	8,884	5,406	8,643

[a]LO, based on low number of potential donors; HI, based on high number of potential donors.

Table 19. Percentage of potential cadaveric organ donors from which organs were procured, 1988–97[a]

Year	Total (%)		Kidney		Liver		Pancreas		Heart		Lung	
	LO	HI	LO	HI	LO	HI	LO	HI	LO	HI	LO	HI
1988	58	38	56	36	27	19	8	5	35	22	3	2
1989	57	37	54	35	34	25	12	7	34	22	4	2
1990	63	41	60	39	41	30	14	9	41	26	5	3
1991	63	41	59	39	45	32	15	10	41	26	8	5
1992	62	41	59	38	47	34	14	9	42	27	10	6
1993	66	43	63	41	52	38	17	11	45	28	15	9
1994	69	45	64	42	56	40	19	12	46	29	17	11
1995	71	47	67	43	59	42	18	11	45	29	17	11
1996	72	47	67	43	60	43	17	11	44	28	14	9
1997	72	47	67	43	61	44	17	11	43	27	15	10

[a]LO, based on low number of potential donors; HI, based on high number of potential donors.

Table 20. Potential supply of cadaveric donor organs by donor type, 1988–97[a]

Year	U.S. population (in millions)	Kidney		Liver		Pancreas		Heart		Lung	
		LO	HI	LO	HI	LO	HI	LO	HI	LO	HI
1988	245.0	13,966	21,414	6,836	9,506	6,836	10,707	5,145	8,134	9,898	15,828
1989	247.3	14,096	21,614	6,900	9,595	6,900	10,807	5,193	8,210	9,990	15,976
1990	249.9	14,244	21,842	6,972	9,696	6,972	10,921	5,248	8,297	10,096	16,144
1991	252.6	14,398	22,078	7,048	9,801	7,048	11,039	5,305	8,386	10,206	16,318
1992	255.4	14,558	22,322	7,126	9,910	7,126	11,161	5,363	8,479	10,318	16,498
1993	258.1	14,712	22,558	7,201	10,014	7,201	11,279	5,420	8,569	10,428	16,674
1994	260.7	14,860	22,786	7,274	10,115	7,274	11,393	5,475	8,655	10,532	16,842
1995	263.2	15,002	23,004	7,343	10,212	7,343	11,502	5,527	8,738	10,634	17,002
1996	265.6	15,140	23,214	7,410	10,305	7,410	11,607	5,578	8,818	10,730	17,158
1997	267.6	15,254	23,388	7,466	10,383	7,466	11,694	5,620	8,884	10,812	17,286

[a] LO, based on low number of potential donors; HI, based on high number of potential donors.

Table 21. Percentage of potential cadaveric donor organs procured, 1988–97[a]

Year	U.S. population (in millions)	Kidney (%)		Liver (%)		Pancreas (%)		Heart (%)		Lung (%)	
		LO	HI	LO	HI	LO	HI	LO	HI	LO	HI
1988	245.0	55	36	27	19	8	5	35	22	2	1
1989	247.3	54	35	34	25	12	7	34	22	3	2
1990	249.9	60	39	41	30	14	9	41	26	5	3
1991	252.6	59	38	45	32	15	10	41	26	7	4
1992	255.4	58	38	47	34	14	9	42	27	9	6
1993	258.1	62	41	52	38	17	11	45	28	14	9
1994	260.7	64	42	56	40	19	12	46	29	16	10
1995	263.2	66	43	59	42	18	11	45	29	16	10
1996	265.6	66	43	60	43	17	11	44	28	13	8
1997	267.6	66	43	62	45	18	11	43	27	14	9

[a] LO, based on low number of potential donors; HI, based on high number of potential donors.

Table 22. Cadaveric kidney transplantation: need, demand, and supply, 1988–97

Year	Estimate							
	Total		Actual transplants	Donor organ supply			Unmet	
	Need	Demand		Actual	Low potential	High potential	Demand	Need
1988	52,382	23,718	7,231	7,712	13,966	21,414	16,487	45,151
1989	55,301	26,033	7,087	7,578	14,096	21,614	18,946	48,214
1990	58,122	28,681	7,784	8,553	14,244	21,842	20,897	50,338
1991	61,340	30,458	7,333	8,481	14,398	22,078	23,125	54,007
1992	65,001	33,662	7,696	8,503	14,558	22,322	25,966	57,305
1993	68,159	37,279	8,170	9,163	14,712	22,558	29,109	59,989
1994	71,734	40,200	8,384	9,531	14,860	22,786	31,816	63,350
1995	75,555	44,530	8,603	9,914	15,002	23,004	35,927	66,952
1996	77,992	48,482	8,571	10,017	15,140	23,214	39,911	69,421
1997	78,806	48,846	8,607	10,080	15,254	23,388	40,239	70,199

Table 23. Cadaveric liver transplantation: need, demand, and supply, 1988–97

Year	Estimate							
	Total		Actual transplants	Donor organ supply			Unmet	
	Need	Demand		Actual	Low potential	High potential	Demand	Need
1990	18,997	4,245	2,677	2,880	6,972	9,696	1,568	16,320
1991	18,702	5,064	2,931	3,173	7,048	9,801	2,133	15,771
1992	18,850	5,880	3,031	3,337	7,126	9,910	2,849	15,819
1993	18,882	6,999	3,404	3,771	7,201	10,014	3,595	15,478
1994	19,435	8,370	3,592	4,112	7,274	10,115	4,778	15,843
1995	19,575	10,422	3,879	4,335	7,343	10,212	6,543	15,696
1996	19,770[a]	12,495	4,013	4,491	7,410	10,305	8,482	15,757[a]
1997	19,968[a]	14,867	4,099	4,651	7,466	10,383	10,768	15,869[a]

[a] Projected.

Table 24. Cadaveric pancreas transplantation: need, demand, and supply, 1988–97

Year	Estimate							
	Total		Actual transplants	Donor organ supply			Unmet	
	Need	Demand		Actual	Low potential	High potential	Demand	Need
1989	7,832	758	413	799	6,900	10,807	345	7,074
1990	8,644	1,020	526	951	6,972	10,921	494	8,118
1991	9,709	1,167	529	1,066	7,048	11,039	638	9,180
1992	10,780	1,507	554	1,044	7,126	11,161	953	10,226
1993	11,464	1,941	772	1,244	7,201	11,279	1,169	10,692
1994	12,531	2,208	840	1,360	7,274	11,393	1,368	11,691
1995	13,752	2,638	1,018	1,288	7,343	11,502	1,620	12,734
1996	14,144	2,903	1,013	1,300	7,410	11,607	1,890	13,131
1997	14,175	3,139	1,055	1,312	7,466	11,694	2,084	13,120

Table 25. Cadaveric heart transplantation: need, demand, and supply, 1988–97

Year	Estimate							
	Total		Actual transplants	Donor organ supply			Unmet	
	Need	Demand		Actual	Low potential	High potential	Demand	Need
1989	50,568	3,543	1,696	1,782	5,193	8,210	1,847	48,872
1990	49,423	4,508	2,095	2,168	5,248	8,297	2,413	47,328
1991	48,955	5,171	2,122	2,198	5,305	8,386	3,049	46,833
1992	48,913	5,640	2,170	2,247	5,363	8,479	3,470	46,743
1993	50,169	5,892	2,295	2,442	5,420	8,569	3,597	47,874
1994	48,881	5,996	2,338	2,526	5,475	8,655	3,658	46,543
1995	48,909	6,597	2,361	2,503	5,527	8,738	4,236	46,548
1996	48,950[a]	6,787	2,342	2,459	5,578	8,818	4,445	46,608[a]
1997	48,965[a]	6,962	2,292	2,421	5,620	8,884	4,670	46,673[a]

[a] Projected.

Table 26. Cadaveric lung transplantation: need, demand, and supply, 1988–97

Year	Estimate							
	Total		Actual transplants	Donor organ supply			Unmet	
	Need	Demand		Actual	Low potential	High potential	Demand	Need
1989	18,382	225	93	334	9,990	15,976	132	18,289
1990	17,693	561	203	461	10,096	16,144	358	17,490
1991	17,971	1,212	401	684	10,206	16,318	811	17,570
1992	17,540	1,695	535	933	10,318	16,498	1,160	17,005
1993	18,531	2,157	660	1,462	10,428	16,674	1,497	17,871
1994	18,297	2,631	708	1,694	10,532	16,842	1,923	17,589
1995	18,358	3,143	848	1,687	10,634	17,002	2,295	17,510
1996	18,500[a]	3,509	790	1,385	10,730	17,158	2,719	17,710[a]
1997	18,450[a]	3,984	911	1,555	10,812	17,286	3,073	17,539[a]

[a]Projected.

Table 27. Cadaveric heart–lung transplantation: need, demand, and supply, 1988–97

Year	Estimate[a]							
	Total		Actual transplants	Donor organ supply			Unmet	
	Need	Demand		Actual	Low potential	High potential	Demand	Need
1988	7,620	341	74	130	4,949	7,914	267	7,546
1989	7,700	381	67	191	4,995	7,988	314	7,633
1990	7,479	343	52	275	5,048	8,072	291	7,427
1991	7,611	246	51	395	5,103	8,159	195	7,560
1992	7,478	271	48	527	5,159	8,249	223	7,207
1993	7,537	313	60	790	5,214	8,337	253	7,477
1994	7,502	322	70	918	5,266	8,421	252	7,432
1995	7,788	306	70	908	5,317	8,501	236	7,718
1996	7,700[b]	324	39	750	5,365	8,579	285	7,671[b]
1997	7,750[b]	354	62	N/A[c]	5,406	8,643	292	7,688[b]

[a]Based on number of lung donors (not donor lungs).
[b]Projected.
[c]NA = not available.

Table 28. Cadaveric transplantation: need, demand, and supply, 1988–97

Year	Estimate							
	Total		Actual transplants	Donor organ supply			Unmet	
	Need	Demand		Actual	Low potential	High potential	Demand	Need
1988	157,124	30,318	10,890	12,161	42,681	65,589	17,530	145,336
1989	159,301	34,252	11,555	12,883	43,079	66,202	20,779	145,828
1990	160,358	39,363	13,337	15,013	43,532	66,900	23,900	144,895
1991	164,288	43,330	13,367	15,602	44,005	67.622	27,129	148,087
1992	168,562	48,679	14,034	16,024	44,491	68,370	32,051	151,934
1993	174,742	54,743	15,361	18,082	44,962	69,094	36,323	156,322
1994	178,380	59,750	15,932	19,223	45,415	69,791	40,708	159,338
1995	183,937	67,681	16,779	19,727	45,849	70,458	47,499	163,755
1996	187,027	74,545	16,768	19,652	46,268	71,102	54,191	166,673
1997	188,052	78,152	17,026	19,960	46,618	71,635	61,126	171,026

Table 29. Cadaveric transplantation: percentage change in estimates from 1988 to 1997

Cadaveric transplant procedure	% change in estimate of the following:							
	Total		Actual transplants	Donor organ supply			Unmet	
	Need	Demand		Actual	Low potential	High potential	Demand	Need
Kidney	50.4	105.9	19.0	30.7	9.2	9.2	144.1	55.5
Liver	2.0	489.0	139.3	152.4	9.2	9.2	122.8	− 11.1
Pancreas	108.9	566.5	332.4	127.0	9.2	9.2	1,104.6	100.6
Heart	− 7.2	117.6	37.3	35.6	9.2	9.2	205.0	8.7
Lung	2.5	3,276.3	2,660.6	5,399.2	9.2	9.2	3,515.3	− 1.9
Heart–lung	1.7	3.8	− 16.2	476.9	9.2	9.2	9.4	1.9
Overall	19.7	157.8	56.3	64.1	9.2	9.2	248.7	17.7

Table 30. Discrepancy between the need for cadaveric transplantation and the supply of cadaveric donor organs, 1997

Cadaveric transplant procedure	Total need	Potential donor organ supply	Differencc
Kidney	78,806	23,388	−55,418
Liver	19,968	10,383	−9,585
Pancreas	14,175	11,694	−2,481
Heart	48,965	8,884	−40,081
Lung	18,450	17,286	−1,164
Heart–lung[a]	7,750	8,643	+893

[a]These figures are deceptive since donor hearts and lungs are required for heart, lung, and heart–lung transplantation. Thus, in effect, the supply of hearts and lungs is inadequate.

REFERENCES

1. **Advisory Group on the Ethics of Xenotransplantation.** 1997. *Animal Tissue into Humans.* Department of Health, London, England.

1a. **Ashraf, H.** 1999. Doctor and patient groups vote for presumed consent. *Lancet* **354:**230.

2. **Associated Press.** 1999. Sickest patients to receive more transplants. *Mod. Healthcare* **29:**4.

3. **Baker, A., A. Dhawan, J. Devlin, G. Mieli-Vergani, J. O'Grady, R. Williams, M. Rela, and N. Heaton.** 1999. Assessment of potential donors for living related liver transplantation. *Br. J. Surg.* **86:**200–205.

4. **Barbers, R. G.** 1998. Cystic fibrosis: bilateral living lobar versus cadaveric lung transplantation (review). *Am. J. Med. Sci.* **315:**155–160.

5. **Barr, M. L., F. A. Schenkel, R. G. Cohen, R. G. Barbers, C. B. Fuller, J. A. Hagen, W. J. Wells, and V. A. Starnes.** 1998. Recipient and donor outcomes in living related and unrelated lobar transplantation. *Transplant. Proc.* **30:**2261–2263.

6. **Bart, K. J., E. J. Macon, and A. L. Humphries.** 1979. A response to the shortage of cadaveric kidneys for transplantation. *Transplant. Proc.* **11:**455-457.

7. **Bart, K. J., E. J. Macon, F. C. Whittier, R. J. Baldwin, and J. H. Blount.** 1981. Cadaveric kidneys for transplantation: a paradox of shortage in the face of plenty. *Transplant. Proc.* **31:**379–382.

8. **Beecham, L.** 1999. BMA wants presumed consent for organ donors. *Br. Med. J.* **319:**141.

9. **Bosch, X.** 1999. Spain leads world in organ donation and transplantation. *JAMA* **282:**17–18.

10. **Bucuvalas, J. C., and F. C. Ryckman** 1999. The long- and short-term outcome of living-donor liver transplantation (editorial). *J. Pediatr.* **134:**259–261.

11. **Burdick, J. F., A. S. Klein, and A. M. Harper.** 1997. The debate over liver allocation in the United States: the UNOS perspective, p. 322–324. *In* J. M. Cecka and P. I. Terasaki (ed.), *Clinical Transplants, 1996.* UCLA Tissue Typing Laboratory, Los Angeles, Calif.

12. **Cattral, M. S., and G. A. Levy.** 1994. Artificial liver support—pipe dream or reality? *N. Engl. J. Med.* **331:**268–269.
13. **Chapman, L. E., T. M. Folks, D. R. Salomon, A. P. Patterson, T. E. Eggerman, and P. D. Noguchi.** 1995. Xenotransplantation and xenogeneic infections. *N. Engl. J. Med.* **333:**1498–1501.
14. **Charatan, F.** 1999. Pennsylvania plans to reward organ donation. *Br. Med. J.* **318:**1371.
15. **Chari, R. S., B. H. Collins, J. C. Magee, J. M. DiMaio, A. D. Kirk, R. C. Harland, R. L. Mccann, J. L. Platt, and W. C. Meyers.** 1994. Brief report: treatment of hepatic failure with ex vivo pig-liver perfusion followed by liver transplantation. *N. Engl. J. Med.* **331:**234–237.
16. **Cho, Y. W., P. I. Terasaki, M. Cecka, and D. W. Gjertson.** 1998. Transplantation of kidneys from donors whose hearts have stopped beating. *N. Engl. J. Med.* **338:**221–225.
17. **Christiansen, C. L., S. L. Gortmaker, J. M. Williams, C. L. Beasley, L. E. Brigham, C. Capossela, M. E. Matthiesen, and S. Gunderson.** 1998. A method for estimating solid organ donor potential by organ precurement region. *Am. J. Public Health* **88:**1645–1650.
18. **Committee on Xenograft Transplantation.** 1996. *Xenotransplantation: Science, Ethics, and Public Policy.* National Academy Press, Washington, D.C.
19. **Committee on Xenotransplantation.** 1998. *Xenotransplantation.* Health Council of the Netherlands, Rijswijk, Netherlands.
20. **Dark, J. H.** 1997. Lung: living-related transplantation (review). *Br. Med. Bull.* **53:**892–903.
21. **Dorling, A., K. Riesbeck, A. Warrens, and R. Lechler.** 1997. Clinical xenotransplantation of solid organs. *Lancet* **349:**867–871.
22. **Durand de Bousingen, D.** 1999. Europe supports moratorium on xenotransplantation. *Lancet* **353:**476.
23. **Editorial.** 1998. Making sense of hepatitis C. *Lancet* **352:**1485.
24. **Editorial.** 1999. Paying respect to organs. *Lancet* **353:**2085.
25. **Evans, R. W.** 1983. Health care technology and the inevitability of resource allocation and rationing decisions, Part I. *JAMA* **249:**2047–2053.
26. **Evans, R. W.** 1983. Health care technology and the inevitability of resource allocation and rationing decisions, Part II. *JAMA* **249:**2208–2219.
27. **Evans, R. W.** 1986. Coverage and reimbursement for heart transplantation. *Int. J. Tech. Assess. Health Care* **2:**425–449.
28. **Evans, R. W.** 1989. Money matters: should ability to pay ever be a consideration in gaining access to transplantation? *Transplant. Proc.* **21:**3419–3423.
29. **Evans, R. W.** 1990. The actual and potential supply of organ donors in the United States, p. 329–341. *In* P. I. Terasaki (ed.), *Clinical Transplants, 1990.* UCLA Tissue Typing Laboratory, Los Angeles, Calif.
30. **Evans, R. W.** 1990. The demand for transplantation in the United States, p. 319–325. *In* P. I. Terasaki (ed.), *Clinical Transplants, 1990.* UCLA Tissue Typing Laboratory, Los Angeles, Calif.
31. **Evans, R. W.** 1992. Need, demand, and supply in kidney transplantation: a review of the data, an examination of the issues, and projections through the year 2000. *Semin. Nephrol.* **12:**234–255.
32. **Evans, R. W.** 1992. Need, demand, and supply in organ transplantation. *Transplant. Proc.* **24:**2152–2154.
33. **Evans, R. W.** 1994. Organ transplantation and the inevitable debate as to what constitutes a basic health care benefit, p. 359–391. *In* P. I. Terasaki and J. M. Cecka (ed.), *Clinical Transplants, 1993.* UCLA Tissue Typing Laboratory, Los Angeles, Calif.
34. **Evans, R. W.** 1995. Liver transplantation in a managed care environment. *Liver Transplant. Surg.* **1:**61–75.
35. **Evans, R. W.** 1995. Need for liver transplantation (letter). *Lancet* **346:**1169.
36. **Evans, R. W.** 1995. Socioeconomic aspects of heart transplantation. *Curr. Opin. Cardiol.* **10:**169–179.
37. **Evans, R. W.** 1997. Left ventricular assist devices—permanent implant versus bridge to transplantation—is either cost-effective? *J. Heart Lung Transplant.* **16:**1180–1185.
38. **Evans, R. W.** 1998. Cardiac replacement: need, demand, and supply estimation, p. 13–24. *In* E. A. Rose and L. W. Stevenson (ed.), *Management of End-Stage Heart Disease.* Lippincott-Raven Press, Boston, Mass.
39. **Evans, R. W., and D. Kitzmann.** 1997. The "arithmetic" of donor liver allocation, p. 338–342. *In* P. I. Terasaki and J. M. Cecka (ed.), *Clinical Transplants, 1996.* UCLA Tissue Typing Laboratory, Los Angeles, Calif.
40. **Evans, R. W., and D. J. Kitzmann.** 1997. Contracting for services: liver transplantation in the era of mismanaged care. *Clin. Liver Dis.* **1:**287–303.
41. **Evans, R. W., and D. J. Kitzmann.** 1998. An economic analysis of kidney transplantation. *Surg. Clin. North Am.* **78:**149–174.

42. **Evans, R. W., C. E. Orians, and N. L. Ascher.** 1992. The potential supply of organ donors: an assessment of the efficiency of organ procurement efforts in the United States. *JAMA* **267:**239–246.
43. **Fishman, J., D. Sachs, and R. Shaikh.** 1998. *Xenotransplantation: Scientific Frontiers and Public Policy.* Academy of Sciences, New York, N.Y.
44. **Forsythe, J. L. R.** 1997. *Transplantation Surgery.* W.B. Saunders, Philadelphia, Pa.
45. **Garrison, R. N., F. R. Bentley, G. H. Raque, H. C. Polk, Jr., L. C. Sladek, M. J. Evanisko, and B. A. Lucas.** 1991. There is an answer to the shortage of organ donors. *Surg. Gynecol. Obstet.* **173:**391–396.
46. **Goldstein, D. J., M. C. Oz, and E. A. Rose.** 1998. Implantable left ventricular assist devices. *N. Engl. J. Med.* **339:**1522–1533.
47. **Gortmaker, S. L., C. L. Beasley, L. E. Brigham, H. G. Franz, R. N. Garrison, B. A. Lucas, R. H. Patterson, A. M. Sobol, N. A. Grenvik, and M. J. Evanisko.** 1996. Organ donor potential and performance: size and nature of the organ donor shortfall. *Crit. Care Med.* **24:**432–439.
48. **Hakim, N. S.** 1997. *Introduction to Organ Transplantation.* Imperial College Press, London, England.
49. **Hauboldt, R. H.** 1993. *Cost Implications of Human Organ Transplantations, An Update: 1993.* Milliman and Robertson, Inc., Brookfield, Wis.
50. **Hauboldt, R. H.** 1996. *Cost Implications of Human Organ and Tissue Transplantation, An Update: 1996.* Milliman & Robertson, Brookfield, Wis.
51. **Hayashi, M., S. Cao, W. Concepcion, H. Monge, O. Ojogho, S. So, and C. Esquivel.** 1998. Current status of living-related liver transplantation. *Pediatr. Transplant.* **2:**16–25.
52. **Hensley, S.** 1999. Panel seeks wider sharing of organs. *Mod. Healthcare* **29:**24.
53. **Hughes, R. D., and R. Williams.** 1995. Evaluation of extracorporeal bioartificial liver devices. *Liver Transplant. Surg.* **1:**200–206.
54. **Inomata, Y., K. Tanaka, S. Uemoto, K. Asonuma, H. Egawa, T. Kiuchi, S. Fujita, and M. Hayashi.** 1999. Living donor liver transplantation: an 8-year experience with 379 consecutive cases. *Transplant. Proc.* **31:**381.
55. **Institute of Medicine.** 1999. *Organ Procurement and Transplantation: Assessing Current Policies and the Potential Impact of the DHHS Final Rule.* National Academy Press, Washington, D.C.
56. **Johnson, E. M., J. S. Najarian, and A. J. Matas.** 1998. Living kidney donation: donor risks and quality of life, p. 231–240. *In* J. M. Cecka and P. I. Terasaki (ed.), *Clinical Transplants, 1997.* UCLA Tissue Typing Laboratory, Los Angeles, Calif.
57. **Julvez, J., P. Tuppin, and S. Cohen.** 1999. Survey in France of response to xenotransplantation. *Lancet* **353:**726.
58. **Kennedy, I., R. A. Sells, A. S. Daar, R. D. Guttmann, R. Hoffenberg, M. Lock, J. Radcliffe-Richards, and N. Tilney.** 1998. The case for "presumed consent" in organ donation. *Lancet* **351:**1650–1652.
59. **Kiuchi, T., Y. Inomata, S. Uemoto, K. Asonuma, H. Egawa, M. Hayashi, S. Fujita, and K. Tanaka.** 1998. Living donor liver transplantation in Kyoto, 1997, p. 191–198. *In* J. M. Cecka and P. I. Terasaki (ed.), *Clinical Transplants, 1997.* UCLA Tissue Typing Laboratory, Los Angeles, Calif.
60. **LifeSource Board of Directors.** 1996. *What Happened to Potential Donors,* 1995–96? LifeSource, Upper Midwest Organ Procurement Organization, Minneapolis, Minn.
61. **Loebe, M., Y. Weng, J. Muller, M. Dandel, R. Halfmann, S. Spiegelsberger, and R. Hetzer.** 1997. Successful mechanical circulatory support for more than two years with a left ventricular assist devide in a patient with dilated cardiomyopathy. *J. Heart Lung Transplant.* **16:**1176–1179.
62. **Mallory, G. B., Jr., and A. H. Cohen.** 1997. Donor considerations in living-related donor lung transplantation. *Clin. Chest Med.* **18:**239–244.
63. **Maximus, Inc.** 1985. *Assessment of the Potential Donor Organ Pool. Assessment of Estimating Potential National Data Sources With Demonstration Estimate.* Maximum, Inc., McLean, Va.
64. **McNamara, P., and C. Beasley.** 1998. Determinants of familial consent to organ donation in the hospital setting, p. 219–229. *In* P. I. Terasaki and J. M. Cecka (ed.), *Clinical Transplants, 1997.* UCLA Tissue Typing Laboratory, Los Angeles, Calif.
65. **Milford, E. L.** 1998. Organ transplantation—barriers, outcomes, and evolving policies. *JAMA* **280:**1184–1185.
66. **Mussivand, T., D. Eng, P. J. Hendry, R. G. Masters, and W. J. Keon.** 1999. Development of a ventricular assist device for out-of-hospital use. *J. Heart Lung Transplant.* **18:**166–171.
67. **Nathan, H. M., B. E. Jarrell, B. Broznik, R. Kochik, B. Hamilton, S. Stuart, T. Ackroyd, and M. Nell.**

1991. Estimation and characterization of the potential renal organ donor pool in Pennsylvania. Report of the Pennsylvania Statewide Donor Study. *Transplantation* **51:**142–149.

68. **National Task Force on Organ Transplantation.** 1986. *Organ Transplantation: Issues and Recommendations.* Office of Organ Transplantation, Health Resources and Services Administration, Department of Health and Human Services, Rockville, Md.
69. **Nuffield Council on Bioethics.** 1996. *Animal-to-Human Transplants: The Ethics of Xenotransplantation.* Nuffield Council on Bioethics, London, England.
70. **Orians, C. E., R. W. Evans, and N. L. Ascher.** 1993. Estimates of organ-specific donor availability for the United States. *Transplant. Proc.* **25:**1541–1542.
71. **Radcliffe-Richards, J., A. S. Daar, R. D. Guttmann, R. Hoffenberg, I. Kennedy, M. Lock, R. A. Sells, and N. Tilney.** 1998. The case for allowing kidney sales. *Lancet* **351:**1950–1952.
72. **Rose, E. A., and L. W. Stevenson.** 1998. *Management of End-Stage Heart Disease.* Lippincott-Raven Press, Boston, Mass.
73. **Ross, L. F., D. T. Rubin, M. Siegler, M. A. Josephson, J. R. Thistlethwaite, Jr., and E. S. Woodle.** 1997. Ethics of a paired-kidney-exchange program. *N. Engl. J. Med.* **336:**1752–1755.
74. **Shelton, D. L.** 1998. Quiet epidemic coming to light. *Am. Med. News* **41:**26.
75. **Shelton, D. L.** 1999. Increasing split livers will decrease organ shortage. *Am. Med. News* **42:**1.
76. **Siminoff, L. A., and K. A. Nelson.** 1999. The accuracy of hospital reports of organ donation eligibility, requests, and consent: a cross-validation study. *Joint Comm. J. Qual. Improve.* **25:**129–136.
77. **Sindhi, R., J. Rosendale, D. Mundy, S. Taranto, P. Baliga, A. Reuben, P. R. Rajagopalan, A. Hebra, E. Tagge, and H. B. Othersen. Jr.** 1999. Impact of segmental grafts on pediatric liver transplantation—a review of the United Network for Organ Sharing Scientific Registry data (1990–1996). *J. Pediatr. Surg.* **34:**107–110.
78. **Skolnick, A. A.** 1998. Using ventricular assist devices as long-term therapy for heart failure. *JAMA* **279:**1509–1510.
79. **Starnes, V. A., M. L. Barr, F. A. Schenkel, M. V. Horn, R. G. Cohen, J. A. Hagen, and W. J. Wells.** 1997. Experience with living-donor lobar transplantation for indications other than cystic fibrosis. *J. Thorac. Cardiovasc. Surg.* **114:**917–921.
80. **Superina, R. A., C. Harrison, E. M. Alonso, and P. F. Whitington.** 1999. Ethical issues in pediatric liver transplantation. *Transplant. Proc.* **31:**1342–1344.
81. **Terasaki, P. I., J. M. Cecka, D. W. Gjertson, and Y. W. Cho.** 1998. Spousal and other living renal donor transplants, p. 269–284. *In* J. M. Cecka and P. I. Terasaki (ed.), *Clinical Transplants, 1997.* UCLA Tissue Typing Laboratory, Los Angeles, Calif.
83. **Touraine, J. L., J. Traeger, H. Betuel, J. M. Dubernard, J. P. Revillard, and C. Dupuy.** 1995. *Organ Shortage: The Solutions.* Kluwer Academic, Boston, Mass.
84. **Ubel, P. A.** 1996. Can we continue to afford organ transplants in an era of managed care? *Am. J. Managed Care* **2:**293–297.
85. **Ubel, P. A., and A. L. Caplan.** 1998. Geographic favoritism in liver transplantation—unfortunate or unfair? *N. Engl. J. Med.* **339:**1322–1325.
86. **United Network for Organ Sharing.** 1998. *1997 Annual Report: The U.S. Scientific Registry of Transplant Recipients and the Organ Procurement and Transplantation Network: Transplant Data 1988–1996.* United Network for Organ Sharing, Richmond, Va.
87. **United Network for Organ Sharing.** 1996. *1996 Annual Report of the U.S. Scientific Registry for Transplant Recipients and the Organ Procurement and Transplantation Network—Transplant Data.* United Network for Organ Sharing and the U.S. Department of Health and Human Services, Richmond, Va.
88. **United Network for Organ Sharing.** 1996. *1995 Annual Report of the U.S. Scientific Registry of Organ Transplant Recipients and the Organ Procurement and Transplantation Network. Transplant Data: 1988–1994.* United Network for Organ Sharing, Richmond, Va.
89. **U.S. Renal Data System.** 1998. *USRDS 1998 Annual Report.* National Institute of Diabetes and Digestive and Kidney Diseases, National Institutes of Health, Bethesda, Md.
90. **U.S. Renal Data System.** 1996. *1996 Annual Data Report.* National Institute of Diabetes and Digestive and Kidney Diseases, National Institutes of Health, Bethesda, Md.
91. **Weiss, R. A.** 1998. Xenotransplantation. *Br. Med. J.* **317:**931–934.
92. **Williams, B. A. H., and M. Sandiford-Guttenbeil.** 1996. *Trends in Organ Transplantation.* Springer Publishing, New York, N.Y.

93. **Williams, N.** 1998. Paving the way for British xenotransplants. *Science* **281:**767.
94. **Woo, M. S., E. F. McLaughlin, M. V. Horn, and P. C. Wong.** 1998. Living donor lobar lung transplantation: the pediatric experience. *Pediatr. Transplant.* **2:**185–190.
95. **Yamaoka, Y., T. Mormoto, Y. Inamoto, A. Tanaka, K. Honda, I. Ikai, K. Tanaka, M. Ichimiya, M. Ueda, and Y. Shimahara.** 1995. Safety of the donor in living-related liver transplantation—an analysis of 100 parental donors. *Transplantation* **59:**224.
96. **Youngner, S. J., R. C. Fox, and L. J. O'Connell.** 1996. *Organ Transplantation: Meaning and Reality.* University of Wisconsin, Madison, Wis.

Section II

IMMUNOLOGICAL HURDLES TO XENOTRANSPLANTATION

Xenotransplantation
Edited by Jeffrey L. Platt

Chapter 3

The Complement System as a Hurdle to Xenotransplantation

Agustin P. Dalmasso

The biology of the complement system is of major interest to xenotransplant investigators because complement activation plays a major role in rejection of solid organ xenografts. A xenograft may trigger complement activation by two general mechanisms. One involves the binding of preexisting or elicited antibodies in the recipient to the vascular endothelium of the graft, and the other involves the direct interaction of the foreign tissue with the recipient's complement (40, 98). In discordant combinations, complement activation occurs immediately, resulting in hyperacute rejection (HAR) of the xenograft. In concordant combinations complement may participate in delayed rejection once antibodies against the graft have been elicited. The role of complement in HAR of a discordant xenograft is prominent as HAR does not occur in complement-deficient recipients and in animals given inhibitors of complement activation. This chapter discusses the role of complement in the pathogenesis of tissue injury in xenograft rejection and reviews methods to inhibit complement activation as part of strategies to achieve xenograft survival. The chapter begins with a brief overview of the complement system; for readers interested in furthering their knowledge of complement, two recently published books are highly recommended as they provide comprehensive reviews of virtually all basic and applied aspects of the complement system (129, 164).

COMPLEMENT ACTIVATION

The complement system is a major effector mechanism that, once activated, may result in various biological processes of great significance in pathophysiology (32, 103, 129, 164). The complement system is composed of 35 plasma and membrane-associated proteins, which include control proteins and receptors on cell membranes that recognize various fragments that result from complement activation (Table 1). Complement may be activated through one of three pathways designated the classical, alternative, and lectin pathways (Fig. 1). Activation by all pathways results in generation of enzyme complexes called

---

Agustin P. Dalmasso • Department of Surgery and Department of Laboratory Medicine and Pathology, University of Minnesota Medical School, Minneapolis, MN 55455.

Table 1. Proteins of the complement system[a]

Soluble proteins
Recognition, activation, and effector proteins:
Classical pathway: C1q, C1r, C1s, C4, C2, C3
Lectin pathway: MBP, MASP-1, MASP-2
Alternative pathway: C3, B, D
Membrane attack complex: C5, C6, C7, C8, C9
Positive regulator: P
Negative regulators: C1 inhibitor, C4-binding protein, H, I, vitronectin, clusterin
Membrane-associated proteins
Negative regulators: CR1, DAF, MCP, CD59
Receptors: C1qR, CR1, CR2, CR3, CR4, C3aR, C5aR

[a]MBP, mannan-binding protein; MASP, MBP-associated serine protease; DAF, decay-accelerating factor; MCP, membrane cofactor protein.

C3 convertases that activate C3, and C5 convertases that activate C5; this is followed by assembly of the membrane attack complex (MAC), which is shared by all pathways.

Activation of the classical pathway (23) begins with C1, a Ca^{2+}-dependent protein complex composed of C1q, C1r, and C1s. The major activators of C1 are antigen-antibody complexes containing IgM or IgG; C1 activation requires that one C1q molecule binds either one IgM molecule or two IgG molecules. The resulting conformational change in C1q leads to the activation of the proenzymes C1r and C1s. C1 can also be activated independently of immune complexes. Examples of direct C1 activators include C-reactive protein, serum amyloid protein, uric acid crystals, endotoxin and other microbial substances, and certain subcellular components of mammalian cells. Within the activated C1 complex, activated C1s cleaves C4 into C4a and C4b, and C2 into C2a and C2b, which is followed by assembly of C4b2a, or classical pathway C3 convertase (Fig. 1). This convertase then cleaves C3 into C3a and C3b; after dissociation of C3a, a highly reactive thiolester bond in C3b undergoes cleavage, exposing reactive groups that result in covalent binding of C3b to free amino or hydroxyl groups. Of the multiple molecules of C3b that are generated, some bind to C4b2a, forming C4b2a3b, or C5 convertase. C5 is cleaved into C5a and C5b, and C5b interacts with the terminal complement proteins, resulting in assembly of the MAC.

Most activators of the alternative pathway are constituents of the cellular surface of many microorganisms; other activators include polymers of IgA. Activation of the alternative pathway (112) involves first a modification of C3 such that its internal thiolester bond is cleaved, with formation of a highly reactive carbonyl that binds covalently to various macromolecules. Modified C3 comprises C3b and $C3H_2O$, which can associate with factor B so that factor B becomes susceptible to cleavage by factor D, yielding fragments Ba and Bb. Bb remains bound to the complex, which now becomes the alternative pathway C3 convertase (Fig. 1); C3bBb cleaves C3 into C3a and C3b, causing an amplification effect on alternative pathway activation. Incorporation of another C3b molecule into a C3bBb complex yields $(C3b)_2Bb$, or alternative pathway C5 convertase, that acts on C5 to produce C5a and C5b. A substance is classified as activator or nonactivator of the alternative pathway depending on whether the acceptor molecule for C3b contains structures that protect bound C3b from the inactivating action of regulatory proteins.

Recently the lectin pathway has been recognized and characterized (93). This pathway is independent of antibody and C1 and is activated by the binding of mannan-binding lectin (MBL) to a microbial surface containing terminal mannose or N-acetylglucosamine.

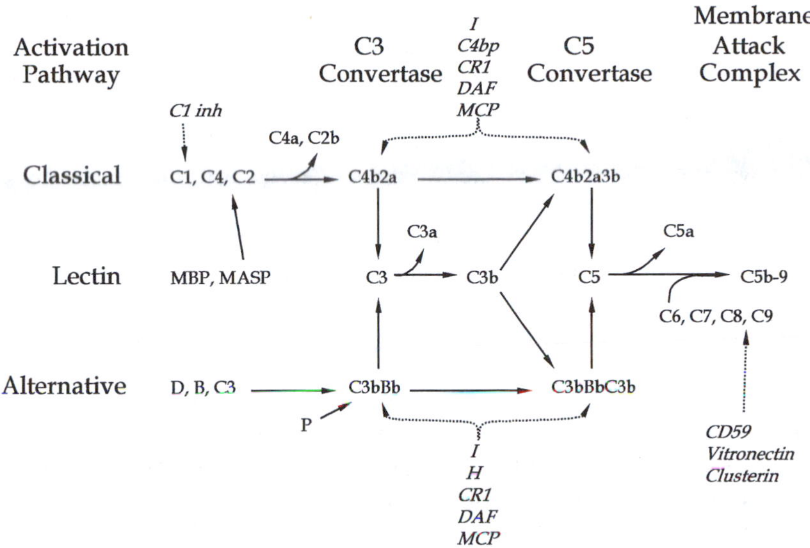

Figure 1. Schematic representation of the main pathways of complement activation. Mechanisms for activator recognition and initiation of activation are unique to each pathway. Classical pathway C3- and C5-convertases are also utilized by the lectin pathway. Sites of action of complement inhibitors are indicated by interrupted lines.

MBL has structural features similar to those of C1q. Bound MBL can activate two C1s-like zymogens called MASP-1 and MASP-2 (MASP for MBL-associated serine protease), which in turn may cleave C2 and C4, forming the classical pathway C3 convertase.

Initiation of MAC assembly follows the generation of C5b, which combines with C6 and C7 to form the C5b-7 complex, which has high affinity for membrane lipid bilayers. Membrane-bound C5b-7 combines with one molecule of C8, forming C5b-8, which then binds multiple molecules of C9. Because of the strong affinity of C5b-8 for phospholipids, the membrane bilayer is disrupted, causing increased permeability, which is further enhanced by incorporation of C9; in addition, a large channel may be formed by polymerized C9 (35). Killing of nucleated cells by the MAC is associated with an increase in intracellular Ca^{2+} and intracellular lipid metabolism, mitochondrial swelling, and hydrolysis of membrane lipids. In contrast to red cells, nucleated cells require multiple MAC deposition for irreversible damage to occur and are able to resist complement-mediated killing by endocytosis and exocytosis of bound MAC (100).

CONTROL OF COMPLEMENT ACTIVATION

Complement activation is regulated by multiple mechanisms that ensure all stages of the complement reaction are under control. Regulation of complement activation has evolved to protect the host against activation that occurs in inflammation and defense against microorganisms. Regulation is accomplished through several plasma and membrane proteins, listed in Table 1. Regulation of the classical pathway is provided by C1 inhibitor (C1 inh), which binds irreversibly to activated C1r and C1s, blocking their enzymatic activity. C1 inh also inhibits activated MASP and controls activation of the contact system of kinin generation and the intrinsic coagulation pathway. The biological significance of C1 inh is highlighted by patients with hereditary angioneurotic edema, a potentially life-threatening condition that is due to a reduced functional activity of C1 inh caused by a heterozygous deficiency or dysfunction of C1 inh (42).

Intensive control of complement activation is centered around the C3 and C5 convertases of both pathways (see Fig. 1). There are two general mechanisms that ensure this control, dissociation from the convertases of the enzymatically active protein moieties C2a and Bb, and proteolytic degradation of C3b and C4b. Some dissociation takes place spontaneously due to the intrinsic unstable nature of the convertase complexes. Enhanced dissociation is provided by the interaction of the convertases with the plasma proteins C4b-binding protein (C4bp) and factor H, or with the membrane proteins decay-accelerating factor (DAF) and complement receptor 1 (CR1) (4, 65, 107). These inhibitors may also prevent the association of C3b or C4b with Bb or C2a, respectively, before they form the complex. On the other hand, the stability and consequent half-life of the alternative pathway C3 convertase are markedly enhanced when properdin is incorporated into the complex. Another control mechanism at the C3-, C5-convertase level consists of the inactivation of C3b and C4b by factor I-mediated proteolysis. Factor I can cleave its substrates only after C3b or C4b binds a protein cofactor from plasma (factor H or C4bp) or from the cell membrane (CR1 and membrane cofactor protein, MCP). Bound C3b that is not part of a convertase can also be cleaved in this manner, yielding C3bi.

Finally, MAC formation is controlled by the membrane-associated protein CD59 (96). CD59 inhibits MAC assembly by blocking binding of C9 to C5b-8 and the additional incorporation of C9 into C5b-9. Successful MAC assembly may also be inhibited by the plasma proteins vitronectin and clusterin, which are multifunctional proteins that interact with late-acting complement components as complexes assemble in plasma.

As will be discussed below, the membrane-associated complement regulators are of great interest to xenotransplantation. DAF, MCP, and CR1, but not CD59, share a similar modular organization of contiguous homologous units called complement control protein modules (CCP) or short consensus repeats (SCR) that consist of approximately 60 amino acid residues. The complement receptor 2 (CR2) and the soluble regulatory proteins factor H and C4bp are also formed to a major extent of CCPs. A few of these CCPs have binding regions for C4b or C3b.

DAF and CD59 act intrinsically, inhibiting the complement reaction only at the membrane sites where they are located, and are anchored to the membrane through a glycosyl phosphatidylinositol moiety. The biological importance of these inhibitors to protect host cells against uncontrolled activation of autologous complement is shown in patients with paroxysmal nocturnal hemoglobinuria, whose erythrocytes and other cells are deficient in phosphatidylinositol-linked complement inhibitors and show enhanced susceptibility to complement lysis (128). This disease highlights the biological significance of these inhibitors as effective protective mechanisms for host tissues against autologous complement.

MCP and CR1 are anchored to the membrane through a hydrophobic peptide. Whereas MCP acts intrinsically, CR1 acts mainly extrinsically as it is a very elongated molecule, with binding sites for C3b and C4b that are relatively remote from the cell membrane where CR1 is anchored (65). Membrane-associated inhibitors are expressed on most cells that are in contact with blood or other biological fluids containing complement. These proteins are inhibitory to homologous complement and may have less inhibitory capacity upon complement from a different species; this is not always the case, as it was recently shown that pig CD59 is equally effective to protect a cell from pig complement or human complement (64, 90).

BIOLOGICAL ACTIVITIES OF COMPLEMENT

The complement system has evolved to provide multiple biological effects that are usually beneficial to the individual. However, at times, due to conditions that lead to excessive or inadequate complement activation, these effects may result in pathologic conditions. Complement participates in four major groups of biological activities, namely, solubilization and removal of immune complexes, enhancement of antibody production, opsonization and killing of microorganisms, and inflammation. To achieve these multiple tasks complement utilizes various protein fragments and complexes that are generated throughout the course of the complement reaction; in many cases these proteins exert their activities after binding to specific cell membrane receptors (Table 1).

The role of complement in prevention of immune complex formation and in solubilization of immune complexes is related to the ability of C1q, C3b, and C4b to bind to immunoglobulin molecules (101). Complement participates in removal of immune complexes through CR1 on red cells that bind C3b deposited on immune complexes, transporting them to the liver and spleen where they are cleared from the circulation. The importance of this process is demonstrated clinically by the high prevalence of immune complex diseases in individuals with certain complement deficiencies. In addition, the classical pathway may play a role in protection against injury to autologous tissues by promoting the elimination of cells after they undergo apoptosis (13, 78). In the absence of an intact classical pathway apoptotic cells may remain in certain tissues such as the kidney, where cytoplasmic and nuclear antigens may be released and give rise to autoimmune diseases.

Complement participates in enhancement of antibody production through interaction of the C3b proteolytic degradation fragments C3d,g/C3d with CR2 on B cells and follicular dendritic cells. In germinal centers follicular dendritic cells with CR2 on their surface are able to display immune complexes containing C3d,g to B lymphocytes. This mechanism is most important in the immune response against low-dose antigen, ensuring a large enhancement in antibody formation through the interaction of C3d,g and antigen with the signaling complex formed by CR2, CD19, and other molecules (45).

Complement is important in defense mechanisms against microorganisms that are mediated by the opsonic activities of C3b and C3bi and by the lytic activity of the MAC (101). Microorganisms coated with C3b and C3bi exhibit enhanced adherence to neutrophils and macrophages through binding to CR1 and complement receptor 3 (CR3), respectively; then the organisms undergo phagocytosis. The significance of this function of complement is shown in C3-deficient patients, who are particularly susceptible to infection with gram-positive bacteria. The MAC mediates killing of gram-negative bacteria and lysis of certain viruses. Patients deficient in a component of the MAC have a higher incidence of neisserial septicemia than normocomplementemic individuals. C3b and C4b may neutralize virus infectivity by blocking attachment sites to host cells. Complement has also been found to participate through several mechanisms in the host response against HIV infection (148).

The role of complement in promotion of inflammation is particularly relevant to xenotransplantation because the mechanisms employed by complement in inflammation also operate in xenograft rejection. Therefore, this topic is discussed in more detail below under "Complement-Mediated Mechanisms of Tissue Injury in Xenograft Rejection." Complement causes increased vascular permeability, attraction of phagocytic cells, enhancement of phagocytosis, cytotoxicity, etc. C3a and C5a induce increased vascular permeability, contraction of smooth muscle, release of mediators from mast cells and polymorphonuclear leukocytes, and generation of oxygen radicals. C5a is a potent chemotactic agent that promotes leukocyte adhesion and stimulates the cyclooxygenase pathway. Bb promotes macrophage spreading and killing efficiency. The terminal components stimulate the conversion of arachidonic acid into various metabolic products, including PGI_2, and production of oxygen radicals. The MAC also induces prothrombinase activity in platelets and endothelial cells. In spite of these powerful proinflammatory effects, individuals with severe complement deficiencies do not have defective inflammatory reactions, due to the redundancy of mechanisms that promote inflammation.

ROLE OF COMPLEMENT IN XENOGRAFT REJECTION

In immediately vascularized discordant organ xenografts rapid and effective complement activation takes place that results in the demise of the organ in minutes or a few hours. The essential role of complement in HAR was first reported 34 years ago by Nelson (105) and Gewurz et al. (56) who showed that complement inactivation with cobra venom factor (CVF) resulted in extended survival of a xenograft. Since then this fundamental observation was extended with numerous studies in several discordant combinations using recipients genetically deficient in a complement component or given inhibitors of complement activation.

Depending on the donor-recipient combination the initial complement activation may take place via the classical pathway or the alternative pathway. When a porcine organ is transplanted into a primate, the classical pathway is activated by preexisting anti-pig IgM antibodies that bind to the vascular endothelium of the graft; in this combination complement is not activated directly by the xenograft (40). Other combinations in which HAR is mediated by activation of the classical pathway are mouse-to-rabbit (74) and rat-to-cynomolgus monkey (5). Although studies with these latter combinations may not be as germane to human xenotransplantation as studies in pig-to-primate, they may offer the opportunity for less expensive experiments with genetically modified rodent donors that are already available or that may be produced at relatively low cost. In certain xenograft models, as in guinea pig-to-rat, complement is activated directly via the alternative pathway by the donor vascular endothelium (98); some strains of rats have anti–guinea pig natural antibodies that contribute to HAR (54). Other combinations in which complement activation is triggered via the alternative pathway are rabbit-to-newborn pig (73) and rat-to-fetal sheep (123).

In the pig-to-primate combination, IgM natural antibodies are very effective in triggering complement activation; however, IgG anti-pig natural antibodies do not activate complement when they bind to porcine endothelial cells (40). Human IgA natural antibodies are able to bind to porcine endothelial cells, and endothelial cell-bound dimeric IgA, but not monomeric IgA, is able to activate complement in vitro via the alternative pathway (136). Because dimeric IgA comprises a small proportion of total serum IgA, IgA is not primarily involved in HAR in pig-to-primate combinations; IgA antibodies, however, may possibly cause complement-dependent damage if a modified recipient is depleted of IgM only.

In addition to the direct evidence provided by the abrogation of HAR in animals with genetic or induced complement deficiencies, the participation of complement in HAR was also suggested by the presence of complement proteins deposited in tissues of the xenograft, together with a very rapid reduction in levels of complement activity and the appearance of complement activation products in the recipient's plasma. Studies to determine deposition of selected complement proteins on the vascular endothelium of a rejecting xenograft have been helpful to define the complement activation pathway involved; e.g., a porcine heart transplanted into non-human primates early during rejection showed deposits of classical pathway proteins along endothelial surfaces, with a distribution similar to that of IgM, but only trace deposits of alternative pathway proteins (40).

When HAR was prevented in complement-deficient recipients, the xenograft was rejected after several days by a process called delayed xenograft rejection or acute vascular rejection (DXR/AVR) (12, 84, 85). An early study in guinea pigs transplanted with a rat heart showed that, while in normocomplemententemic animals rejection occurred in 22 min, in C4-deficient guinea pigs rejection was delayed until day 3.5; the histology of the hearts undergoing delayed rejection showed cellular infiltration (70). This process was then studied in more detail in the guinea pig-to-rat combination. In rats given CVF to maintain complete complement deficiency for several days the mean survival time of the guinea pig cardiac xenograft was prolonged to 3.7 days from 19 min in controls (84). These rats developed increasing levels of anti–guinea pig antibodies, and the grafts showed leukocyte margination along blood vessels, beginning at 12 h posttransplant, and progressive cell infiltration, interstitial hemorrhage, and necrosis over the next 72 h. The grafts showed deposition of IgM, IgG, and fibrin along blood vessels, but no C3 deposition (85). Similar results were obtained with pig hearts transplanted in CVF-treated baboons, with graft survival of 3.5 days compared with less than 90 min in controls (84, 86).

The histology of organs that underwent this type of rejection was similar to that of vascular rejection, with infiltration of mononuclear cells but with minimal presence of T cells. The mechanism of DXR/AVR is likely multifactorial, with certain molecular incompatibilities between donor and recipient possibly playing a role. Antibodies are thought to play a major pathogenic role, as antibody depletion prolonged graft survival for several days (87). Although antibodies may have a direct action (159), they may be more important as mediators of antibody-dependent cell cytotoxicity by NK cells and monocytes (52, 53). Antibodies may also initiate complement activation, as suggested by the observation that, when complement was inactivated with CVF in conjunction with antibody depletion, graft survival was further extended to a few weeks; rejection was accompanied by intravascular coagulation and fibrin deposition triggered by the xenograft (67, 86).

Although the participation of the MAC is not an absolute requirement for the production of DXR/AVR because this form of rejection takes place in C6-deficient animals (14, 74), products from earlier stages of complement activation may be important. When the classical pathway is activated, as in pig-to-human combinations, cell-bound antibodies bind C1q, which may be pathogenic; then activation of C1 leads to production of C4a, which, although functionally weak, over many hours might be pathogenic. Small amounts of C3 and C5 convertases may be formed due to incomplete antibody depletion or suppression, or insufficient complement inhibition, and also due to local synthesis of complement proteins by the endothelium of the donor organ where the injury takes place. Accordingly, some level of complement activation may induce endothelial cell activation, with stimulation of proinflammatory and procoagulant changes that would contribute to AVR/DXR. This view is supported by extensive in vitro studies on the effects of complement activation fragments and complexes upon donor endothelial cells and recipient leukocytes and platelets, as reviewed in the following section.

COMPLEMENT-MEDIATED MECHANISMS OF TISSUE INJURY IN XENOGRAFT REJECTION

The vascular endothelium is the first target of the immediate, humoral, immune attack on a solid organ xenograft. Although antibodies in the absence of complement are able to induce activation of endothelial cells (159), several products of complement activation have a much stronger stimulating effect on endothelial cells than antibodies alone (33, 34, 131). Complement activation results in generation of biologically active fragments and complexes derived from several complement proteins that may cause injury to the xenograft, either by acting directly on the endothelium of the graft or by recruiting and activating effector cells and plasma proteins of the recipient (Table 2). The consequences of complement activation to a xenograft in a discordant unmodified recipient are loss of the endothelial cell barrier function, vasoconstriction, and promotion of coagulation, which result in interstitial edema, hemorrhage, and thrombosis, the hallmarks of HAR.

Table 2. Effects of complement activation products on endothelial cells and vessels of the xenograft and blood cells of the recipient

Complement activation product	Endothelial cells of the graft	Blood cells of the recipient
C1q	Expression of E-selectin, ICAM-1, VCAM-1	Platelets: Activation of glycoproteins IIb-IIIa Increased expression of P-selectin
C3bi	PMN adhesion	
Anaphylatoxins	Increased permeability Expression of P-selectin Synthesis of oxygen radicals and enzymes Increased adhesiveness for leukocytes Vessel contraction Release of heparan sulfate (C5a)	Neutrophil and macrophage activation Neutrophils: Chemotaxis Generation of oxygen radicals Expression of elastase Aggregation and release of granular contents Platelets: Aggregation and release of granular contents
C5b-7, C5b-8, and C5b-9	Cell retraction and formation of intercellular gaps	
C5b-9	Synthesis and secretion of IL-1α, IL-8, and MCP-1 Expression of P-selectin and E-selectin Enhanced response to TNF-α Synthesis of PGI_2 and TxA_2 Release of basic fibroblast growth factor, PAF, and PDGF Expression of tissue factor and von Willebrand factor Membrane vesiculation Cell death	Platelets: Assembly of prothrombinase complex Membrane vesiculation

The identification of the activation products of complement that are important for xenograft rejection has been accomplished with experiments in recipient animals with well-defined genetic complement deficiencies. These studies demonstrated that the MAC is the major mediator of HAR, which was first suggested by the prolonged survival of a xenogeneic heart transplanted into C6-deficient rabbits (20, 173). More recent studies showed that a guinea pig heart survived for 1 to 2 days in C6-deficient rats, in contrast to less than 20 min in controls; rejection was associated with granulocyte and monocyte infiltration (14). The shorter xenograft survival in C6-deficient rats (1 to 2 days) in comparison to normal rats treated with CVF (3 to 4 days) is due to the ability of C6-deficient rats to generate C3a and C5a; if C6-deficient rats are given CVF to destroy C3 and C5, graft survival was prolonged to 3 to 4 days, with less cell infiltration (71). Results similar to those with CVF were obtained with C6-deficient rats receiving recombinant neutrophil-inhibiting factor, a hookworm glycoprotein that inhibits CR3 (CD11b/CD18) and blocks binding of neutrophils and macrophages to endothelial cell-bound C3bi (72). The role of leukocyte adhesion in xenograft rejection was also demonstrated using a leumedin to block adhesion in C6-deficient rats (43).

Studies with an ex vivo perfusion model of pig-to-human transplantation suggested that also in humans C5a and the MAC would play the predominant role in HAR of a porcine heart (80). Whereas a porcine heart that was perfused with unmodified human blood survived only 25 min, with histologic and immunopathologic characteristics of HAR, addition of a monoclonal antibody against human C5 to the human blood extended heart survival for at least 6 h, without evidence of HAR or tissue deposition of MAC.

An understanding of which biological effects of complement are most relevant in the induction of HAR has been difficult because HAR develops very rapidly; it seems obvious that HAR results from a few of the effects of complement that have been found in vitro to be most injurious to the integrity of an endothelial cell monolayer. If there is intense complement activation, endothelial cell killing and detachment may occur, with exposure of the subendothelial matrix; however, before endothelial cell killing takes place or when limiting amounts of antibody or complement prevail, endothelial cell activation precedes cytotoxicity and may mediate tissue injury without complement-induced cytotoxicity (117).

Numerous studies have been performed with an in vitro model system consisting of cultured porcine endothelial cell monolayers as targets incubated with human natural antibodies and complement, either as purified proteins or in serum. With this model it was shown that normal human serum is cytotoxic to porcine endothelial cells through complement activation via the classical pathway. Binding of complement components to the endothelial cells and cytotoxicity required the presence of IgM natural antibodies and components of the classical pathway; the alternative pathway did not appear to be primarily involved (40); it has also been shown that dimeric IgA natural antibodies are able to cause endothelial cell killing via the alternative pathway (136).

Although HAR is mediated by the MAC, products of complement activation that are generated at earlier stages of the complement reaction may potentially cause injury to a xenograft when HAR is avoided. Accordingly, complement activation may contribute to vascular injury, focal ischemia, and thrombosis in DXR/AVR. Extensive in vitro studies suggested that complement products can stimulate the endothelial cells to become activated, proinflammatory, and procoagulant, and concomitantly complement can activate and recruit leukocytes and platelets to the graft (33, 34, 131). When complement is activated on the endothelium of a xenograft, the complement fragments that are released into the fluid phase may bind to various blood cells of the recipient as blood circulates through the foreign organ. These effects of complement (summarized in Table 2) can potentially cause tissue damage at any time during the life of a xenograft whenever complement activation takes place, triggered by antibodies or other complement activators originating in damaged tissues of the graft. The majority of the known effects of complement on endothelial cells are described below; however, not all these studies have been performed with pig endothelial cells and human complement, the model that is most relevant to pig-to-human transplantation.

Effects of C1q

Endothelial cells possess several receptors that are able to bind distinct areas of a C1q molecule that is associated with antibody. Expression of some of these receptors is upregulated by exposure of endothelial cells to TNF-α or INF-γ (58), and binding of aggregated C1q to endothelial cells leads to expression of adhesion molecules on the cell membrane (58, 88), which in turn may cause the recruitment and activation of leukocytes. Because platelets possess C1q receptors they may also be activated by interaction with modified C1q as they circulate through the graft, resulting in expression of adhesion molecules and binding to the endothelium (114).

Effects of C3bi

Endothelial cell-bound C3b is rapidly cleaved by factor I with the collaboration of MCP or factor H, yielding C3bi. C3bi causes neutrophils to adhere to the endothelium through CR3, the neutrophil integrin CD11b/CD18 (161). On the other hand, leukocyte CR3 may be activated through a conformational modification following leukocyte stimulation with C5a or other substances (111, 162).

Effects of C5a and Other Anaphylatoxins

Although C5a is the most powerful of the anaphylatoxins, C3a also has significant biological activities and both proteins may play a role in xenograft rejection. Not only is there a difference in the intensity of the effects that are common to all anaphylatoxins, but there are certain effects that are specific for individual anaphylatoxins. Both C3a and C5a can cause vasoconstriction, but a role for C4a as an anaphylatoxin in humans or pigs has not been clearly established. The presence of a specific receptor for C5a has been documented in leukocytes and endothelial cells (62, 104). C5a stimulates the expression of adhesion molecules and the synthesis of oxygen products in endothelial cells (50, 51, 104).

C5a induces activation of an enzyme that cleaves heparan sulfate from porcine endothelial cells (68, 118), a loss that may result in tissue damage as heparan sulfate contributes to blood vessel barrier functions, maintenance of an anticoagulant environment, and inhibition of injury by oxygen and free radicals. Incubation of porcine endothelial cells with natural antibody and complement in human serum caused rapid release of a large proportion of the endothelial cell-associated heparan sulfate chains; the release preceded cell death and was dependent on complement activation for generation of C5a (116). C5a can induce tissue factor activity in human umbilical vein endothelial cells (69).

C3a and C5a are able to activate neutrophils and monocytes to express adhesion molecules, resulting in generation of oxygen radicals and in adhesion of these cells to the endothelium (50, 160). C5a promotes expression of elastase in neutrophils and release of their granular contents (110). These effects strongly indicate that the anaphylatoxins, especially C5a, may be an important mechanism of injury to a xenogeneic endothelium.

Effects of Terminal Components

The biologic effect of the terminal complement components that usually first comes to mind is the ability to induce cell cytotoxicity. Complement-mediated killing of endothelial cells certainly can take place and in certain instances may occur during HAR. However, like all nucleated cells, endothelial cells exhibit resistance to the lytic effects of complement, a property that has facilitated the study of the action of sublytic amounts of MAC on many cell types (100, 106). It has been found that sublytic MAC has multiple effects on endothelial cells, which, in conjunction with those the MAC can exert on recipient blood cells, have been implicated in the production of tissue damage to xenografts.

Deposition of C5b-7, C5b-8, and C5b-9 on a porcine endothelial cell monolayer was found to cause endothelial cell retraction in vitro, with formation of transient gaps between endothelial cells, through which blood cells and macromolecules could escape (132). This process may expose the subendothelium and allow platelets to adhere to collagen. Recovery of monolayer integrity required assembly of the complete MAC, in conjunction with a substance secreted by the endothelial cells. This effect of the terminal complement complexes inducing endothelial cell retraction and intercellular pore formation may be important for the development of intercellular hemorrhage that is characteristic of HAR.

The MAC in sublytic amounts may cause Ca^{2+} influx and cell activation, resulting in release of reactive oxygen products, eicosanoids, and cytokines. The MAC was found to induce endothelial cell expression of MCP-1 and IL-8, within 3 h of incubation, which did not require de novo protein synthesis; it also induced a late phase of MCP-1, IL-8, and RANTES gene expression, which in part required production of IL-1α as an intermediate step (75, 140). Endothelial cell production of basic fibroblast growth factor and platelet-activating factor is also stimulated by the MAC (10). Among the effects of terminal complement components on endothelial cells is the release of vasoactive PGE_2 and TXA_2, which cause vasoconstriction and disruption of cytoskeletal actin microfilaments with widening of interendothelial junctions and increased permeability (150). The MAC may also contribute to injury by reducing vascular endothelium-dependent relaxation, as has been shown for coronary arteries (146). Pig endothelial cells can be stimulated by human complement to produce IL-1α, which acts as an autocrine factor on the endothelial cells to induce cyclooxygenase-2 and thromboxane synthase (16), resulting in release of PGE_2 and TXA_2; complement also causes increased release of PGI_2 (16). The MAC can also activate endothelial cells to express adhesion molecules on the cell membrane (61).

The MAC may promote thrombosis by inducing endothelial cell membrane vesiculation, expression of von Willebrand factor, and assembly of the prothrombinase complex (59, 61); additionally, the MAC stimulates porcine endothelial cells to synthesize tissue factor, which occurred over a period of 16 to 42 h and was secondary to complement-induced release of IL-1α (130). The completely assembled MAC may cause endothelial cell detachment and exposure of the subendothelium, with consequent platelet deposition and activation.

These biological effects of the MAC result from the insertion of the complex into the cell membrane. However, during complement activation the terminal components also assemble in the fluid phase; these complexes are unable to insert in a cell membrane due to a conformational loss of the binding region in the C7 moiety of C5b-7 that is essential for membrane insertion. This C5b-7 remains in the fluid phase where it binds C8 and C9. Recent studies have shown that this complex retains biological activity upon endothelial cells, as it is able to stimulate human umbilical vein endothelial cells to express tissue factor and the adhesion molecules VCAM-1, ICAM-1, and ELAM-1 (153). Therefore, it is possible that in a xenogeneic organ transplant C5b-9 may be formed in the fluid phase after losing its membrane-inserting capacity and contribute to the mechanisms that result in xenograft tissue injury.

COMPLEMENT AND ACCOMMODATION

Accommodation of a grafted organ refers to the survival of the organ in the presence of anti-graft antibodies and normal complement levels in the recipient (7). Discussed below are only a few points pertaining to the association of complement with accommodation. Accommodation was first observed in human renal allotransplantation across the ABO barrier. It was known that a proportion of ABO-incompatible renal allografts did not undergo HAR, mainly in cases with low antibody levels; in these cases the expression of complement regulators on the graft endothelium may have contributed to prevent HAR. It was then observed that HAR could be prevented in additional cases by removal of antibodies before and during a short time following engraftment (2, 143). Accommodation was thought to have developed if the transplant was not rejected when antibody levels returned after discontinuation of antibody removal, in spite of normal complement and persistence of donor antigen on the vascular endothelium of the graft (8). In these cases of allografts in humans it is possible that complement regulators of the graft may have played a role in preventing complement-mediated rejection while the levels of antibodies were low, permitting the development of accommodation.

Accommodation has been demonstrated in the hamster-to-rat model of concordant cardiac xenotransplantation. In this model, if complement-dependent graft rejection is prevented by complement inactivation with CVF, continuous immunosuppression with cyclosporine allows graft survival in the majority of recipients (60). The tissues of the accommodated heart overexpress genes for protective antioxidant and antiapoptotic proteins, where heme oxygenase-1 is thought to play a prominent role (6, 144). During induction of accommodation it was critical to temporarily inactivate complement with CVF to prevent injury by complement-fixing antibodies. However, it has recently been found that the only requirement to permit induction of accommodation is suppression of the complement effects that are due to the MAC. In C6-deficient rats, as well as in normocomplementemic rats given anti-C6 antibodies, accommodation was induced without administration of CVF to the same extent as in normal rats receiving CVF (149). This implies that the only role of CVF in induction of accommodation is the inactivation of MAC proteins; induction of accommodation does not require CVF-induced inactivation of C3, other components of the alternative pathway, or C5. These results also exclude the possibility that CVF might participate in induction of accommodation as an activator of protective mechanisms either directly or through its effects generating complement activation products or affecting other processes.

The current understanding of mechanisms of induction and maintenance of accommodation in the hamster-to-rat model suggests that induction of accommodation in pig-to-primate combinations would require, in addition to recipient modifications that have not as yet been delineated in primates, inhibition of complement activation and development of protective mechanisms against injury in the tissues of the graft, especially in the vascular endothelium. In this regard resistance against MAC-mediated injury has been induced in pig endothelial cells in vitro. Prolonged exposure of pig endothelial cells to human anti-pig natural antibodies rendered the cells resistant to the cytotoxic effects of complement (37, 44).

Recent studies suggested that binding of the antibodies to αgal mediates this effect, as resistance against complement could be induced more readily with the αgal-binding lectin from *Bandeiraea simplicifolia* than with antibodies (36). The incubation with antibody or lectin did not impair complement activation or the binding of complement components to the endothelial cells; instead, it induced endothelial cell activation that required protein synthesis and tyrosine protein kinase activity. At the time of maximal resistance the cells had regained a normal morphology and metabolic activity and the state of resistance lasted at least 3 days. It is possible that the protective changes against xenograft rejection that have been described in the organ graft in rodent models have a counterpart in this protection of porcine endothelial cells against the effects of the MAC. These changes induced in vitro may represent an important component for induction of accommodation in pig-to-primate models.

INHIBITION OF COMPLEMENT ACTIVATION IN XENOTRANSPLANTATION

Because complement activation takes place immediately after engraftment of a xenogeneic organ, causing its rejection, there is great interest in investigating methods to interfere with this activation. This strategy would prevent both the direct effects of complement on the vascular endothelium of the xenograft and the injurious effects of the blood cells of the recipient upon the xenograft to the extent that these cells are recruited and activated through complement-mediated mechanisms. Obviously the best strategy to prevent the effects of complement is to eliminate the factors that trigger complement activation. One approach is to remove anti-porcine natural antibodies, especially those against αgal, and then inhibit the production of elicited antibodies (3, 57). Alternatively, antibody binding to the endothelium of the graft may be blocked by using small antigen-binding fragments of humanized antibodies against the relevant antigens.

Another approach consists of reducing the number of antigen sites on the endothelium of the donor organ that are the target of antibodies in the recipient. This has been accomplished by genetic manipulation of donor mice to disable the gene for the αgalactosyl transferase that synthesizes endothelial cell αgal, the main target for natural antibodies (135, 152); however, it has not yet been possible to accomplish this in pigs. Transgenic pigs have been prepared that express the human gene for fucosyl transferase, also called H-transferase (109, 141). This enzyme competes favorably with αgalactosyl transferase to attach fucose instead of galactose to a common acceptor sugar.

In spite of the merits of these approaches to reduce deposition of antibodies on the endothelium, it is likely that residual antigens or antibodies may still result in antibody binding to the endothelium, which would trigger complement-dependent mechanisms of tissue injury. Therefore methods to inhibit progression of the complement reaction will still be necessary, either through administration of fluid phase complement inhibitors or by expression of membrane-associated complement regulators in the donor organ.

Complement Inhibition by Expression of Membrane-Associated Complement Regulators

Membrane complement regulators such as DAF, MCP, and CD59 are important to limit the extent of complement activation and to protect autologous tissues from harmful effects of activated complement (4, 65). Therefore, it was thought that with proper expression of membrane-associated inhibitors in the graft, complement inhibition could be achieved selectively in the graft, without compromising the role of systemic complement against infectious agents. Moreover, this approach could provide a long-term safeguard against complement-mediated tissue injury, as complement activation might occur even late during the life of the graft, through antibody-dependent or -independent mechanisms.

The membrane-associated complement regulators are considered to be very efficient to protect a cell from complement of the same species and less efficient against complement of other species, a concept that is referred to as homologous restriction. Accordingly, a complement regulator such as pig DAF on pig cells might not be able to efficiently prevent damage to those cells by human complement. Homologous restriction is the foundation of the proposal to engineer donor pigs that express human complement regulators so that a pig organ would be protected against primate complement when transplanted into a primate. The potential for that approach was initially demonstrated by incorporating human DAF into porcine endothelial cell membranes, which resulted in protection of the cells from the cytotoxic effects of human complement (41).

Because of its implications to xenotransplantation, the ability of pig complement regulators to function with human complement has recently been investigated. It was found that pig MCP and CD59 indeed can efficiently inhibit human complement (156, 157). Moreover, with the recent isolation, cloning, and expression of porcine CD59, it was shown that pig CD59 is as effective against human complement as it is against porcine complement (64, 90). With regard to DAF, it has not been determined whether porcine DAF is effective against human complement, but this information should be forthcoming once the gene for porcine DAF is cloned and expressed. The findings that porcine MCP and CD59 are functionally equivalent to their human counterparts are of great interest to xenotransplantation. Application of this development requires achieving continuous overexpression of the pig complement inhibitors in a donor pig or the development of a detection mechanism on the vascular endothelium of the graft that would trigger overexpression when needed. Optimal expression may require the use of transgenesis.

Early studies to test the hypothesis that inhibitors of the recipient species are protective against recipient complement showed that nonhuman cells transfected with cDNA for human complement regulators expressed the corresponding proteins on the cell membrane and were also protected from attack by human complement (1, 19, 108, 172). This approach was useful for the initial comparison of different inhibitors and to evaluate the combination of various inhibitors expressed on the same cell. In addition to the evaluation of human DAF, MCP, and CD59 on pig endothelial cells, studies have also been done to test the efficacy of C4bp engineered to express a phosphatidylinositol for anchoring to the cell membrane (97); using a similar approach it would be of interest to investigate the efficacy of C1 inh.

Following these initial studies, transgenic donor mice and pigs were prepared that express human complement inhibitors (29, 49, 94, 127, 145, 154). The inhibitors were generally found to have broad tissue distribution, with variable level of expression, and at times high expression was achieved. Often the initial evaluation of the functional capacity of the expressed inhibitor to protect against xenogeneic hyperacute injury was carried out by ex vivo perfusion of an organ from the transgenic animal with xenogeneic blood (17, 95, 142). Perfusion of a pig organ with human blood was considered a model of great interest because it would permit testing events that might occur in the few hours following engraftment of such an organ in a patient. When perfused with human blood, solid organs like hearts, kidneys, and lungs from transgenic pigs expressing appropriate amounts of DAF, MCP, or CD59 on the vascular endothelium demonstrated extended survival, lower levels of tissue damage, and reduced deposition of complement proteins distal to the site of the complement reaction where the inhibitor is known to act (27, 31, 79, 138, 139, 168).

In vivo experiments with transgenic pig organs transplanted into non-human primates have shown that organs expressing the inhibitors do not undergo HAR; critically, protection has been demonstrated in the absence of other modifications of the donor or recipient (18, 30, 87). This protection is usually incomplete as the organ in hours or a few days undergoes injury that may at least in part be complement-dependent. These studies clearly demonstrate that, similar to the relative resistance of human organ allografts against HAR in the presence of anti-A or anti-B antibodies, expression of complement inhibitors of the recipient species in the xenograft affords protection against HAR. The results also confirm that, to achieve long xenograft survival, a combination of methods to avert HAR, DXR/AVR, and cell-mediated rejection will be required. Results of published studies using organs from transgenic pigs transplanted into primates that were unmodified or underwent various forms of antibody depletion and immunosuppression have been recently reviewed (82). Non-human primates on various treatment protocols that were recipients of a life-supporting transgenic pig heart or kidney transplant survived a few weeks (137, 170). Kidneys from transgenic pigs that express human DAF appear to provide adequate function when transplanted into a primate; maintenance of appropriate hemoglobin levels required administration of human erythropoietin (169).

Research efforts continue directed at improving protection of a donor organ against complement attack. As expected, organs from transgenic animals that express two complement inhibitors are better protected than organs expressing only one inhibitor (18, 26, 102). Recent studies evaluated the combinatorial effect of expression of a membrane complement inhibitor plus reduced expression of endothelial αgal on susceptibility of mouse cells to cytotoxicity by human serum (24). It was found that lymphocytes from mice that are transgenic for both CD59 and H-transferase are better protected from lysis by human serum than cells from mice expressing only one of those proteins. Interestingly, cells expressing CD59 and reduced levels of αgal (from mice transgenic for human H-transferase) were equally protected as cells that expressed CD59 and no αgal (from αgal knockout mice). As protection with cells expressing no αgal was not complete, the study also confirms the importance of antibodies against antigens other than αgal in xenograft injury. The degree of protection from combining transgenic expression of complement inhibitors and reduction of αgal expression was also studied in a perfusion model of xenotransplantation (25, 158). It was found that reduction in αgal expression extended the function of a mouse heart perfused with human plasma beyond that in hearts expressing the complement inhibitors only. This effect was similar whether reduction of αgal expression was complete or partial.

Technologies are being developed to improve the expression of complement regulators. For example, it is thought that the use of yeast artificial chromosomes would allow the preparation of constructs that contain the regulatory regions as they exist in the human chromosome and possibly genes of several inhibitors; however, this method may have important limitations (30). The use of promoters such as that from the ICAM-2 gene that direct expression preferentially to endothelial cells also appears to be very attractive (27, 28). Another approach of interest is the development of chimeric complement inhibitors that act at different points in the complement reaction, such as the hDAF-CD59 molecule that contains the functional domains of DAF and CD59 (48).

With regard to the production of transgenic animals, it is of interest that the expression of significant quantities of transgenic hDAF on porcine spermatozoa does not compromise the breeding potential of these animals (155). Another consideration is that human membrane inhibitors are able to interact with certain infectious agents, often to specifically serve as receptors for microbial entry into a host cell (113, 154). For example, human MCP serves as a receptor for the measles virus and *Streptococcus pyogenes*. Therefore, these interactions raise the possibility that transgenic animals that express human inhibitors may become susceptible to certain human pathogens. Accordingly, when vaccines for the relevant pathogen are available, these animals may have to be vaccinated against those organisms.

Inhibition of Complement Activation with Soluble Molecules

A soluble complement inhibitor, CVF, has been an important tool to investigate xenograft rejection mechanisms, as its use to inactivate complement permitted establishment that HAR is mediated by complement activation (56, 105), and subsequently that, with maintenance of undetectable complement levels for several days, abrogation of HAR is followed by DXR/AVR (84, 85). With regard to potential clinical applications of soluble inhibitors, they may be useful especially in the early period following engraftment, even in a recipient of an organ xenograft that has been modified for optimal expression of membrane-associated complement inhibitors. Immediately after revascularization the soluble inhibitor may contribute to protect the organ from reperfusion injury and then to ensure protection from the initial complement activation due to binding of antibodies that still may occur in an organ with reduced xenoantigen expression or when a recipient had a large portion of the natural antibodies removed; this would ensure protection at a time when complement activation may be relatively intense.

In recent years, due to the recognition of the role of complement in the pathophysiology of tissue injury in many diseases, several inhibitors have been prepared and others are currently being developed that may have a potential for clinical applications (91, 165). Various groups of soluble complement inhibitors of interest to xenotransplantation are listed in Table 3. A potentially useful novel approach may consist of preparing transgenic donor pigs that, in addition to expressing a membrane complement inhibitor, also synthesize and secrete appropriate amounts of a soluble complement inhibitor in the local environment of the graft to provide added safeguard against complement injury. For example, a kidney or liver from such an engineered donor may overexpress DAF on the endothelial surface and also secrete sufficient sCR1 to contribute an additional protective layer against complement activation. In this regard transgenic mice have been developed that overexpress a complement inhibitor as a soluble protein; these mice are protected from antibody-induced glomerular injury (122). However, a problem with this approach, as well as with the use of soluble complement inhibitors in general, is that a balance may be difficult to obtain so

Table 3. Soluble inhibitors of complement activation used in models of xenotransplantation

Soluble proteins derived from membrane-associated complement inhibitors
sCR1, sDAF, sCD59, CAB-2
Other physiologic proteins
C1 inhibitor, IVIG, CVF
Antibodies against complement proteins
anti-C5, anti-C8, Fv anti-C5
Other inhibitors tested
Compstatin, heparin
Other inhibitors of potential interest
Ig peptides, C1q-binding peptides, aptamers

that systemic inhibition does not compromise the protective role of complement against infectious agents and persistence of immune complexes.

Soluble Forms of Membrane-Associated Complement Inhibitors

These soluble proteins, devoid of membrane anchor, have been obtained by recombinant technology. Soluble human CR1 (sCR1) was the first of this group of inhibitors to be prepared and successfully evaluated for efficacy to protect against complement-mediated tissue injury in a large number of experimental models. sCR1 inhibits activation of both the classical and alternative pathways through its decay-accelerating and cofactor activities (166). Since sCR1 inhibits complement in several species in addition to primates, initial studies in rats showed that administration of sCR1 caused a dose-dependent prolongation of the survival of a guinea pig cardiac transplant (119, 167). Administration of a single dose (15 mg/kg) of sCR1 to cynomolgus monkeys prolonged the survival of a pig cardiac xenograft to 48 to 90 h, in comparison to rejection in less than 1 h in untreated controls (121). Continuous infusion of sCR1 (40 mg/kg/day) in cynomolgus monkeys maintained low levels of complement activity and prolonged the survival of a porcine heart up to 7 days, while sCR1 together with immunosuppression could extend survival for several weeks (120). sCR1 may also be useful to protect a xenogeneic organ from complement-dependent damage in reperfusion injury since it has been shown that sCR1 reduced reperfusion injury in a pig lung allotransplant model (115). Human recombinant MCP has been found to function as an inhibitor of both complement pathways (21, 22). Soluble recombinant DAF has also been tested as a complement inhibitor (99). Recently a single molecule has been developed that consists of sCR1 covalently modified by sialyl Lewis x glycosylation (66). This hybrid molecule that inhibits both complement activation and selectin-mediated adherence may be able to localize the complement inhibition to a site of interest, such as a xenograft. The modified sCR1 has been shown to reduce tissue injury in a mouse model of cerebral ischemia to a larger extent than unmodified sCR1 (66). Therefore, this inhibitor is of great interest for xenotransplantation.

CAB-2, a recombinant soluble chimeric protein derived from human DAF and MCP, has been shown to inhibit complement activation, markedly reducing tissue injury in models of pig-to-human xenotransplantation. CAB-2 combines the inhibitory activities of DAF and MCP upon C3- and C5-convertases of both complement activation pathways (63). CAB-2 does not mediate the secondary cleavage of C3bi to C3d,g, suggesting that CAB-2 may preserve antimicrobial defense mechanisms by retaining the opsonization properties of C3bi (63). CAB-2 inhibits the pathologic effects of complement activation triggered by immune complexes in both the Arthus reaction and Forssman shock models (63), as well as in a model of cardiopulmonary bypass (124). Addition of CAB-2 in vitro to human serum inhibited cytotoxicity and the deposition of C4b and C3bi on porcine endothelial cells (81). In an ex vivo perfusion model, addition of CAB-2 to human blood prolonged survival of a pig heart in a dose-dependent manner, retarded the onset of increased coronary vascular resistance, and markedly inhibited the generation of C3a and SC5b-9 (81). Hearts surviving $>$240 min demonstrated trace or no deposition of C9 and normal tissue architecture. In an in vivo model of pig-to-rhesus monkey heterotopic cardiac transplantation graft, survival of up to 4 days was obtained with a single dose of 15 mg/kg CAB-2 or with multiple doses, in the absence of immunosuppression (134). CAB-2 markedly reduced the generation of C3a and SC5b-9 and tissue deposition of C3 and C9 at rejection, suggesting that CAB-2 may be a useful therapeutic agent for xenotransplantation.

A fusion protein that may have potential for xenotransplantation would be one that targets a complement inhibitor to the endothelial cell surface by means of an antibody that recognizes an epitope of relevance for triggering xenogeneic injury. The antibody fragment would be such that blocks binding of anti-pig antibodies against that epitope but does not activate complement or bind to Fc receptors on recipient cells, while the complement inhibitor would function as the analogous molecule in its membrane-associated form. In fact, a model for this approach has recently been developed that employs soluble CD59 fused to an antibody-combining site at the end of the CH1γ fragment of IgG with specificity for the dansyl hapten (171). It was found that the fusion protein specifically bound to dansyl-labeled Chinese hamster ovary cells and provided protection against complement-mediated lysis.

Other Physiologic Proteins

The use of physiologic proteins of the same species in which complement inhibition is desired has the advantage that those proteins are nonantigenic and thus can be used repeatedly. C1 inh is of interest for pig-to-primate transplantation because it selectively inhibits the classical pathway, leaving the alternative pathway intact for protection of the recipient. Addition of C1 inh to human serum in vitro was found to inhibit activation and cytotoxicity of porcine endothelial cells (39). Large amounts of C1 inh were needed for complete inhibition of cytotoxicity, due to the fact that C1 inh is only moderately effective when C1 activation is triggered by strong activators like antigen-antibody complexes. On the other hand, C1 inh in combination with heparin inhibited complement activation much more effectively than either agent alone (38). Deposition of C4b on porcine endothelial cells incubated with human serum was strongly suppressed by addition of C1 inh plus heparin to the serum, suggesting that this approach may be effective to avert HAR mediated by the classical pathway. C1 inh was found to reduce tissue injury of a pig kidney perfused ex vivo with human blood (47). C1 inh may also protect the xenograft against reperfusion injury, as it was shown that C1 inh reduces damage to the myocardium in a model of reperfusion injury following a period of ischemia (15).

Intravenous IgG (IVIG), when administered in large doses, is an effective complement inhibitor, especially of the classical pathway, by providing a high concentration of IgG that functions as acceptor for binding of C3b and C4b (9). This IgG in the vessels of the xenograft may thus compete with the endothelium for binding of activated complement proteins. IVIG has been shown to prolong graft survival in guinea pig-to-rat cardiac transplantation (55, 83). When IVIG was used with conventional immunosuppression in pig-to-primate combinations, graft survival was extended up to 10 days (89). Addition of IgG in vitro to human serum reduced the binding of C3b to porcine endothelial cells, likely through decreased formation of C3 convertase on the cells. IVIG may also offer additional protection of the graft by mechanisms other than inhibition of complement activation, as IVIG is thought to induce blockade of Fc receptors and modulate cytokine production (165).

CVF, a cobra glycoprotein analogous to C3b, strongly activates the alternative pathway when added to mammalian plasma; it binds factor B, which is then activated by factor D to Bb. Bb remains firmly bound to CVF, resulting in a very effective alternative pathway C3 convertase (163). Because CVF in the complex is resistant to inactivation by factor I, it causes massive complement activation and the consequent inactivation of C3, C5, and terminal components, with generation of C3a and C5a that may result in tissue injury. Although these anaphylatoxins may cause severe pulmonary injury and other complications, especially in rodents, they have not been a significant problem in baboons (84). CVF is highly immunogenic and elicits antibodies that make it ineffective several days after its administration (151). Although CVF is not a candidate for use in humans, it has been invaluable to demonstrate the role of complement in HAR and for defining xenograft AVR/DXR when complement was effectively inhibited.

Antibodies against Complement Proteins

Antibodies against certain components or activation fragments of complement may have a role in protecting a xenograft, especially recombinant humanized derivatives of monoclonal antibodies (92). With an anti-human C5 monoclonal antibody it was possible to suppress HAR in an ex vivo model of pig-to-human xenografting (80), and a monoclonal antibody against C8 protected a rat heart from damage caused by perfusion with human blood (126). These antibodies are likely less effective than inhibitors that act earlier in the complement reaction; thus, in contrast to CAB-2, which blocks the generation of C3-convertase, the occurrence of monocyte activation in a simulated extracorporeal circulation model could not be prevented with an anti-C5 antibody (124).

Recently a single-chain anti-C5 was used in patients undergoing cardiopulmonary bypass (125). With doses of 0.2 to 2.0 mg/kg the $T_{1/2}$ was 10 to 31 h, and with the highest doses there was complete inhibition of SC5b-9 generation and reduction in cardiopulmonary bypass-induced release of cardiac-specific phosphokinase. The results suggest that a single-chain inhibiting antibody against C5 may have a place for the treatment of clinical conditions where the MAC plays a predominant pathophysiologic role.

Other Inhibitors

Compstatin, a 13-amino acid cyclic peptide that was selected from a phage-displayed random peptide library, inhibits activation of both classical and alternative pathways through binding reversibly to native C3, preventing cleavage of C3 by the C3 convertases (133). In an ex vivo kidney perfusion model of pig-to-human transplantation, compstatin was found to prolong organ survival and effectively inhibit generation of activation products of C3 and terminal components, and prevent tissue deposition of C3 and MAC (46).

The effect of heparin was tested in vivo for protection against complement-mediated loss of heparan sulfate that may play a role in HAR. A nonanticoagulant, heparin, was studied to ascertain if it would alter the fate of heparan sulfate in guinea pig hearts radioactively labeled with [^{35}S]-sulfate and transplanted into rats (147). Heparin administration inhibited the release of heparan sulfate from the transplanted heart, prolonged the survival of the transplant, and reduced the amount of C3b bound to the heart, in comparison to control animals.

A recent report indicates that a hexadecemeric multiple peptide of the C1q-binding site (residues 282–292) from human IgG_1 inhibits lysis of pig red cells by human serum, with an I_{50} value of 1 μM (77). This study suggests that peptides derived from the C1q binding region of immunoglobulins could hold promise to inhibit activation of the classical complement pathway. The alternative approach, i.e., using a C1q fragment to block the binding of IgM and IgG to C1q, is also currently under investigation (76). An advantage of these approaches is that they attempt to prevent classical pathway complement activation at its earliest stage. A new approach to specifically inhibit C5 activation is currently being pursued with the derivation of RNA aptamers that bind C5, inhibiting cleavage of C5 by the convertases of both pathways (11). One aptamer with a kD of 2.5 nM was produced that retained functional inhibitory activity.

CONCLUSION

A major area of xenotransplantation research has focused on the mechanisms by which complement participates in rejection. Rapid progress has been possible, due to the existing large body of knowledge about the biochemistry, molecular biology, and pathophysiologic role of complement. While the MAC alone is responsible for HAR, the role of various complement fragments and complexes in the production of injury to the vascular endothelium and other constituents of an organ xenograft is being defined. Because complement participates in multiple ways in causing xenograft injury, the use of complement inhibitors is a major part of strategies to protect a xenograft. Although soluble complement inhibitors that can be used in vivo are beginning to be developed, small nontoxic molecules that inhibit complement efficiently are not yet available. Some of the large molecules that have been successful to abrogate HAR in experimental animals may be useful, at least temporarily, to reduce reperfusion injury and prevent HAR. On the other hand, the usefulness of transgenic donor pigs that express membrane-associated complement regulators has been firmly documented; clearly this approach provides considerable protection to the xenograft. It is likely that some form of molecular engineering to express membrane complement inhibitors and to suppress expression of important membrane antigens will be part of protocols to achieve prolonged graft survival, together with induction of immunological tolerance or accommodation, and the administration of immunosuppressive agents that are safer and more selective than those currently available. Therefore, as in the past, xenotransplantation research will continue to include a strong participation of studies on the pathophysiologic role of complement in graft rejection and accommodation, as well as on the development of new approaches to more effectively inhibit complement activation.

Acknowledgments. Work performed in the author's laboratory has been supported by the Department of Veterans Affairs Medical Research; the National Heart, Lung, and Blood Institute of the National Institutes of Health (grant ROI-HL62195); and the Minnesota Medical Foundation. The author is indebted to Barbara A. Benson for her assistance in the preparation of the manuscript.

REFERENCES

1. **Akami, T., R. Sawada, N. Minato, M. Naruto, A. Yamada, J. Imanishi, M. Mitsuo, I. Nakai, M. Okamoto, H. Nakajima, K. Arakawa, and T. Oka.** 1992. Cytoprotective effect of CD59 antigen on xenotransplantation immunity. *Transplant. Proc.* **24:**485–487.

2. **Alexandre, G. P. J., J. P. Squifflet, M. De Bruyère, D. Latinne, R. Reding, P. Gianello, M. Carlier, and Y. Pirson.** 1987. Present experiences in a series of 26 ABO-incompatible living donor renal allografts. *Transplant. Proc.* **19:**4538–4542.
3. **Alwayn, I. P. J., M. Basker, L. Buhler, and D. K. C. Cooper.** 1999. The problem of anti-pig antibodies in pig-to-primate xenografting: current and novel methods of depletion and/or suppression of production of anti-pig antibodies. *Xenotransplantation* **6:**157–168.
4. **Atkinson, J. P., T. J. Oglesby, D. White, E. A. Adams, and M. K. Liszewski.** 1991. Separation of self from non-self in the complement system: a role for membrane cofactor protein and decay accelerating factor. *Clin. Exp. Immunol.* **86**(S1)**:**27–30.
5. **Azimzadeh, A., P. Wolf, A. P. Dalmasso, M. Odeh, J. P. Beller, M. Fabre, B. Charreau, K. Thibaudeau, J. Cinqualbre, J. P. Soulillou, and I. Anegon.** 1996. Assessment of hyperacute rejection in a rat-to-primate cardiac xenograft model. *Transplantation* **61:**1305–1313.
6. **Bach, F. H., C. Ferran, P. Hechenlettner, W. Mark, N. Koyamada, T. Miyatake, H. Winkler, A. Badrichani, D. Candinas, and W. W. Hancock.** 1997. Accommodation of vascularized xenografts: expression of "protective genes" by donor endothelial cells in a host TH2 cytokine environment. *Nature Med.* **3:**196–204.
7. **Bach, F. H., M. A. Turman, G. M. Vercellotti, J. L. Platt, and A. P. Dalmasso.** 1991. Accommodation: a working paradigm for progressing toward clinical discordant xenografting. *Transplant. Proc.* **23:**205–207.
8. **Bannett, A. D., R. F. McAlack, M. Morris, M. W. Chopek, and J. L. Platt.** 1989. ABO incompatible renal transplantation: a qualitative analysis of native endothelial tissue ABO antigens after transplantation. *Transplant. Proc.* **21:**783–785.
9. **Basta, M., L. F. Fries, and M. M. Frank.** 1991. High doses of intravenous Ig inhibit in vitro uptake of C4 fragments onto sensitized erythrocytes. *Blood* **77:**376–380.
10. **Benzaquen, L. R., A. Nicholson-Weller, and J. A. Halperin.** 1994. Terminal complement proteins C5b-9 release basic fibroblast growth factor and platelet-derived growth factor from endothelial cells. *J. Exp. Med.* **179:**985–992.
11. **Biesecker, G., L. Dihel, K. Enney, and R. A. Bendele.** 1999. Derivation of RNA aptamer inhibitors of human complement C5. *Immunopharmacology* **42:**219–230.
12. **Blakely, M. L., W. J. Van der Werf, M. C. Berndt, A. P. Dalmasso, F. H. Bach, and W. W. Hancock.** 1994. Activation of intragraft endothelial and mononuclear cells during discordant xenograft rejection. *Transplantation* **58:**1059–1066.
13. **Botto, M., C. Dell'Agnola, A. E. Bygrave, E. M. Thompson, H. T. Cook, F. Petry, M. Loos, P. P. Pandolfi, and M. J. Walport.** 1998. Homozygous C1q deficiency causes glomerulonephritis associated with multiple apoptotic bodies. *Nature Genet.* **19:**56–59.
14. **Brauer, R. B., W. M. I. Baldwin, M. R. Daha, S. K. Pruitt, and F. Sanfilippo.** 1993. Use of C6-deficient rats to evaluate the mechanism of hyperacute rejection of discordant cardiac xenografts. *J. Immunol.* **151:**7240–7248.
15. **Buerke, M., D. Prufer, M. Dahm, H. Oelert, J. Meyer, and H. Darius.** 1998. Blocking of classical complement pathway inhibits endothelial adhesion molecule expression and preserves ischemic myocardium from reperfusion injury. *J. Pharmacol. Exp. Ther.* **286:**429–438.
16. **Bustos, M., T. M. Coffman, S. Saadi, and J. L. Platt.** 1997. Modulation of eicosanoid metabolism in endothelial cells in a xenograft model. Role of cyclooxygenase-2. *J. Clin. Invest.* **100:**1150–1158.
17. **Byrne, G. W., K. R. McCurry, D. Kagan, C. Quinn, M. J. Martin, J. L. Platt, and J. S. Logan.** 1995. Protection of xenogeneic cardiac endothelium from human complement by expression of CD59 or DAF in transgenic mice. *Transplantation* **60:**1149–1156.
18. **Byrne, G. W., K. R. McCurry, M. J. Martin, S. M. McClellan, J. L. Platt, and J. S. Logan.** 1997. Transgenic pigs expressing human CD59 and decay-accelerating factor produce an intrinsic barrier to complement-mediated damage. *Transplantation* **63:**149–155.
19. **Charreau, B., A. Cassard, L. Tesson, B. Le Mauff, J. M. Navenot, D. Blanchard, D. Lublin, J. P. Soulillou, and I. Anegon.** 1994. Protection of rat endothelial cells from primate complement-mediated lysis by expression of human CD59 and/or decay-accelerating factor. *Transplantation* **58:**1222 1229.
20. **Chartrand, C., S. O'Regan, P. Robitaille, and M. Pinto-Blonde.** 1979. Delayed rejection of cardiac xenografts in C6-deficient rabbits. *Immunology* **38:**245–248.

21. **Christiansen, D., J. Milland, B. R. Thorley, I. F. McKenzie, and B. E. Loveland.** 1996. A functional analysis of recombinant soluble CD46 in vivo and a comparison with recombinant soluble forms of CD55 and CD35 in vitro. *Eur. J. Immunol.* **26:**578–585.
22. **Christiansen, D., J. Milland, B. R. Thorley, I. F. McKenzie, P. L. Mottram, L. J. Purcell, and B. E. Loveland.** 1996. Engineering of recombinant soluble CD46: an inhibitor of complement activation. *Immunology* **87:**348–354.
23. **Cooper, N. R.** 1985. The classical complement pathway: activation and regulation of the first complement component. *Adv. Immunol.* **37:**151–216.
24. **Costa, C., L. Zhao, S. Decesare, and W. L. Fodor.** 1999. Comparative analysis of three genetic modifications designed to inhibit human serum-mediated cytolysis. *Xenotransplantation* **6:**6–16.
25. **Cowan, P. J., C. G. Chen, T. A. Shinkel, N. Fisicaro, E. Salvaris, A. Aminian, M. Romanella, M. J. Pearse, and A. J. d'Apice.** 1998. Knock out of alpha1,3-galactosyltransferase or expression of alpha1,2-fucosyltransferase further protects CD55- and CD59-expressing mouse hearts in an ex vivo model of xenograft rejection. *Transplantation* **65:**1599–1604.
26. **Cowan, P. J., T. A. Shinkel, A. Aminian, M. Romanella, P. L. Wigley, A. J. Lonie, M. B. Nottle, M. J. Pearse, and A. J. d'Apice.** 1998. High-level co-expression of complement regulators on vascular endothelium in transgenic mice: CD55 and CD59 provide greater protection from human complement-mediated injury than CD59 alone. *Xenotransplantation* **5:**184–190.
27. **Cowan, P. J., C. A. Somerville, T. A. Shinkel, M. Katerelos, A. Aminian, M. Romanella, M. J. Tange, M. J. Pearse, and A. J. d'Apice.** 1998. High-level endothelial expression of human CD59 prolongs heart function in an ex vivo model of xenograft rejection. *Transplantation* **65:**826–831.
28. **Cowan, P. J., D. Tsang, C. M. Pedic, L. R. Abbott, T. A. Shinkel, A. J. d'Apice, and M. J. Pearse.** 1998. The human ICAM-2 promoter is endothelial cell-specific in vitro and in vivo and contains critical Sp1 and GATA binding sites. *J. Biol. Chem.* **273:**11737–11744.
29. **Cozzi, E., A. W. Tucker, G. A. Langford, G. Pino-Chavez, L. Wright, M. J. O'Connell, V. J. Young, R. Lancaster, M. McLaughlin, K. Hunt, M. C. Bordin, and D. J. White.** 1997. Characterization of pigs transgenic for human decay-accelerating factor. *Transplantation* **64:**1383–1392.
30. **Cozzi, E., N. Yannoutsos, G. A. Langford, G. Pino-Chavez, J. Wallwork, and D. J. G. White.** 1997. Effect of transgenic expression of human decay-accelerating factor on the inhibition of hyperacute rejection of pig organs, p. 665–682. *In* D. K. C. Cooper, E. Kemp, J. L. Platt, and D. J. G. White (ed.), *Xenotransplantation. The Transplantation of Organs and Tissues Between Species*, 2nd ed. Springer-Verlag, Berlin, Germany.
31. **Daggett, C. W., M. Yeatman, A. J. Lodge, E. P. Chen, P. Van Trigt, G. W. Byrne, J. S. Logan, J. H. Lawson, J. L. Platt, and R. D. Davis.** 1997. Swine lungs expressing human complement-regulatory proteins are protected against acute pulmonary dysfunction in a human plasma perfusion model. *J. Thoracic Cardiovasc. Surg.* **113:**390–398.
32. **Dalmasso, A. P.** 1986. Complement in the pathophysiology and diagnosis of human diseases. *Crit. Rev. Clin. Lab. Sci.* **24:**123–183.
33. **Dalmasso, A. P.** 1992. The complement system in xenotransplantation. *Immunopharmacology* **24:**149–160.
34. **Dalmasso, A. P.** 1997. Role of complement in xenograft rejection, p. 38–60. *In* D. K. C. Cooper, E. Kemp, J. L. Platt, and D. J. G. White (ed.), *Xenotransplantation. The Transplantation of Organs and Tissues Between Species*, 2nd ed. Springer-Verlag, Berlin, Germany.
35. **Dalmasso, A. P., and B. A. Benson.** 1988. Pore size of lesions induced by complement on red cell membranes and its relation to C5b-8, C5b-9 and poly C9, p. 207–219. *In* E. R. Podack (ed.), *Cytolytic Lymphocytes and Complement: Effectors of the Immune System*, vol. 1. CRC Press, Boca Raton, Fla.
36. **Dalmasso, A. P., B. A. Benson, J. S. Johnson, C. Larcto, and M. Abrahamsen.** 2000. Resistance against the membrane attack complex of complement induced in porcine endothelial cells with a Galα(1–3) Gal binding lectin: up-regulation of CD59 expression. *J. Immunol.* **164:**3764–3773.
37. **Dalmasso, A. P., T. He, and B. A. Benson.** 1996. Human IgM xenoreactive natural antibodies can induce resistance of porcine endothelial cells to complement-mediated injury. *Xenotransplantation* **3:**54–62.
38. **Dalmasso, A. P., and J. L. Platt.** 1994. Potentiation of C1 inhibitor plus heparin in prevention of complement-mediated activation of endothelial cells in a model of xenograft hyperacute rejection. *Transplant. Proc.* **26:**1246–1247.
39. **Dalmasso, A. P., and J. L. Platt.** 1993. Prevention of complement-mediated activation of xenogeneic endothelial cells in an in vitro model of xenograft hyperacute rejection by C1 inhibitor. *Transplantation* **56:**1171–1176.

40. **Dalmasso, A. P., G. M. Vercellotti, R. J. Fischel, R. M. Bolman, F. H. Bach, and J. L. Platt.** 1992. Mechanism of complement activation in the hyperacute rejection of porcine organs transplanted into primate recipients. *Am. J. Pathol.* **140:**1157–1166.
41. **Dalmasso, A. P., G. M. Vercellotti, J. L. Platt, and F. H. Bach.** 1991. Inhibition of complement-mediated endothelial cell cytotoxicity by decay accelerating factor. Potential for prevention of xenograft hyperacute rejection. *Transplantation* **52:**530–533.
42. **Davis, A. E.** 1988. C1 inhibitor and hereditary angioneurotic edema. *Annu. Rev. Immunol.* **6:**595–628.
43. **Davis, E. A., T. T. Lam, Z. Qian, S. Ibrahim, W. M. Baldwin, 3rd, and F. P. Sanfilippo.** 1995. Inhibition of neutrophil adhesion and the membrane attack complex of complement synergistically prolongs cardiac xenograft survival. *J. Heart Lung Transplant.* **14:**973–980.
44. **Dorling, A., C. Stocker, T. Tsao, D. O. Haskard, and R. I. Lechler.** 1996. In vitro accommodation of immortalized porcine endothelial cells: resistance to complement mediated lysis and down-regulation of VCAM expression induced by low concentrations of polyclonal human IgG antipig antibodies. *Transplantation* **62:**1127–1136.
45. **Fearon, D. T., and R. H. Carter.** 1995. The CD19/CR2/TAPA-1 complex of B lymphocytes: linking natural to acquired immunity. *Annu. Rev. Immunol.* **13:**127–149.
46. **Fiane, A. E., T. E. Mollnes, V. Videm, T. Hovig, K. Høgåsen, O. J. Melbye, L. Spruce, W. T. Moore, A. Sahu, and J. D. Lambris.** 1999. Compstatin, a peptide inhibitor of C3, prolongs survival of ex vivo perfused pig xenografts. *Xenotransplantation* **6:**52–65.
47. **Fiane, A. E., V. Videm, H. T. Johansen, O. J. Mellbye, E. W. Nielsen, and T. E. Mollnes.** 1999. C1-inhibitor attenuates hyperacute rejection and inhibits complement, leukocyte and platelet activation in an ex vivo pig-to-human perfusion model. *Immunopharmacology* **42:**231–243.
48. **Fodor, W. L., S. A. Rollins, E. R. Guilmette, E. Setter, and S. P. Squinto.** 1995. A novel bifunctional chimeric complement inhibitor that regulates C3 convertase and formation of the membrane attack complex. *J. Immunol.* **155:**4135–4138.
49. **Fodor, W. L., B. L. Williams, L. A. Matis, J. A. Madri, S. A. Rollins, J. W. Knight, W. Velander, and S. P. Squinto.** 1994. Expression of a functional human complement inhibitor in a transgenic pig as a model for the prevention of xenogeneic hyperacute organ rejection. *Proc. Natl. Acad. Sci. USA* **91:**11153–11157.
50. **Foreman, K. E., M. M. Glovsky, R. L. Warner, S. J. Horvath, and P. A. Ward.** 1996. Comparative effect of C3a and C5a on adhesion molecule expression on neutrophils and endothelial cells. *Inflammation* **20:**1–9.
51. **Friedl, H. P., G. O. Till, U. S. Ryan, and P. A. Ward.** 1989. Mediator-induced activation of xanthine oxidase in endothelial cells. *FASEB J.* **3:**2512–2518.
52. **Fryer, J., J. R. Leventhal, A. P. Dalmasso, P. Simone, S. Chen, L. H. Sun, J. Jesserun, N. Reinsmoen, and A. Matas.** 1994. Cellular rejection in a discordant xenograft when hyperacute rejection is prevented: analysis using adoptive and passive transfer. *Transplant Immunol.* **2:**87–93.
53. **Fryer, J. P., J. R. Leventhal, A. P. Dalmasso, S. Chen, P. A. Simone, J. J. Goswitz, N. L. Reinsmoen, and A. J. Matas.** 1995. Beyond hyperacute rejection. Accelerated rejection in a discordant xenograft model by adoptive transfer of specific cell subsets. *Transplantation* **59:**171–176.
54. **Gambiez, L., B. J. Weill, C. Chereau, Y. Calmus, and D. Houssin.** 1990. The hyperacute rejection of guinea pig to rat heart xenografts is mediated by preformed IgM. *Transplant. Proc.* **22:**1058.
55. **Gautreau, C., T. Kojima, G. Woimant, J. Cardoso, P. Devillier, and D. Houssin.** 1995. Use of intravenous immunoglobulin to delay xenogeneic hyperacute rejection. An in vivo and in vitro evaluation. *Transplantation* **60:**903–907.
56. **Gewurz, H., D. S. Clark, M. D. Cooper, R. L. Varco, and R. A. Good.** 1967. Effect of cobra venom-induced inhibition of complement activity on allograft and xenograft rejection reactions. *Transplantation* **5:**1296–1303.
57. **Good, A. H., D. K. C. Cooper, A. J. Malcolm, R. M. Ippolito, E. Koren, F. A. Neethling, Y. Ye, N. Zuhdi, and L. R. Lamontagne.** 1992. Identification of carbohydrate structures that bind human antiporcine antibodies: implications for discordant xenografting in humans. *Transplant. Proc.* **24:**559–562.
58. **Guo, W. X., B. Ghebrehiwet, B. Weksler, K. Schweitzer, and E. I. Peerschke.** 1999. Up-regulation of endothelial cell binding proteins/receptors for complement component C1q by inflammatory cytokines. *J. Lab. Clin. Med.* **133:**541–550.
59. **Hamilton, K. K., R. Hattori, C. T. Esmon, and P. J. Sims.** 1990. Complement proteins C5b-9 induce vesiculation of the endothelial plasma membrane and expose catalytic surface for assembly of the prothrombinase enzyme complex. *J. Biol. Chem.* **265:**3809–3814.

60. **Hasan, R., J. Van den Bogaerde, J. Forty, L. Wright, J. Wallwork, and D. J. G. White.** 1992. Xenograft adaptation is dependent on the presence of antispecies antibody, not prolonged residence in the recipient. *Transplant. Proc.* **24:**531–532.

61. **Hattori, R., K. K. Hamilton, R. P. McEver, and P. J. Sims.** 1989. Complement proteins C5b-9 induce secretion of high molecular weight multimers of endothelial von Willebrand factor and translocation of granule membrane protein GMP-140 to the cell surface. *J. Biol. Chem.* **264:**9053–9060.

62. **Haviland, D. L., R. L. McCoy, W. T. Whitehead, H. Akama, E. P. Molmenti, A. Brown, J. C. Haviland, W. C. Parks, D. H. Perlmutter, and R. A. Wetsel.** 1995. Cellular expression of the C5a anaphylatoxin receptor (C5aR): demonstration of C5aR on nonmyeloid cells of the liver and lung. *J. Immunol.* **154:**1861–1869.

63. **Higgins, P. J., J. L. Ko, R. Lobell, C. Sardonini, M. K. Alessi, and C. G. Yeh.** 1997. A soluble chimeric complement inhibitory protein that possesses both decay-accelerating and factor I cofactor activities. *J. Immunol.* **158:**2872–2881.

64. **Hinchliffe, S. J., N. K. Rushmere, S. M. Hanna, and B. P. Morgan.** 1998. Molecular cloning and functional characterization of the pig analogue of CD59: relevance to xenotransplantation. *J. Immunol.* **160:**3924–3932.

65. **Hourcade, D., V. M. Holers, and J. P. Atkinson.** 1989. The regulators of complement activation (RCA) gene cluster. *Adv. Immunol.* **45:**381–416.

66. **Huang, J., L. J. Kim, R. Mealey, H. C. Marsh, Y. Zhang, A. J. Tenner, E. S. Connolly, and D. J. Pinsky.** 1999. Neuronal protection in stroke by an sLe^{x}-glycosylated complement inhibitory protein. *Science* **285:**595–599.

67. **Ierino, F. L., T. Kozlowski, J. B. Siegel, A. Shimizu, R. B. Colvin, P. T. Banerjee, D. K. Cooper, A. B. Cosimi, F. H. Bach, D. H. Sachs, and S. C. Robson.** 1998. Disseminated intravascular coagulation in association with the delayed rejection of pig-to-baboon renal xenografts. *Transplantation* **66:**1439–1450.

68. **Ihrcke, N. S., and J. L. Platt.** 1996. Shedding of heparan sulfate proteoglycan by stimulated endothelial cells: evidence for proteolysis of cell-surface molecules. *J. Cell. Physiol.* **168:**625–637.

69. **Ikeda, K., K. Nagasawa, T. Horiuchi, T. Tsuru, H. Nishizaka, and Y. Niho.** 1997. C5a induces tissue factor activity on endothelial cells. *Thromb. Haemost.* **77:**394–398.

70. **Jefferson, K. P., K. S. Tyerman, M. McLeish, D. S. J. Collier, and S. Thiru.** 1991. Donor pretreatment prolongs survival of discordant xenografts. *Transplant. Proc.* **23:**2280–2281.

71. **Johnson, E. M., J. Leventhal, A. P. Dalmasso, J. Goswitz, P. Simone, S. Chen, M. Moyle, and A. J. Matas.** 1996. Inactivation of C3 and C5 prolongs cardiac xenograft survival and decreases leukocyte infiltration in a model of delayed xenograft rejection. *Transplant. Proc.* **28:**603.

72. **Johnson, E. M., J. Leventhal, A. P. Dalmasso, J. Goswitz, P. Simone, S. Chen, M. Moyle, and A. J. Matas.** 1996. Use of a novel CD11b/CD18 inhibitory agent in a C6 deficient rat to evaluate delayed xenograft rejection. *Transplant. Proc.* **28:**728.

73. **Johnston, P. S., S. M. L. Lim, M. W. Wang, L. Wright, and D. J. G. White.** 1991. Hyperacute rejection of xenografts in the complete absence of antibody. *Transplant. Proc.* **23:**877–879.

74. **Kerr, S. R., A. P. Dalmasso, E. V. Apasova, S. S. Chen, M. Kirschfink, and A. J. Matas.** 1999. Mouse-to-rabbit xenotransplantation: a new small animal model of hyperacute rejection mediated by the classical complement pathway. *Transplantation* **67:**360–365.

75. **Kilgore, K. S., C. M. Flory, B. F. Miller, V. M. Evans, and J. S. Warren.** 1996. The membrane attack complex of complement induces interleukin-8 and monocyte chemoattractant protein-1 secretion from human umbilical vein endothelial cells. *Am. J. Pathol.* **149:**953–961.

76. **Kishore, U., M. V. Perdikoulis, P. Strong, and K. B. M. Reid.** 1998. A homotrimer of the B-chain globular head region of Clq is an inhibitor of Clq-mediated complement activation. *Mol. Immunol.* **35:**375.

77. **Kojima, T., C. A. Del Carpio, H. Tajiri, K. Yoshikawa, S. Saga, and I. Yokoyama.** 1999. Inhibition of complement-mediated immune hemolysis by peptides derived from the constant domain of immunoglobulin. *Transplantation 67:*637–638.

78. **Korb, L. C., and J. M. Ahearn.** 1997. C1q binds directly and specifically to surface blebs of apoptotic human keratinocytes: complement deficiency and systemic lupus erythematosus revisited. *J. Immunol.* **158:**4525–4528.

79. **Kroshus, T. J., R. M. Bolman, A. P. Dalmasso, S. A. Rollins, E. R. Guilmette, B. L. Williams, S. P. Squinto, and W. L. Fodor.** 1996. Expression of human CD59 in transgenic pig organs enhances organ survival in an ex vivo xenogeneic perfusion model. *Transplantation* **61:**1513–1521.

80. **Kroshus, T. J., S. A. Rollins, A. P. Dalmasso, E. A. Elliot, L. A. Matis, S. P. Squinto, and R. M. Bolman.** 1995. Complement inhibition with an anti-C5 monoclonal antibody prevents acute cardiac tissue injury in an ex vivo model of pig-to-human xenotransplantation. *Transplantation* **60:**1194–1202.

81. **Kroshus, T. J., C. T. Salerno, C. G. Yeh, P. J. Higgins, R. M. Bolman, and A. P. Dalmasso.** 2000. A recombinant soluble chimeric complement inhibitor composed of human CD46 and CD55 reduces acute cardiac tissue injury in models of pig-to-human heart transplantation. *Transplantation* **69:**2282–2289.

82. **Lambrigts, D., D. H. Sachs, and D. K. Cooper.** 1998. Discordant organ xenotransplantation in primates: world experience and current status. *Transplantation* **66:**547–561.

83. **Latremouille, C., N. Haeffner-Cavaillon, N. Goussef, C. Mandet, N. Hinglais, P. Bruneval, J. Bariety, A. Carpentier, and D. Glotz.** 1994. Normal human polyclonal immunoglobulins for intravenous use significantly delay hyperacute xenograft rejection. *Transplant. Proc.* **26:**1285.

84. **Leventhal, J. R., A. P. Dalmasso, J. W. Cromwell, J. L. Platt, C. J. Manivel, R. M. Bolman, and A. J. Matas.** 1993. Prolongation of cardiac xenograft survival by depletion of complement. *Transplantation* **55:**857–865.

85. **Leventhal, J. R., A. J. Matas, L. H. Sun, S. Reif, R. M. Bolman, A. P. Dalmasso, and J. L. Platt.** 1993. The immunopathology of cardiac xenograft rejection in the guinea pig-to-rat model. *Transplantation* **56:**1–8.

86. **Leventhal, J. R., P. Sakiyalak, J. Witson, P. Simone, A. J. Matas, R. M. Bolman, and A. P. Dalmasso.** 1994. The synergistic effect of combined antibody and complement depletion on discordant cardiac xenograft survival in nonhuman primates. *Transplantation* **57:**974–978.

87. **Lin, S. S., B. C. Weidner, G. W. Byrne, L. E. Diamond, J. H. Lawson, C. W. Hoopes, L. J. Daniels, C. W. Daggett, W. Parker, R. C. Harland, R. D. Davis, R. R. Bollinger, J. S. Logan, and J. L. Platt.** 1998. The role of antibodies in acute vascular rejection of pig-to-baboon cardiac transplants. *J. Clin. Invest.* **101:**1745–1756.

88. **Lozada, C., R. I. Levin, M. Huie, R. Hirschhorn, D. Naime, M. Whitlow, P. A. Recht, B. Golden, and B. N. Cronstein.** 1995. Identification of C1q as the heat-labile serum cofactor required for immune complexes to stimulate endothelial expression of the adhesion molecules E-selectin and intercellular and vascular cell adhesion molecules 1. *Proc. Natl. Acad. Sci. USA* **92:**8378–8382.

89. **Magee, J. C., B. H. Collins, R. C. Harland, B. J. Lindman, R. R. Bollinger, M. M. Frank, and J. L. Platt.** 1995. Immunoglobulin prevents complement-mediated hyperacute rejection in swine-to-primate xenotransplantation. *J. Clin. Invest.* **96:**2404–2412.

90. **Maher, S. E., D. L. Pflugh, N. J. Larsen, M. F. Rothschild, and A. L. Bothwell.** 1998. Structure/function characterization of porcine CD59: expression, chromosomal mapping, complement-inhibition, and costimulatory activity. *Transplantation* **66:**1094–1100.

91. **Makrides, S. C.** 1998. Therapeutic inhibition of the complement system. *Pharmacol. Rev.* **50:**59–87.

92. **Matis, L. A., and S. A. Rollins.** 1995. Complement-specific antibodies: designing novel anti-inflammatories. *Nat. Med.* **1:**839–841.

93. **Matsushita, M.** 1996. The lectin pathway of the complement system. *Microbiol. Immunol.* **40:**887–893.

94. **McCurry, K. R., D. L. Kooyman, C. G. Alvarado, A. H. Cotterell, M. J. Martin, J. S. Logan, and J. L. Platt.** 1995. Human complement regulatory proteins protect swine-to-primate cardiac xenografts from humoral injury. *Nat. Med.* **1:**423–427.

95. **McCurry, K. R., D. L. Kooyman, L. E. Diamond, G. W. Byrne, J. S. Logan, and J. L. Platt.** 1995. Transgenic expression of human complement regulatory proteins in mice results in diminished complement deposition during organ xenoperfusion. *Transplantation* **59:**1177–1182.

96. **Meri, S.** 1994. Protectin (CD59). Complement lysis inhibitor and prototype domain in a new protein superfamily. *Immunologist* **2:**149–155.

97. **Mikata, S., S. Miyagawa, K. Iwata, S. Nagasawa, M. Hatanaka, M. Matsumoto, W. Kamiike, H. Matsuda, R. Shirakura, and T. Seya.** 1998. Regulation of complement-mediated swine endothelial cell lysis by a surface-bound form of human C4b binding protein. *Transplantation* **65:**363–368.

98. **Miyagawa, S., H. Hirose, R. Shirakura, Y. Naka, S. Nakata, Y. Kawashima, T. Seya, M. Matsumoto, A. Uenaka, and H. Kitamura.** 1988. The mechanism of discordant xenograft rejection. *Transplantation* **46:**825–830.

99. **Moran, P., H. Beasley, A. Gorrell, E. Martin, P. Gribling, H. Fuchs, N. Gillett, L. E. Burton, and I. W. Caras.** 1992. Human recombinant soluble decay accelerating factor inhibits complement activation in vitro and in vivo. *J. Immunol.* **149:**1736–1743.

100. **Morgan, B. P.** 1993. Cellular responses to the membrane attack complex, p. 325–351. *In* K. Whaley,

M. Loos, and J. M. Weiler (ed.), *Complement in Health and Disease*, vol. 20. Kluwer Academic Publishers, Boston, Mass.

101. **Morgan, B. P.** 1995. Physiology and pathophysiology of complement: progress and trends. *Crit. Rev. Clin. Lab. Sci.* **32:**265–298.
102. **Mulder, L. C. F., M. Mora, M. Lazzeri, M. Boschi, E. Ciccopiedi, C. Melli, P. Bruzzone, D. Alfani, R. Cortesini, and M. Rossini.** 1996. Human MCP and DAF double transgenic mice are protected from human complement attack in an *in vivo* model. *Transplant. Proc.* **28:**589.
103. **Müller-Eberhard, H. J.** 1992. Complement: chemistry and pathways, p. 33–61. *In* J. I. Gallin, I. M. Goldstein, and R. Snyderman (ed.), *Inflammation. Basic Principles and Clinical Correlates.* Raven Press, New York, N.Y.
104. **Murphy, H. S., J. A. Shayman, G. O. Till, M. Mahrougui, C. B. Owens, U. S. Ryan, and P. A. Ward.** 1992. Superoxide responses of endothelial cells to C5a and TNF-alpha: divergent signal transduction pathways. *Am. J. Physiol.* **263:**L51–59.
105. **Nelson, R. A.** 1966. A new concept of immunosuppression in the hypersensitivity reactions and in transplantation immunity. *Surv. Ophthalmol.* **11:**498–505.
106. **Nicholson-Weller, A., and J. A. Halperin.** 1993. Membrane signaling by complement C5b-9, the membrane attack complex. *Immunol. Res.* **12:**244–257.
107. **Nicholson-Weller, A., and C. Wang.** 1994. Structure and function of decay accelerating factor CD55. *J. Lab. Clin. Med.* **123:**485–491.
108. **Oglesby, T. J., C. J. Allen, M. K. Liszewski, D. J. G. White, and J. P. Atkinson.** 1992. Membrane cofactor protein (CD46) protects cells from complement-mediated attack by an intrinsic mechanism. *J. Exp. Med.* **175:**1547–1551.
109. **Osman, N., I. F. McKenzie, K. Ostenried, Y. A. Ioannou, R. J. Desnick, and M. S. Sandrin.** 1997. Combined transgenic expression of α-galactosidase and α1,2-fucosyltransferase leads to optimal reduction in the major xenoepitope Galα(1,3)Gal. *Proc. Natl. Acad. Sci. USA* **94:**14677–14682.
110. **Owen, C. A., M. A. Campbell, P. L. Sannes, S. S. Boukedes, and E. J. Campbell.** 1995. Cell surface-bound elastase and cathepsin G on human neutrophils: a novel, non-oxidative mechanism by which neutrophils focus and preserve catalytic activity of serine proteinases. *J. Cell Biol.* **131:**775–789.
111. **Oxvig, C., C. Lu, and T. A. Springer.** 1999. Conformational changes in tertiary structure near the ligand binding site of an integrin I domain. *Proc. Natl. Acad. Sci. USA* **96:**2215–2220.
112. **Pangburn, M. K., and H. J. Müller-Eberhard.** 1984. The alternative pathway of complement. *Springer Semin. Immunopathol.* **7:**163–203.
113. **Pascual, M., and L. E. French.** 1995. Complement in human diseases: looking towards the 21st century. *Immunol. Today* **16:**58–61.
114. **Peerschke, E. I., K. B. Reid, and B. Ghebrehiwet.** 1993. Platelet activation by C1q results in the induction of αIIb/β3 integrins (GPIIb-IIIa) and the expression of P-selectin and procoagulant activity. *J. Exp. Med.* **178:**579–587.
115. **Pierre, A. F., A. M. Xavier, M. Liu, S. D. Cassivi, T. F. Lindsay, H. C. Marsh, A. S. Slutsky, and S. H. Keshavjee.** 1998. Effect of complement inhibition with soluble complement receptor 1 on pig allotransplant lung function. *Transplantation* **66:**723–732.
116. **Platt, J. L., A. P. Dalmasso, B. J. Lindman, N. S. Ihrcke, and F. H. Bach.** 1991. The role of C5a and antibody in the release of heparan sulfate from endothelial cells. *Eur. J. Immunol.* **21:**2887–2890.
117. **Platt, J. L., G. M. Vercellotti, A. P. Dalmasso, A. J. Matas, R. M. Bolman, J. S. Najarian, and F. H. Bach.** 1990. Transplantation of discordant xenografts: a review of progress. *Immunol. Today* **11:**450–456.
118. **Platt, J. L., G. M. Vercellotti, B. Lindman, T. R. Oegema, Jr., F. H. Bach, and A. P. Dalmasso.** 1990. Release of heparan sulfate from endothelial cells: implications for pathogenesis of hyperacute rejection. *J. Exp. Med.* **171:**1363–1368.
119. **Pruitt, S. K., W. M. Baldwin, H. C. Marsh, Jr., S. S. Lin, C. G. Yeh, and R. R. Bollinger.** 1991. The effect of soluble complement receptor type 1 on hyperacute xenograft rejection. *Transplantation* **52:**868–873.
120. **Pruitt, S. K., R. R. Bollinger, B. H. Collins, H. C. Marsh, Jr., J. L. Levin, A. R. Rudolph, W. M. Baldwin, 3rd, and F. Sanfilippo.** 1997. Effect of continuous complement inhibition using soluble complement receptor type 1 on survival of pig-to-primate cardiac xenografts. *Transplantation* **63:**900–902.
121. **Pruitt, S. K., A. D. Kirk, R. R. Bollinger, H. C. Marsh, Jr., B. H. Collins, J. L. Levin, J. R. Mault, J. S. Heinle, S. Ibrahim, A. R. Rudolph, W. M. Baldwin, III., and F. Sanfilippo**. 1994. The effect of soluble complement receptor type 1 on hyperacute rejection of porcine xenografts. *Transplantation* **57:**363–370.

122. **Quigg, R. J., C. He, A. Lim, D. Berthiaume, J. J. Alexander, D. Kraus, and V. M. Holers.** 1998. Transgenic mice overexpressing the complement inhibitor crry as a soluble protein are protected from antibody-induced glomerular injury. *J. Exp. Med.* **188:**1321–1331.
123. **Rajasinghe, H. A., V. M. Reddy, W. W. Hancock, M. H. Sayegh, and F. L. Hanley.** 1996. Key role of the alternate complement pathway in hyperacute rejection of rat hearts transplanted into fetal sheep. *Transplantation* **62:**407–411.
124. **Rinder, C. S., H. M. Rinder, K. Johnson, M. Smith, D. L. Lee, J. Tracey, G. Polack, P. Higgins, C. G. Yeh, and B. R. Smith.** 1999. Role of C3 cleavage in monocyte activation during extracorporeal circulation. *Circulation* **100:**553–558.
125. **Rollins, S. A., J. C. K. Fitch, S. Shernan, C. S. Rinder, H. M. Rinder, B. R. Smith, C. D. Collard, G. L. Stahl, B. L. Alford, L. Li, and L. A. Matis.** 1998. Anti-C5 single chain antibody therapy blocks complement and leukocyte activation and reduces myocardial tissue damage in CPB patients. *Mol. Immunol.* **35:**397.
126. **Rollins, S. A., L. A. Matis, J. P. Springhorn, E. Setter, and D. W. Wolff.** 1995. Monoclonal antibodies directed against human C5 and C8 block complement-mediated damage of xenogeneic cells and organs. *Transplantation* **60:**1284–1292.
127. **Rosengard, A. M., N. R. B. Cary, G. A. Langford, A. W. Tucker, J. Wallwork, and D. J. G. White.** 1995. Tissue expression of human complement inhibitor, decay-accelerating factor, in transgenic pigs: a potential approach for preventing xenograft rejection. *Transplantation* **59:**1325–1333.
128. **Rosse, W. F., and R. E. Ware.** 1995. The molecular basis of paroxysmal nocturnal hemoglobinuria. *Blood* **86:**3277–3286.
129. **Rother, K., G. O. Till, and G. M. Hansch (ed.).** 1998. *The Complement System.* Springer, Berlin, Germany.
130. **Saadi, S., R. A. Holzknecht, C. Patte, D. M. Stern, and J. L. Platt.** 1995. Complement-mediated regulation of tissue factor activity in endothelium. *J. Exp. Med.* **182:**1807–1814.
131. **Saadi, S., and J. L. Platt.** 1998. Endothelial cell responses to complement activation, p. 335–353. *In* J. E. Volanakis and M. M. Frank (ed.), *The Human Complement System in Health and Disease.* Marcel Dekker, Inc., New York, N.Y.
132. **Saadi, S., and J. L. Platt.** 1995. Transient perturbation of endothelial integrity induced by natural antibodies and complement. *J. Exp. Med.* **181:**21–31.
133. **Sahu, A., B. K. Kay, and J. D. Lambris.** 1996. Inhibition of human complement by a C3-binding peptide isolated from a phage-displayed random peptide library. *J. Immunol.* **157:**884–891.
134. **Salerno, C. T., A. P. Dalmasso, T. J. Kroshus, C. A. Svendsen, D. M. Kulick, S. J. Park, S. J. Shumway, M. Guzman, C. G. Yeh, P. J. Higgins, A. A. Kreasy, and R. M. Bolman.** 1997. A recombinant soluble chimeric complement inhibitor CAB-2.0 prolongs xenograft survival in a heterotopic model of pig-to-primate cardiac transplantation. *Surg. Forum* **48:**265–267.
135. **Sandrin, M. S., H. A. Vaughan, P. L. Dabkowski, and I. F. C. McKenzie.** 1993. Anti-pig IgM antibodies in human serum react predominantly with Gal(α1-3)Gal epitopes. *Proc. Natl. Acad. Sci. USA* **90:**11391–11395.
136. **Schaapherder, A. F. M., H. G. Gooszen, M. T. J. W. Te Bulte, and M. R. Daha.** 1995. Human complement activation via the alternative pathway on porcine endothelium initiated by IgA antibodies. *Transplantation* **60:**287–291.
137. **Schmoeckel, M., F. N. Bhatti, A. Zaidi, E. Cozzi, P. D. Waterworth, M. J. Tolan, G. Pino-Chavez, M. Goddard, R. G. Warner, G. A. Langford, J. J. Dunning, J. Wallwork, and D. J. G. White.** 1998. Orthotopic heart transplantation in a transgenic pig-to-primate model. *Transplantation* **65:**1570–1577.
138. **Schmoeckel, M., G. Nollert, M. Shahmohammadi, J. Muller-Hocker, V. K. Young, W. Kasper-Konig, D. J. White, C. Hammer, and B. Reichart.** 1997. Transgenic human decay accelerating factor makes normal pigs function as a concordant species. *J. Heart Lung Transplant.* **16:**758–764.
139. **Schmoeckel, M., G. Nollert, M. Shahmohammadi, Y. V. K., G. Chavez, W. Kasper-Konig, D. J. G. White, J. Muller-Hocker, R. M. Arendt, U. Wilbert-Lampen, C. Hammer, and B. Reichart.** 1996. Prevention of hyperacute rejection by human decay accelerating factor in xenogeneic perfused working hearts. *Transplantation* **62:**729–734.
140. **Selvan, R. S., H. B. Kapadia, and J. L. Platt.** 1998. Complement-induced expression of chemokine genes in endothelium: regulation by IL-1-dependent and -independent mechanisms. *J. Immunol.* **161:**4388–4395.
141. **Sharma, A., J. Okabe, P. Birch, M. S. B., M. J. Martin, J. L. Platt, and J. S. Logan.** 1996. Reduction in the level of Gal(α1,3)Gal in transgenic mice and pigs by the expression of an α(1,2)fucosyltransferase. *Proc. Natl. Acad. Sci. USA* **93:**7190–7195.

142. **Shinkel, T. A., P. J. Cowan, H. Barlow, A. Aminian, M. Romanella, D. M. Lublin, M. J. Pearse, and A. J. d'Apice.** 1998. Expression and functional analysis of glycosyl-phosphatidyl inositol-linked CD46 in transgenic mice. *Transplantation* **66:**1401–1406.

143. **Slapak, M., N. Digard, M. Ahmed, T. Shell, and F. Thompson.** 1990. Renal transplantation across the ABO barrier: a 9-year experience. *Transplant. Proc.* **22:**1425–1428.

144. **Soares, M. P., Y. Lin, J. Anrather, E. Csizmadia, K. Takigami, K. Sato, S. T. Grey, R. B. Colvin, A. M. Choi, K. D. Poss, and F. H. Bach.** 1998. Expression of heme oxygenase-1 can determine cardiac xenograft survival. *Nature Med.* **4:**1073–1077.

145. **Somerville, C. A., A. G. Kyriazis, A. McKenzie, J. Allison, M. J. Pearse, and A. J. F. D'Apice.** 1994. Functional expression of human CD59 in transgenic mice. *Transplantation* **58:**1430–1435.

146. **Stahl, G. L., W. R. Reenstra, and G. Frendl.** 1995. Complement-mediated loss of endothelium-dependent relaxation of porcine coronary arteries. Role of the terminal membrane attack complex. *Circ. Res.* **76:**575–583.

147. **Stevens, R. B., Y. L. Wang, H. Kaji, J. Lloveras, A. Dalmasso, F. H. Bach, P. Rubinstein, D. E. R. Sutherland, and J. L. Platt.** 1993. Administration of nonanticoagulant heparin inhibits the loss of glycosaminoglycans from xenogeneic cardiac grafts and prolongs graft survival. *Transplant. Proc.* **25:**382.

148. **Stoiber, H., A. Clivio, and M. Dierich.** 1997. Role of complement in HIV infection. *Ann. Rev. Immunol.* **15:**649–674.

149. **Suhr, B. D., M. Guzman-Paz, E. P. Apasova, A. J. Matas, and A. P. Dalmasso.** Induction of accommodation in the hamster-to-rat model requires inhibition of the membrane attack complex of complement. *Transplant. Proc.*, in press.

150. **Suttorp, N., W. Seeger, S. Zinsky, and S. Bhakdi.** 1987. Complement complex C5b-8 induced PGI2 formation in cultured endothelial cells. *Am. J. Physiol.* **253:**C13–C21.

151. **Taniguchi, S., T. Kobayashi, F. A. Neethling, Y. Ye, M. Niekrasz, D. J. White, and D. K. Cooper.** 1996. Cobra venom factor stimulates anti-alpha-galactose antibody production in baboons. Implications for pig-to-human xenotransplantation. *Transplantation* **62:**678–681.

152. **Tearle, R. G., M. J. Tange, Z. L. Zannettino, M. Katerelos, T. A. Shinkel, B. J. W. van Denderen, A. J. Lonie, I. Lyons, M. B. Nottle, T. Cox, C. Becker, A. M. Peura, P.L. Wigley, R. J. Crawford, A. J. Robins, M. J. Pearse, and A. J. F. d'Apice.** 1996. The α-1,3-galactosyltransferase knockout mouse. Implications for xenotransplantation. *Transplantation* **61:**13–19.

153. **Tedesco, F., M. Pausa, E. Nardon, M. Introna, A. Mantovani, and A. Dobrina.** 1997. The cytolytically inactive terminal complement complex activates endothelial cells to express adhesion molecules and tissue factor procoagulant activity. *J. Exp. Med.* **185:**1619–1627.

154. **Thorley, B. R., J. Milland, D. Christiansen, M. B. Lanteri, B. McInnes, I. Moeller, P. Rivailler, B. Horvat, C. Rabourdin-Combe, D. Gerlier, I. F. McKenzie, and B. E. Loveland.** 1997. Transgenic expression of a CD46 (membrane cofactor protein) minigene: studies of xenotransplantation and measles virus infection. *Eur. J. Immunol.* **27:**726–734.

155. **Tucker, A. W., H. S. Davies, C. A. Carrington, A. C. Richards, K. Elsome, and D. J. G. White.** 1996. The fertility and breeding potential of boars expressing a functional regulator of human complement activation. *Transplant. Proc.* **28**:642.

156. **van den Berg, C. W., and B. P. Morgan.** 1994. Complement-inhibiting activities of human CD59 and analogues from rat, sheep and pig are not homologously restricted. *J. Immunol.* **152:**4095–4101.

157. **van den Berg, C. W., J. M. Perez de la Lastra, D. Llanes, and B. P. Morgan.** 1997. Purification and characterization of the pig analogue of human membrane cofactor protein (CD46/MCP). *J. Immunol.* **158:**1703–1709.

158. **van Denderen, B. J., E. Salvaris, M. Romanella, A. Aminian, M. Katerelos, M. J. Tange, M. J. Pearse, and A. J. d'Apice.** 1997. Combination of decay-accelerating factor expression and alpha1,3-galactosyltransferase knockout affords added protection from human complement-mediated injury. *Transplantation* **64:**882–888.

159. **Vanhove, B., R. de Martin, J. Lipp, and F. H. Bach.** 1994. Human xenoreactive natural antibodies of the IgM isotype activate pig endothelial cells. *Xenotransplantation* **1:**17–23.

160. **Varani, J., I. Ginsburg, L. Schuger, D. F. Gibbs, J. Bromberg, K. J. Johnson, U. S. Ryan, and P. A. Ward.** 1989. Endothelial cell killing by neutrophils. Synergistic interaction of oxygen products and proteases. *Am. J. Pathol.* **135:**435–438.

161. **Vercellotti, G. M., J. L. Platt, F. H. Bach, and A. P. Dalmasso.** 1991. Neutrophil adhesion to xenogeneic endothelium via iC3b. *J. Immunol.* **146:**730–734.
162. **Vetvicka, V., B. P. Thornton, and G. D. Ross.** 1996. Soluble beta-glucan polysaccharide binding to the lectin site of neutrophil or natural killer cell complement receptor type 3 (CD11b/CD18) generates a primed state of the receptor capable of mediating cytotoxicity of iC3b-opsonized target cells. *J. Clin. Invest.* **98:**50–61.
163. **Vogel, C. W., and H. J. Müller-Eberhard.** 1982. The cobra venom factor-dependent C3 convertase of human complement. *J. Biol. Chem.* **257:**8292–8299.
164. **Volanakis, J. E., and M. M. Frank (ed.).** 1998. *The Human Complement System in Health and Disease.* Marcel Dekker, Inc., New York, N.Y.
165. **Wagner, E., and M. M. Frank.** 1998. Development of clinically useful agents to control complement-mediated tissue damage, p. 527–546. *In* J. E. Volanakis and M. M. Frank (ed.), *The Human Complement System in Health and Disease.* Marcel Dekker, Inc., New York, N.Y.
166. **Weissman, H. F., T. Bartow, M. K. Leppo, H. C. Marsh, Jr., G. R. Carson, M. F. Concino, M. P. Boyle, K. H. Roux, M. L. Weisfeldt, and D. T. Fearon.** 1990. Soluble human complement receptor type 1: in vivo inhibitor of complement suppressing post-ischemic myocardial inflammation and necrosis. *Science* **249:**146–151.
167. **Xia, W., D. T. Fearon, F. D. Moore, Jr., F. J. Schoen, F. Ortiz, and R. L. Kirkman.** 1992. Prolongation of guinea pig cardiac xenograft survival in rats by soluble human complement receptor type 1. *Transplant. Proc.* **24:**479–480.
168. **Yeatman, M., C. W. Daggett, C. L. Lau, G. W. Byrne, J. S. Logan, J. L. Platt, and R. D. Davis.** 1999. Human complement regulatory proteins protect swine lungs from xenogeneic injury. *Ann. Thorac. Surg.* **67:**769–775.
169. **Zaidi, A., F. Bhatti, M. Schmoeckel, E. Cozzi, G. Chavez, J. Wallwork, D. White, and P. Friend.** 1998. Kidneys from HDAF transgenic pigs are physiologically compatible with primates. *Transplant Proc.* **30:**2465–2466.
170. **Zaidi, A., M. Schmoeckel, F. Bhatti, P. Waterworth, M. Tolan, E. Cozzi, G. Chavez, G. Langford, S. Thiru, J. Wallwork, D. White, and P. Friend.** 1998. Life-supporting pig-to-primate renal xenotransplantation using genetically modified donors. *Transplantation* **65:**1584–9150.
171. **Zhang, H., J. Yu, E. Bajawa, S. L. Morrison, and S. Tomlinson.** 1999. Targeting of functional antibody-CD59 fusion proteins to a cell surface. *J. Clin. Invest.* **103:**55–61.
172. **Zhao, J., S. A. Rollins, S. E. Maher, A. L. Bothwell, and P. J. Sims.** 1991. Amplified gene expression in CD59-transfected Chinese hamster ovary cells confers protection against the membrane attack complex of human complement. *J. Biol. Chem.* **266:**13418–13421
173. **Zhow, X. J., N. Niesen, I. Pawlowski, G. Biesecker, G. Andres, J. Brentjens, and F. Milgrom.** 1990. Prolongation of survival of discordant kidney xenografts by C6 deficiency. *Transplantation* **50:**896–898.

Xenotransplantation
Edited by Jeffrey L. Platt

Chapter 4

NK Cells as a Barrier to Xenotransplantation

Thierry Berney, Antonello Pileggi, and Luca Inverardi

The use of heterologous species for clinical transplantation has attracted increasing interest in recent years due to the shortage of human donors, resulting in significant progress toward the understanding of the mechanisms leading to recognition and rejection of xenogeneic grafts. Many unanswered questions, however, still exist concerning the pathogenesis of xenograft rejection and the definition of strategies aimed at prolonging graft survival.

While it is now accepted that rejection of discordant xenogeneic organs is characterized by an intricate interplay of humoral and cellular immune mechanisms, the hallmark is the occurrence of hyperacute rejection, due to the presence of xenoreactive natural antibodies that recognize the carbohydrate epitope Galα1-3Gal (Gal epitope), expressed on the endothelial cell surface of all mammals except humans and Old World primates. This phenomenon leads to the loss of vascularized grafts within minutes to hours of transplantation, but when its occurrence is prevented, a second type of rejection can be observed, which has been termed delayed xenograft rejection (DXR). Analysis of the leukocyte infiltrates found in tissues undergoing DXR has led to the identification of natural killer (NK) lymphocytes as an important effector cell subset.

This paper focuses on the role of NK cells in xenogeneic graft rejection, on the biology of NK cells, and on NK-cell receptors in particular.

ROLE AND ONTOGENY OF NK CELLS

NK cells are a bone marrow–derived subpopulation of phenotypically identifiable lymphocytes ($CD16^+$, $CD56^+$, $CD3^-$) that share a common progenitor with T cells (reviewed in reference 4). NK cells contribute to the natural host defense mechanisms, both by exerting cytotoxicity on certain virally infected (79) or tumor cells (85) and by releasing cytokines that promote an inflammatory response, such as γ-interferon (IFN), tumor necrosis factor (TNF), granulocyte/macrophage-colony stimulating factor, and macrophage colony-stimulating factor. These critical functions enable NK cells to provide resistance against microorganisms, to control malignant growth, to modulate other immune cells, and to regulate hematopoietic cell differentiation. NK cells mediate target lysis without the need for

Thierry Berney, Antonello Pileggi, and Luca Inverardi • Diabetes Research Institute, University of Miami School of Medicine, 1450 NW 10th Ave., Miami, FL 33136.

prior sensitization and without restriction by major histocompatibility complex (MHC) gene products. Human NK cells comprise 10 to 15% of peripheral blood lymphocytes. They are also present in all central and peripheral lymphoid organs (60, 73, 85).

NK cells originate in the bone marrow (BM), but at present their progenitors and lineage development have not been fully characterized. BM contains mononuclear stem cells, characterized by the expression of the surface antigen CD34, that have the ability of self-renewal, proliferation, and differentiation toward both myeloid and lymphoid lineages upon stimulation by stem cell factor (SCF). Stromal BM cells probably play a role in NK-cell differentiation from $CD34^+$ progenitors by the production of stimulating cytokines and growth factors (IL-1, IL-2, IL-15, SCF) and inhibition of differentiation toward other cellular lineages. During NK-cell ontogeny, the CD34 surface antigen is lost and cells acquire the expression of membrane markers characteristic of mature NK cells (CD2, CD16, CD56) (4, 71).

NK cells are non–T-cell lymphocytes that share selected morphologic, functional, and phenotypic characteristics with cytotoxic T lymphocytes (CTL), possibly because of a common early lymphoid differentiation pathway. Both these cells are phenotypically mature lymphocytes with cytoplasmic granules and express a number of cell surface antigens that are not present on mature B cells or myeloid cells; they also have common effector functions such as cytolytic activity and lymphokine production. Furthermore, they likely originate from a common precursor, as suggested by the fact that human fetal NK cells express CD3 and by the observation that patients with severe combined immunodeficiency lack both T and NK cells but have normal numbers of B lymphocytes and myeloid cells. The thymus has been shown to contain progenitors capable of evolving along either the T or NK differentiation pathway that lose the CD34 marker during differentiation to become noncytotoxic committed NK progenitors (62, 63). Acquisition of the $CD56^+$ surface marker characterizes mature and cytotoxic NK cells. The presence of IL-2, IL-7, and SCF is essential for successful functional maturation along this pathway (4, 71). However, evidence of the presence of NK cells in the human fetal liver before thymus development and in athymic mice suggests that the thymus is not essential for NK-cell development (18).

The "Missing Self" Hypothesis

A major step forward in the understanding of the molecular mechanisms underlying target recognition by NK cells came from the observation of an inverse correlation between surface MHC class I expression by target cells and their sensitivity to lysis by NK lymphocytes. This observation led to the formulation of the "missing self" hypothesis, which postulates that NK cells survey tissues for normal expression of MHC class I molecules and lyse targets with aberrant or absent MHC class I expression. This is at profound variance with the well-known requirement for class I restriction in the cognate recognition of specific antigens by cytolytic $CD8^+$ T lymphocytes (46, 68). The missing self hypothesis has been supported by several independent findings demonstrating that allotypic MHC class I products actually protect cells from lysis by NK lymphocytes, apparently by delivering negative regulatory signals that inhibit NK-cell cytotoxic function (36). Further evidence in favor of this hypothesis originated from the observation that cells from mice lacking MHC class I expression owing to disruption of the β_2-microglobulin gene are more susceptible to NK-cell lysis than are cells from normal mice, and that the defect can be reversed by transfection of target cells with MHC class I (8). Definitive verification of the missing self theory has been provided by the recent identification, cloning, and characterization of increasing numbers of human and murine NK-lymphocyte receptors involved in MHC class I recognition. These receptors deliver, upon binding, inhibitory signals, which temporarily switch off the NK-cell lytic potential.

NK-Cell Inhibitory Receptors Recognizing MHC Class I Molecules

Two families of NK-cell receptors are able to recognize and bind MHC class I molecules, and serve similar functions in transmitting inhibitory signals (reviewed in reference 60). The first comprises the Ly-49 family of receptors in mice and the KIRs (killer inhibitory receptors) in humans. The second includes the CD94/NKG2 family.

Ly-49

In mice, the Ly-49 family of NK-cell receptors is responsible for H-2 recognition on potential target cells and subsequent inhibition of NK-cell–mediated cytotoxicity. Ly-49 receptors are type II integral membrane glycoproteins of the C-type (calcium-dependent) lectin superfamily. They are expressed as disulfide-linked homodimers. As yet, several Ly-49 receptors have been identified and cloned. Several strain-specific alleles have been recognized, and different specificities for selected MHC class I molecules have been shown to characterize different receptors. At least nine genes encoding for Ly-49 have been identified in the "NK gene complex" located on mouse chromosome 6 that are responsible for the diversity of Ly-49 receptors (70). Products of several Ly-49 genes are expressed in overlapping subsets of NK cells in each individual and define a repertoire of Ly-49 receptors with distinct patterns of recognition of MHC class I molecules (11). As a result of the array of Ly-49 receptors expressed on the surface of each NK lymphocyte, a single NK cell can recognize targets expressing a variety of MHC class I specificities. Engagement of any Ly-49 receptor will deliver an inhibitory signal to the NK cell. This might partly explain the relatively minor role played by NK cells in allogeneic transplant rejection, since sharing of one MHC class I antigen between donor and recipient might suffice to cause a proportion of recipient NK lymphocytes to recognize donor cells as self, thus preventing their lysis by inhibiting NK-cell cytotoxicity triggering. This has been illustrated by the fact that bone marrow isolated from mice deficient in β_2-microglobulin is rejected more efficiently than wild-type allogeneic bone marrow (8). Another cornerstone observation pointing to a crucial role of the missing self as a triggering event for NK-cell activation derives from experiments of bone marrow transplantation in a parent to F1 combination. Selected subsets of NK cells from F1 recipient mice, in fact, appear capable of rejecting bone marrow transplants from parental H-2-homozygous donors. The 5E6 subset of NK cells expressing the Ly-49C receptor, which recognizes H-2^b, can lyse marrow cells from Balb/c donors transplanted into (Balb/c $\times$ B6) F1 recipients. Conversely, Ly-49 G2-positive NK cells, which recognize H-2^d, from the same recipients, can reject bone marrow grafts from B6 donors (59, 88). Thus, cross-reactivity of NK-inhibitory receptors and MHC class I antigens (or its absence) appears to be the central mechanism responsible for both the secondary role of NK lymphocytes in allogeneic rejection and their prevailing role in the phenomenon of "hybrid resistance," as rejection of parental bone marrow by F1 hybrids has been named. Although this observation suggests a dynamic, quantitative equilibrium between NK-cell Ly-49 repertoire and target H-2 expression, it fails to explain the target tissue selectivity of

NK-cell lysis. Nonhematopoietic tissue and organ grafts performed across the same strain combination (parents to F1) are, in fact, consistently accepted. Selection and acquisition of the Ly-49 expression repertoire are still not fully understood but appear to be subject to MHC class I–dependent modulation in vivo. Experimental systems of adoptive transfer of spleen cells or peripheral T lymphocytes have provided recent evidence that Ly-49 expression levels are highly dynamic after the education and maturation process and can be modulated in mature NK cells exposed to an altered MHC class I environment (35, 37).

KIRs

In humans, NK-cell–inhibitory receptors that bind MHC class I molecules have been termed KIRs and are membrane glycoproteins belonging to the immunoglobulin (Ig) superfamily. The KIR genes are located on human chromosome 19, and 12 different, as yet unidentified, loci are believed to contribute to the KIR genome (75). KIRs are expressed on the cell surface either as monomers or as homodimers bound by a disulfide link. Their extracellular portion consists of two or three Ig-like domains defining two subfamilies of receptors, named KIR2D and KIR3D, respectively. Further, their intracytoplasmic domains have either long (L) or short (S) sequences, defining distinct functions for the receptors. Members of these subfamilies display loose specificity for particular HLA loci products, notably KIR2DL for HLA-C, KIR3DL monomer for HLA-B, and KIR3DL dimer for HLA-A; KIR2D and KIR3D are able to broadly cross-react with many different HLA-B (17, 55, 86) and HLA-C allotypes. Conversely, several MHC class I allotypes do not seem to have a corresponding KIR, indicating that the KIR repertoire might not be all-inclusive (40). HLA-C molecules bind to KIRs with association and dissociation rates among the fastest of the immune system, which seems essential for the biological NK function of rapid immune surveillance of cells with abnormal expression of MHC class I antigens (80).

CD94/NKG2

The paradigm of C-type lectin for murine and Ig superfamily molecules for human NK inhibitory receptors was broken when CD94 and CD94/NKG2 disulfide-bound heterodimers were shown to recognize and apparently bind with broad specificity HLA class I molecules and deliver inhibitory signals to NK cells (12, 41, 56). For example, results from cytotoxicity assays using anti-CD94/NKG2A monoclonal antibodies have implicated this receptor in the recognition of a throng of HLA-A, -B, -C, and -G ligands (reviewed in reference 40). The CD94/NKG2 complex is a member of the C-type lectin superfamily, composed of the invariant CD94 subunit, a glycoprotein lacking a cytoplasmic portion and thus signaling capacity, and the product of a gene of the NKG2 family. NKG2 gene products are transmembrane glycoproteins with an intracytoplasmic domain encoded by one of four genes (29), and they are not expressed on the cell membrane unless they are bound to CD94 (12, 41). The NKG2 gene is not unique to humans since it has recently been cloned in the mouse. It is located in the NK gene complex, and its product has been shown to associate with CD94 to form an MHC class I–binding receptor with inhibitory function (81, 82). Direct experimental binding of the CD94/NKG2 complex to MHC class I molecules was recently demonstrated, indicating that the nonclassical MHC class I HLA-E and -G are the predominant ligands of CD94/NKG2 (10, 73). Nonclassical MHC class I products need to bind peptides derived from HLA-A, -B, or -C in order to be stabilized and expressed. The binding of CD94/NKG2 receptor to these HLA complexes clarifies the apparent broad reactivity of this class of receptors. Similarly, in the mouse the ligand for the

CD94/NKG2A heterodimer has been recently demonstrated to be the Qa-1(b) molecule, a murine equivalent of nonclassical class I molecules (81).

Mechanisms of Inhibition

In spite of the considerable overall structural differences between the described families of NK inhibitory receptors, a common mechanism is used to inhibit the cytolytic activity of NK lymphocytes. The basis of this common mechanism is to be recognized in the highly conserved intracellular domains of the inhibitory receptors. These comprise short sequences (six amino acids, among which is a tyrosine), called ITIM (immunoreceptor tyrosine-based inhibitory motif), and are found on all inhibitory receptors except the CD94 monomer; the ITIM can be redundant with up to three repeated sequences in the endodomain of the transmembrane protein. Upon phosphorylation of the tyrosine residues, the endodomain binds to and recruits the protein-tyrosine phosphatase SHP-1, which is associated with inhibition of activation pathways in hematopoietic cells (13, 52). SHP-1 further inhibits tyrosine-kinase activation, which blocks NK-cell positive signaling (reviewed in reference 42).

Activating Receptors

The missing self hypothesis is not sufficient to explain NK-cell activation; if lack of MHC class I expression were, in fact, sufficient to lead to lysis of MHC null targets, the survival of red blood cells (class I negative) would represent a paradox. NK-cell–activating receptors must exist in a finely regulated dynamic relationship with KIRs to provide a comprehensive explanation of NK-cell target specificity.

The array of NK-cell–activating receptors is even more heterogeneous than that of inhibitory receptors. The most widely studied of them is the low-affinity Fcγ receptor, CD16 or FcγRIIIA. This receptor is responsible for antibody-dependent cellular cytotoxicity (ADCC), a major mechanism of NK-cell killing. ADCC is initiated when CD16 binds the Fc fragment of an IgG that has recognized and bound an antigen on a target cell. CD16 is the α subunit of a receptor complex, in noncovalent association with homo- or heterodimers of the ζ subunit of the T-cell receptor (TCR) and/or the γ subunit of the high-affinity IgE receptor (FcεRI).

As outlined above, KIRs can be found in either of two forms, depending on the length of their cytoplasmic domain. KIR2DS (p50) and KIR3DS lack ITIM sequences in their short cytoplasmic tails. Interestingly, they bind MHC class I similarly to the forms of the molecules with long cytoplasmic domains (L) but activate rather than inhibit NK-cell function (50), and are, therefore, termed KARs (killer activatory receptors). Other members of the KAR group include receptors of both the Ly-49 and CD94/NKG2 families that lack ITIM sequences on their intracytoplasmic portion, such as Ly49-D and -H, and CD94/NKG2C and E (11, 29, 48).

The mechanism of NK activation via CD16 and KARs is similar and involves signal transduction through immunoreceptor tyrosine-based activation motifs (ITAMs). ITAMs are short tyrosine-containing amino acid sequences that, upon phosphorylation, bind to and activate selected protein tyrosine kinases (PTK). The intracytoplasmic ITAMs of CD16 are found in the ζ and γ subunits of the complex (51, 87), while ITIM-lacking KARs depend on a lysine residue on their short intracytoplasmic portion for assembly with intracellular ITAM-containing subunits. DAP12, a disulfide-linked ITAM-containing homodimer, has been recently identified as complexed with the short tail of glycoproteins of the KIR family and capable of activating PTK (39). A 16-kDa phosphoprotein has been described as a murine equivalent that associates with Ly49-D (49).

The simultaneous existence of NK inhibitory and activating receptors for MHC class I molecules seems contradictory and remains somewhat mysterious. The existence of activating NK receptors with MHC class I specificity goes against the missing self hypothesis for NK recognition and subsequent killing. It is as yet not known whether KARs are expressed in individuals with the same specificities as their inhibitory counterparts, or whether KAR receptors exhibiting alloreactivity are preferentially expressed.

The NKR-P1 activating receptor is another member of the C-type lectin superfamily and was initially described in the rat (22). Homologs of its encoding gene, located in the NK gene complex, and its products have been identified in the human (CD161) and in the mouse (NK1.1). It is expressed as a disulfide-bound homodimer on all NK cells (40). The stimulatory function of CD161 has been deduced by the observation that cross-linking of NKR-P1 activates NK-cell cytotoxic function and promotes release of γ-IFN (1); the ligand on target cells has not yet been identified. However, in vitro binding of rat NKR-P1 with various oligosaccharides containing mannose and galactose residues has been shown to activate NK-cell cytotoxicity (5). The mechanism of NK-cell activation by engagement of NKR-P1 is poorly understood but requires the presence of the FcRγ-chain, a component of IgG and IgE Fc receptors (2). Other NK-cell–activating surface markers include the CD2 and CD28 molecules, the role of which has been well described in T-cell–APC interaction and in the costimulatory pathways of T-cell activation.

NK CELLS AS A BARRIER TO XENOTRANSPLANTATION

The first and major obstacle to discordant xenotransplantation is the occurrence of hyperacute rejection due to the presence of preformed xenogeneic natural antibodies (XNAs) in the recipient of a vascularized graft (19, 57). XNAs bind to the surface of endothelial cells of the grafted organ and lead to complement activation, activation of the coagulation cascade, thrombosis, and hemorrhage. The specificity of human XNA has been characterized, with prevalent recognition of the carbohydrate epitope Galα1-3Gal (Gal epitope). The Gal epitope is expressed on the surface of selected cell lineages (in particular endothelial cells and hemolymphopoietic elements) in all mammals except Old World primates and humans. In these species a nonsense or missense mutation has silenced the galactosyl transferase, now present in the genome as a pseudogene. Absence of Gal epitope expression on the cell surface leads during ontogeny to the emergence of anti-Gal antibody-producing B lymphocytes. Recent generation and analysis of α-Gal transferase knockout (KO) mice have confirmed this hypothesis. α-Gal transferase KO mice have, in fact, detectable levels of anti-Gal antibodies. While anti-Gal antibodies preexist to sensitization with xenogeneic cells, their titer can rise significantly upon challenge (21). Recent analysis of patients treated with porcine hepatocyte-based bioartificial liver and of patients who received pig islets of Langerhans (3, 25) has demonstrated a vigorous xenoantibody response with predominance of Gal specificity and toxicity toward endothelial cells; no major new xenoantibody specificities have emerged after xenogeneic exposure, since XNAs showed a similar molecular pattern of recognition on porcine aortic endothelial cells (PAEC) before and after challenge (3). XNAs lead to hyperacute rejection of all vascularized discordant xenografts and of some concordant xenografts. When hyperacute rejection occurs, the transplanted organ is lost within minutes of transplantation (26, 61). The treatment of discordant xenograft recipients with XNA depletion or complement-depleting/blocking compounds, such as cobra venom factor (CVF) or soluble complement receptor 1, overcomes these early events and prolongs graft survival by a few days (15, 58). Whenever hyperacute rejection is avoided or suppressed in a xenograft, by antibody depletion or complement blockade, a second set of immune responses, termed delayed xenograft rejection (DXR) or acute vascular rejection, is revealed. Histologically, DXR is characterized by platelet aggregation and fibrin deposition, endothelial cell activation, and tissue infiltration by activated macrophages and NK cells (9, 28). The occurrence of typical histological and clinical DXR in nude rats provides evidence that T-cell–independent immune responses are involved (14). Because few cells bearing an NK-cell phenotype are seen in xenografts undergoing hyperacute rejection (43, 61), these findings indicate that NK cells might play a major role in the occurrence of DXR. The xenotransplantation community has recently focused increasingly on this subject, and major advances have allowed a better understanding of the mechanisms involved.

The role of NK cells in the xenogeneic transplantation setting first became apparent when it was reported that NK-cell depletion was necessary, in addition to irradiation and T-cell depletion, for bone marrow to engraft and donor-specific tolerance to occur in a rat-to-mouse model (68). Since then, the effects of NK depletion or NK impairment (such as in the beige mouse) have been studied in a number of solid organ xenogeneic transplantation models. Mice bearing the *beige* mutation, an analog of the human Chediak-Higashi syndrome, are characterized by a lack of NK-cell activity and exhibit significant delay in the rejection of concordant skin and heart xenografts (53, 74). Depletion of NK cells by an anti-asialoglycoprotein receptor (asialo-GM1) antiserum prolongs the survival of hamster heart transplants in leflunomide-treated nude rats, lacking operational B- and T-lymphocyte compartments (45). In a hamster-to-rat skin transplantation model, NK-cell depletion by a monoclonal antibody directed against the NKR-P1A–activating receptor significantly potentiated the effects on graft survival of T-cell suppression by a combined treatment with antilymphocyte serum and rapamycine (24). However, NK-cell depletion alone was less effective, in terms of survival time, than T-cell suppression alone, perhaps because of the transient functional inhibition induced by the monoclonal antibody. Along the same line, NK-cell depletion of human peripheral blood lymphocytes by anti-CD16 and anti-CD56 monoclonal antibody (mAb) was not sufficient to prevent lysis of porcine target cells in vitro but necessitated additional anti-CD8 treatment (16).

The role of NK cells in the rejection of vascularized grafts has been further characterized in several experiments dealing with adhesion to, activation, and lysis of xenogeneic endothelial cells (EC), which are the first target that recipient lymphocytes encounter. We have in the past utilized an experimental model of ex vivo perfusion of an isolated xenogeneic organ (rat heart) with human peripheral blood lymphocytes to try to characterize the role of NK cells in the early events of graft recognition. We could show that preferential adhesion of NK cells on the endothelium occurred. When enriched preparations of NK cells were used, up to 90% of NK cells were retained in the organ within 60 min in the presence of human IgG, a proportion that dropped to 40% after IgG removal (33). These experiments indicated the existence of two interaction pathways between NK lymphocytes and endothelium: one involving direct recognition of endothelial surface markers and adhesion molecules by NK receptors and ligands, the other necessitating the presence of recipient IgG antibodies, "bridging" NK and EC, by immunological recognition of xenogeneic targets on the endothelium followed by engagement of the receptor for the Fc fragment of IgGs (FcγRIII, of which CD16 is the main component) expressed on all NK cells. The first mechanism was further defined by observing a near-total inhibition of cellular adhesion after LFA-1 and Mac-1 functional inactivation by mAb, designating these leukocyte integrins as important players in this process. Similarly, significant inhibition of adhesion was obtained after blockade of the FcγRIII molecule by anti-CD16 antibody pretreatment of NK cells (33). Consistently, 25% of peripheral human blood lymphocytes adhered to PAEC, half the adherent cells being NK cells. The major adhesion molecules involved were CD11a, the α-chain of LFA-1, and CD49d, the α-chain of VLA-4 (6, 7).

Basically, NK cells can kill their target by either direct cytotoxicity or antibody-dependent cell-mediated cytotoxicity (ADCC) (4, 16, 31, 33, 42, 65). Incubation of human NK cells with PAEC induces rapid cell damage and the appearance of gaps between cells (47). Both mechanisms seem to be involved in xenogeneic cell destruction, since in vitro cytotoxicity experiments displayed the same characteristics as the ex vivo adhesion experiments outlined above, i.e., direct and antibody-mediated lysis, with partial inhibition after anti-LFA-1 and anti-Mac-1 mAb treatment (33). Further, in another series of experiments, direct in vitro cytolysis of PAEC by human blood lymphocytes was enhanced by addition of human serum, and this increase in cytotoxicity was blocked by anti FcγRIII mAb (84). There is conflicting evidence regarding the relative contribution of each of these two cytotoxicity pathways. Direct, IL-2-activated cytolysis of porcine endothelium cells by baboon NK cells was shown to be slightly more efficient than ADCC but highly dependent on the interactions between accessory molecules (CD2, CD49d) expressed on NK cells and their ligands on the endothelium (34). A somewhat less prominent involvement of ADCC was also observed in human NK cytotoxicity experiments against fetal porcine islet cells, since NK could kill porcine islet cells directly, whereas ADCC was not observed in the presence of natural antibodies but required the addition of xenoimmune serum (38). Somehow contrasting results were observed by another group that reported little or no in vitro cytotoxic activity of purified human NK cells against various porcine target cells, unless decomplemented human plasma or purified anti-Gal antibodies were added (66). When cytokine-stimulated NK cells from Fas-ligand-mutated *gld* mice were incubated with human target cells, they exhibited the same cytotoxicity as NK cells from immunocompetent animals. In contrast, NK cells from perforin-knockout mice had low cytotoxic activity against the same targets, suggesting a predominant mediation of xenocytolysis by the perforin pathway (72). The effector mechanisms of NK-cell–dependent ADCC have been linked to the ability of causing apoptosis (DNA damage), as well as cell membrane damage in vitro, in a model of incubation of human NK cells and IgG with a porcine kidney cell line (PK15). Consistent with the above-mentioned results, target cell lysis was inhibited by chemically blocking the perforin/granzyme but not the Fas/FasL pathway (20).

Contact and adhesion of recipient NK cells and donor endothelium also induce activation of EC, as demonstrated in a model of coincubation of PAEC with human NK cells. This interaction induces increased expression of E-selectin and IL-8 by EC, a phenomenon accentuated by the addition of human IgG, confirming the importance of antibody-mediated recognition (23). The activation of EC has been shown to be initiated by ligation of NK membrane-bound lymphotoxin with the TNF receptor 1 expressed on EC (83).

The dichotomy of hyperacute rejection and DXR, occurring as two sequential, distinct, and unrelated phenomena, has been recently challenged by the observation that adhesion to and lysis of PAEC by cocultured human NK cells could be inhibited by the presence in the culture medium of various carbohydrates, among which is Galα1-3Gal. Direct recognition of the Gal epitope by NK cells was demonstrated by selective inhibition of NK cell adhesion to porcine endothelium by saturating concentrations of XNA $F(ab')_2$ fragments and by demonstration of selective adherence of human NK cells to an Old World monkey cell line (COS-7) transfected to express the porcine Gal epitope (32). Another series of experiments used an allogeneic model of heterotopic vascularized heart transplantation, in which hearts from wild-type mice were transplanted into α1,3galactosyltransferase knockout (Gal KO) mice. The Gal KO mice, like humans, develop variable titers of antibodies directed against Gal. When animals with high titers of anti-Gal antibodies were transplanted, grafts were rejected in 8 to 13 days, with histological features very similar to those of DXR, i.e., cellular infiltrates consisting principally of macrophages (80 to 90%) and NK cells (10%). In contrast, recipients with low anti-Gal titers demonstrated prolonged graft survival (54). Although the receptors on NK cells responsible for direct recognition have not been identified, it is tempting to confront these observations with the in vitro binding of the rat NKR-P1 receptor to various mannose- and galactose-containing oligosaccharides, which has been shown to activate NK cell cytotoxicity (5).

These results suggest a comprehensive model of xenogeneic recognition by the human immune system, in which both xenoreactive natural antibodies and NK cells, through a common evolutionary pathway, recognize overlapping, species-specific, carbohydrate targets. In turn, recognition of the Gal or other carbohydrate epitopes by NK cells can be mediated either by a putative carbohydrate NK receptor or via IgG-mediated "bridging" and subsequent engagement of the FcγRIII NK receptor in a fashion similar to ADCC (30, 31).

The missing self hypothesis as the basis for NK-cell immune surveillance is a simple, or maybe simplistic, model for the explanation of the more powerful role NK lymphocytes play in xenorejection, as compared to allogeneic rejection. It is easy to figure that cross-reactivity with MHC molecules on allogeneic foreign cells is more likely to occur, notably in the case of shared MHC antigens, than with xenogeneic targets, where none is expected to take place. The extent of cross-reactivity sufficient to inhibit NK cytotoxicity against a foreign cell is not known, but a qualitative "receptor calibration" model has been proposed to account for how NK cells can interact with self as well as non-self MHC and adapt their receptors to perform optimally. This model states that three conditions must be met for inhibition to take place: a critical amount of receptors on the NK cells, a critical amount of MHC ligands on the target cells, and a critical affinity between receptor and MHC molecule (67). The lack of recognition of MHC class I molecules by the recipient NK cells as an activating mechanism has been demonstrated in the xenogeneic transplantation setting by transfection experiments on an immortalized bone marrow–derived porcine cell line with different human MHC class I allelic genes. The cytotoxic activity of certain NK-cell clones (GL183+) was inhibited by the expression of HLA-Cw3 by the porcine cells. The cytotoxicity of these clones was conserved on cells expressing HLA-B27 or HLA-A2 molecules, whereas GL183− clones were cytotoxic toward HLA-Cw3–transfected cells (65). A parallel approach has been used with PAECs transfected to express HLA-G, a nonclassical MHC class I molecule and a preferential ligand for CD94/NKG2 (73). This method conferred significant protection against human NK-mediated lysis in vitro (64). The possibility of MHC class I recognition by NK receptors across species barriers has been explored by cloning and molecular characterization of MHC class I loci obtained from three haplotypes of inbred miniature swine. Comparison of amino acid sequences recognized by human NK inhibitory receptors revealed that the residues critical for recognition by these receptors were altered in the porcine genes. This provides a likely explanation for the inefficiency of porcine MHC class I molecules to inhibit human NK-cell lysis (76).

Control of NK-cell–dependent mechanisms of xenograft immune recognition has resulted in significant improvement of primary graft survival in animal models but does not seem to be the ultimate step in immunosuppression in the xenogeneic setting. The variety of B-, T-, and NK-cell–deleting experiments in models of xenotransplantation has led to the emergence of macrophages as an immune-competent cell population with a meaningful role in xenograft rejection. The presence of numerous macrophages in the cellular infiltrates seen in DXR has already been mentioned (9, 26, 28, 54). Hamster-to-rat heart transplantation experiments have shown that treatment with L-NAME, a blocking agent for macrophage nitric oxide synthesis, of B-, T-, and NK-cell–depleted rats significantly prolonged graft survival. Rejection still occurred after 11 days, with persisting presence of macrophages in the cellular infiltrates, with high expression of TNF, and P- and E-selectin (44). Macrophages seem to be a difficult cell population to control, since treatment with deoxyspergualin, a macrophage-depleting drug, prolonged guinea pig-to-rat heart graft survival in otherwise B-, T-, and NK-cell–depleted animals but could not alter macrophage infiltration or macrophage-lectin induction (27).

CONCLUSIONS

In clinical transplantation, there is no doubt that if xenografts are to be accepted, strategies aimed at turning off NK cells have to be devised, although this might represent only one aspect of a multifaceted approach. Engagement of killer inhibitory receptors by xenogeneic cells to prevent their lysis by NK lymphocytes has been successfully obtained via expression of classical or nonclassical MHC class I molecules (64, 65). The generation of tailor-made transgenic donors, expressing human class I histocompatibility antigens specific for the recipient, could be envisioned. Alternatively, one could attempt to block the NK-activating receptors, either the ADCC-mediating CD16 or other receptors responsible for direct cytotoxicity. Anti-CD16 monoclonal antibodies have been efficiently used to that effect in animal models (33). Also, monoclonal antibody–targeting of adhesion molecules (LFA-1, VLA-4) critical for NK-target cell–cell interaction represents another possibility (6, 33). Chimerism induced by donor-specific bone marrow transplantation has been shown to produce allo- and xenotolerance, even across a discordant barrier, with evidence of NK as well as T- and B-cell tolerance (77, 78). However, it seems likely that more than one of the approaches briefly outlined above might be eventually necessary to efficiently prevent NK-cell–mediated xenograft damage.

REFERENCES

1. **Arase, H., N. Arase, and T. Saito.** 1995. Interferon gamma production by natural killer (NK) cells and NK1.1+ T cells upon NKR-P1 cross-linking. *J. Exp. Med.* **183:**2391–2396.
2. **Arase, N., H. Arase, S. Y. Park, H. Ohno, C. Ra, and T. Saito.** 1997. Association with FcRgamma is essential for activation signal through NKR-P1 (CD161) in natural killer (NK) cells and NK1.1+ T cells. *J. Exp. Med.* **186:**1957–1963.
3. **Baquerizo, A., A. Mhoyan, M. Kearns-Jonker, W. S. Arnaout, C. Schackleton, R. W. Busuttil, A. A. Demetriou, and D. V. Cramer.** 1999. Characterization of human xenoreactive antibodies in liver failure

patients exposed to pig hepatocytes after bioartificial liver treatment: an ex vivo model of pig to human xenotransplantation. *Transplantation* **56:**5–18.

4. **Barao, I., and J. L. Ascensao.** 1998. Human natural killer cells. *Arch. Immunol. Ther. Exp.* **46:**213–229.
5. **Bezouska, K., C. T. Yuen, J. O'Brien, R. A. Childs, W. Chai, A. M. Lawson, K. Drbal, A. Fiserova, M. Pospisil, and T. Feizi.** 1994. Oligosaccharide ligands for NKR-P1 protein activate NK cells and cytotoxicity. *Nature* **372:**150–157.
6. **Birmele, B., G. Thibault, H. Nivet, Y. Gruel, P. Bardos, and Y. Lebranchu.** 1996. Human lymphocyte adhesion to xenogeneic porcine endothelial cells: modulation by human TNF-alpha and involvement of VLA-4 and LFA-1. *Transplant. Immunol.* **4:**265–270.
7. **Birmele, B., G. Thibault, H. Watier, I. Vallee, Y. Gruel, H. Nivet, H. Salmon, P. Bardos, and Y. Lebranchu.** 1994. Human peripheral blood lymphocyte adhesion to xenogeneic porcine aortic endothelial cells: preferential adhesion of CD3-CD16+ NK cells. *Transplant. Proc.* **26:**1150–1151.
8. **Bix, M., N. S. Liao, M. Zijlstra, J. Loring, R. Jaenisch, and D. Raulet.** 1991. Rejection of class I MHC-deficient hematopoietic cells by irradiated MHC-matched mice. *Nature* **349:**329–331.
9. **Blakely, M. L., W. J. Van der Werf, M. C. Berndt, A. P. Dalmasso, F. H. Bach, and W. W. Hancock.** 1994. Activation of intragraft endothelial and mononuclear cells during discordant xenograft rejection. *Transplantation* **58:**1059–1066.
10. **Braud, V. M., D. S. Allan, C. A. O'Callaghan, K. Soderstrom, A. D'Andrea, G. S. Ogg, S. Lazetic, N. T. Young, J. I. Bell, J. H. Phillips, L. L. Lanier, and A. J. McMichael.** 1998. HLA-E binds to natural killer cell receptors CD94/NKG2A, B and C. *Nature* **391:**795–799.
11. **Brennan, J., D. Mager, W. Jefferies, and F. Takei.** 1994. Expression of different members of the Ly-49 gene family defines distinct natural killer cell subsets and cell adhesion properties. *J. Exp. Med.* **180:**2287–2295.
12. **Brooks, A. G., P. E. Posch, C. J. Scorzelli, F. Borrego, and J. E. Colinga.** 1997. NKG2A complexed with CD94 defines a novel inhibitory natural killer cell receptor. *J. Exp. Med.* **185:**795–800.
13. **Burshtyn, D. N., W. Yang, T. Yi, and E. O. Long.** 1997. A novel phosphotyrosine motif with a critical amino acid at position −2 for the SHE2 domain-mediated activation of the tyrosine phosphatase SHP-1. *J. Biol. Chem.* **272:**13066–13072.
14. **Candinas, D., S. Belliveau, N. Koyamada, T. Miyatake, P. Hechenleitner, W. Mark, F. H. Bach, and W. W. Hancock.** 1996. T cell independence of macrophage and natural killer cell infiltration, cytokine production, and endothelial activation during delayed xenograft rejection. *Transplantation* **62:**1920–1927.
15. **Candinas, D., B. A. Lesnikoski, S. C. Robson, T. Miyatake, S. M. Scesney, H. C. Marsh, Jr., U. S. Ryan, A. P. Dalmasso, W. W. Hancock, and F. H. Bach.** 1995. Effect of repetitive high-dose treatment with soluble complement receptor type 1 and cobra venom factor on discordant xenograft survival. *Transplantation* **62:**336–342.
16. **Chan, D. V., and H. Auchincloss, Jr.** 1996. Human anti-pig cell-mediated cytotoxicity in vivo involves non-T as well as T cell components. *Xenotransplantation* **3:**158–165.
17. **Colonna, M., and J. Samaridis.** 1995. Cloning of immunoglobulin-superfamily members associated with HLA-C and HLA-B recognition by human natural killer cells. *Science* **268:**405–408.
18. **Cook, J. L., D. N. Ikle, and B. A. Routes.** 1995. Natural killer cell ontogeny in the athymic rat. Relationship between functional maturation and acquired resistance to E1A oncogene-expressing sarcoma cells. *J. Immunol.* **155:**5512–5518.
19. **Dalmasso, A. P., G. M. Vercellotti, R. J. Fischel, R. M. Bolman, F. H. Bach, and J. L. Platt.** 1992. Mechanism of complement activation in the hyperacute rejection of porcine organs transplanted into primate recipients. *Am. J. Pathol.* **140:**1157–1166.
20. **Fujiwara, I., H. Nakajima, H. Yamagishi, T. Matsuda, N. Mizuta, and T. Okta.** 1998. The molecular mechanism of apoptosis induced by xenogeneic cytotoxicity. *Xenotransplantation* **5:**50–56.
21. **Galili, U.** 1993. Interaction of the natural anti-Gal antibody with alpha-galactosyl epitopes: a major obstacle for xenotransplantation in humans. *Immunol. Today* **14:**480–482.
22. **Giorda, R., W. A. Rudert, C. Vavassori, W. H. Chambers, J. C. Hiserodt, and M. Trucco.** 1990. NKR-P1, a signal transduction molecule on natural killer cells. *Science* **249:**1298–1300.
23. **Goodman, D. J., M. Von Albertini, A. Willson, M. T. Millan, and F. H. Bach.** 1996. Direct activation of porcine endothelial cells by human natural killer cells. *Transplantation* **61:**763–771.
24. **Gourlay, W. A., W. H. Chambers, A. P. Monaco, and T. Maki.** 1998. Importance of natural killer cells in the rejection of hamster skin xenografts. *Transplantation* **65:**727–734.

25. **Groth, C. G., O. Korsgren, A. Tibell, J. Tollemar, E. Moller, J. Bolinder, J. Ostman, F. P. Reinholt, C. Hellerstrom, and A. Andersson.** 1994. Transplantation of porcine fetal pancreas to diabetic patients. *Lancet* **344:**1402–1404.
26. **Hancock, W. W., M. L. Blakely, W. Van der Werf, and F. H. Bach.** 1993. Rejection of guinea pig cardiac xenografts post-cobra venom factor therapy is associated with infiltration by mononuclear cells secreting interferon-gamma and diffuse endothelial activation. *Transplant. Proc.* **25:**2932.
27. **Hancock, W. W., T. Miyatake, N. Koyamada, J. P. Kut, M. Soares, M. E. Russell, F. H. Bach, and M. H. Sayegh.** 1997. Effects of leflunomide and deoxyspergualin in the guinea pig → rat cardiac model of delayed xenograft rejection: suppression of B cell and C-C chemokine responses but not induction of macrophage lectin. *Transplantation* **64:**696–704.
28. **Hancock, W. W.** 1997. Delayed xenograft rejection. *World J. Surg.* **21:**917–923.
29. **Houchins, J. P., T. Yabe, C. McSherry, and F. H. Bach.** 1991. DNA sequence analysis of NKG2, a family of related cDNA clones encoding type II integral membrane proteins on human natural killer cells. *J. Exp. Med.* **173:**1017–1029.
30. **Inverardi, L., and R. Pardi.** 1996. Human natural killer cells and natural antibodies recognize overlapping molecular structures on discordant xenogeneic endothelium, p. 104–125. *In* E. Kemp, K. Reemtsma, D. White, J. Platt, and D. K. C. Cooper (eds.), *Xenotransplantation*, Springer Scientific Publication, Berlin, Germany.
31. **Inverardi, L., B. Clissi, and R. Pardi.** 1997. Xenorecognition by NK cells and natural antibodies: a common evolutionary pathway? *Xenotransplantation* **5:**9–11.
32. **Inverardi, L., B. Clissi, A. L. Stolzer, J. R. Bender, M. S. Sandrin, and R. Pardi.** 1997. Human natural killer lymphocytes directly recognize evolutionarily conserved oligosaccharide ligands expressed by xenogeneic tissues. *Transplantation* **63:**1318–1330.
33. **Inverardi, L., M. Samaja, R. Motterlini, F. Mangili, J. R. Bender, and R. Pardi.** 1992. Early recognition of a discordant xenogeneic organ by human circulating lymphocytes. *J. Immunol.* **149:**1416–1423.
34. **Itescu, S., P. Kwiatkowski, J. H. Artrip, S. F. Wang, J. Ankersmit, O. P. Minanov, and R. E. Michler.** 1998. Role of natural killer cells, macrophages, and accessory molecule interactions in the rejection of pig-to-primate xenografts beyond the hyperacute period. *Hum. Immunol.* **59:**275–286.
35. **Kase, A., M. H. Johansson, M. Y. Olsson-Alheim, K. Karre, and P. Hoglund.** 1998. External and internal calibration of the MHC class I-specific receptor Ly49A on murine natural killer cells. *J. Immunol.* **161:**6133–6138.
36. **Kaufman, D. S., R. A. Schoon, and P. J. Leibson.** 1993. MHC class I expression on tumor targets inhibits natural killer cell-mediated cytotoxicity without interfering with target recognition. *J. Immunol.* **150:**1429–1436.
37. **Khoo, N. K., L. Fahlen, and C. L. Sentman.** 1998. Modulation of Ly49A receptors on mature cells to changes in major histocompatibility complex class I molecules. *Immunology* **95:**126–131.
38. **Kumagai-Braesch, M., M. Satake, Y. Qian, J. Holgersson, and E. Moller.** 1998. Human NK cell and ADCC reactivity against xenogeneic porcine target cells including fetal porcine islet cells. *Xenotransplantation* **5:**132–145.
39. **Lanier, L. L., B. C. Corliss, J. Wu, C. Leong, and J. H. Phillips.** 1998. Immunoreceptor DAP12 bearing a tyrosine-based activation motif is involved in activating NK cells. *Nature* **391:**703–707.
40. **Lanier, L. L.** 1998. NK cell receptors. *Annu. Rev. Immunol.* **16:**359–393.
41. **Lazetic, S., C. Chang, J. P. Houchins, L. L. Lanier, and J. H. Phillips.** 1996. Human natural killer cell receptors involved in MHC class I recognition are disulfide-linked heterodimers of CD94 and NKG2 subunits. *J. Immunol.* **157:**4741–4745.
42. **Leibson, P. J.** 1997. Signal transduction during natural killer cell activation: inside the mind of a killer. *Immunity* **6:**655–661.
43. **Leventhal, J. R., A. J. Matas, L. H. Sun, S. Reif, R. M. Bolman, 3d, A. P. Dalmasso, and J. L. Platt.** 1993. The immunopathology of cardiac xenograft rejection in the guinea pig-to-rat model. *Transplantation* **56:**1–8.
44. **Lin, Y., M. Vandeputte, and M. Waer.** 1997. Contribution of activated macrophages to the process of delayed xenograft rejection. *Transplantation* **64:**1677–1683.
45. **Lin, Y., M. Vandeputte, and M. Waer.** 1997. Natural killer cell- and macrophage-mediated rejection of concordant xenografts in the absence of T and B cell responses. *J. Immunol.* **158:**5658–5667.
46. **Ljunggren, H. G., and K. Karre.** 1985. Host resistance directed selectively against H-2-deficient lymphoma variants. Analysis of the mechanism. *J. Exp. Med.* **162:**1745–1759.

47. **Malyguine, A. M., S. Saadi, J. L. Platt, and J. R. Dawson.** 1996. Human natural killer cells induce morphologic changes in porcine endothelial cell monolayers. *Transplantation* **61:**161–164.
48. **Mason, L. H., S. K. Anderson, W. M. Yokoyama, H. R. Smith, R. Winkler-Pickett, and J. R. Ortaldo.** 1996. The Ly-49D receptor activates murine natural killer cells. *J. Exp. Med.* **184:**2119–2128.
49. **Mason, L. H., J. Willette-Brown, S. K. Anderson, P. Gosselin, E. W. Shores, P. E. Love, J. R. Ortaldo, and D. W. McVicar.** 1998. Characterization of an associated 16kDa tyrosine phosphoprotein required for Ly-49D signal transduction. *J. Immunol.* **160:**4148–4152.
50. **Moretta, A., S. Sivori, M. Vitale, D. Pende, L. Morelli, R. Augugliaro, C. Bottino, and L. Moretta.** 1995. Existence of both inhibitory (p58) and activatory (p50) receptors for HLA-C molecules in human natural killer cells. *J. Exp. Med.* **182:**875–884.
51. **O'Shea, J. J., A. M. Weissman, I. C. Kennedy, and J. R. Ortaldo.** 1991. Engagement of the natural killer cell IgG Fc receptor results in tyrosine phosphorylation of the zeta chain. *Proc. Natl. Acad. Sci. USA* **88:**350–354.
52. **Olcese, L., P. Lang, F. Vely, A. Cambiaggi, D. Marguet, M. Blery, K. L. Hippen, R. Biassoni, A. Moretta, L. Moretta, J. C. Cambier, and E. Vivier.** 1996. Human and mouse killer-cell inhibitory receptors recruit PTP1C and PTP1D protein tyrosine phosphatases. *J. Immunol.* **156:**4531–4534.
53. **Patselas, T., F. Thomas, D. Araneda, and W. Marchman.** 1995. Role of natural killer and killer cells in concordant xenograft rejection. *Transplant. Proc.* **27:**262–263.
54. **Pearse, M. J., E. Witort, P. Mottram, W. Han, L. Murray-Segal, M. Romanella, E. Salvaris, T. A. Shinkel, D. J. Goodman, and A. J. d'Apice.** 1998. Anti-Gal antibody-mediated allograft rejection in alpha 1,3-galactosyltransferase gene knockout mice: a model of delayed xenograft rejection. *Transplantation* **66:**748–754.
55. **Pende, D., R. Biassoni, C. Cantoni, S. Verdiani, M. Falco, C. di Donato, L. Accame, C. Bottino, A. Moretta, and L. Moretta.** 1996. The natural killer cell receptor specific for HLA-A allotypes: a novel member of the p58/p70 family of inhibitory receptors that is characterized by three immunoglobulin-like domains and is expressed as a 140-kD disulphide-linked dimer. *J. Exp. Med.* **184:**505–518.
56. **Phillips, J. H., C. Chang, J. Mattson, J. E. Gumperz, P. Parham, and L. L. Lanier.** 1996. CD94 and a novel associated protein (94AP) form a NK cell receptor involved in the recognition of HLA-A, HLA-B and HLA-C allotypes. *Immunity* **5:**163–172.
57. **Platt, J. L., R. J. Fischel, A. J. Matas, S. A. Reif, R. M. Bolman, and F. H. Bach.** 1991. Immunopathology of hyperacute xenograft rejection in a swine-to-primate model. *Transplantation* **52:**214–220.
58. **Pruitt, S. K., W. M. Baldwin, 3d, H. C. Marsh, Jr., S. S. Lin, C. G. Yeh, and R. R. Bollinger.** 1991. The effect of soluble complement receptor type 1 on hyperacute xenograft rejection. *Transplantation* **52:**868–873.
59. **Raziuddin, A., D. L. Longo, L. Mason, J. R. Ortaldo, and W. J. Murphy.** 1996. Ly-49 G2+ NK cells are responsible for mediating the rejection of H-2b bone marrow allografts in mice. *Int. Immunol.* **8:**1833–1839.
60. **Reynolds, C. W., and J. R. Ortaldo.** 1987. Natural killer activity: the definition of a function rather than a cell type. *Immunol. Today* **8:**172–174.
61. **Saadi, S., and J. L. Platt.** 1998. Immunology of xenotransplantation. *Life Sci.* **62:**365–387.
62. **Sanchez, M. J., M. O. Muench, M. G. Roncarolo, L. L. Lanier, and J. H. Phillips.** 1994. Identification of a common T/natural killer cell progenitor in human fetal thymus. *J. Exp. Med.* **180:**569–576.
63. **Sanchez, M. J., H. Spits, L. L. Lanier, and J. H. Phillips.** 1993. Human natural killer cell committed thymocytes and their relation to the T cell lineage. *J. Exp. Med.* **178:**1857–1866.
64. **Sasaki, H., X. C. Xu, D. M. Smith, T. Howard, and T. Mohanakumar.** 1999. HLA-G expression protects porcine endothelial cells against natural killer cell-mediated xenogeneic cytotoxicity. *Transplantation* **67:**31–37.
65. **Seebach, J. D., C. Comrack, S. Germana, C. LeGuern, D. H. Sachs, and H. DerSimonian.** 1997. HLA-Cw3 expression on porcine endothelial cells protects against xenogeneic cytotoxicity mediated by a subset of human NK cells. *J. Immunol.* **159:**3655–3661.
66. **Seebach, J. D., K. Yamada, I. M. McMorrow, D. H. Sachs, and H. DerSimonian.** 1996. Xenogeneic human anti-pig cytotoxicity mediated by activated natural killer cells. *Xenotransplantation* **3:**188–197.
67. **Sentman, C. L., M. Y. Olsson, and K. Karre.** 1995. Missing self recognition by natural killer cells in MHC class I transgenic mice. A 'receptor calibration' model for how effector cells adapt to self. *Semin. Immunol.* **7:**109–119.
68. **Sharabi, Y., I. Aksentijevich, T. M. Sundt, 3d, D. H. Sachs, and M. Sykes.** 1990. Specific tolerance induction across a xenogeneic barrier: production of mixed rat/mouse lymphohematopoietic chimeras using a nonlethal preparative regimen. *J. Exp. Med.* **172:**195–202.

69. **Shimizu, Y., and R. DeMars.** 1989. Demonstration by class I gene transfer that reduced susceptibility of human cells to natural killer cell-mediated lysis is inversely correlated with HLA class I antigen expression. *Eur. J. Immunol.* **19:**447–451.
70. **Silver, E. T., J. F. Elliott, and K. P. Kane.** 1995. Alternatively spliced Ly-49D and H transcripts are found in IL-2-activated NK cells. *Immunogenetics* **44:**478–482.
71. **Sivakumar, P. V., I. Puzanov, N. S. Williams, M. Bennett, and V. Kumar.** 1998. Ontogeny and differentiation of murine natural killer cells and their receptors, p. 161–192. *In* K. Karre and M. Colonna (eds.), *Specificity, Function and Development of NK Cells.* Springer, Berlin, Germany.
72. **Smyth, M. J., K. Y. T. Thia, and M. H. Kershaw.** 1997. Xenogeneic mouse anti-human NK cytotoxicity is mediated via perforin. *Xenotransplantation* **4:**78–84.
73. **Soderstrom, K., B. Corliss, L. L. Lanier, and J. H. Phillips.** 1997. CD94/NKG2 is the predominant inhibitory receptor involved in recognition of HLA-G by decidual and peripheral blood NK cells. *J. Immunol.* **159:**1072–1075.
74. **Spritz, R. A.** 1998. Genetic defects in Chediak-Higashi syndrome and the beige mouse. *J. Clin. Immunol.* **18:**97–105.
75. **Steffens, U., Y. Vyas, B. Dupont, and A. Selvakumar.** 1998. Nucleotide and amino acid sequence alignment for human killer cell inhibitory receptors (KIR). *Tissue Antigens* **51:**398–413.
76. **Sullivan, J. A., H. F. Oettinger, D. H. Sachs, and A. S. Edge.** 1997. Analysis of polymorphism in porcine MHC class I genes: alterations in signals recognized by human cytotoxic lymphocytes. *J. Immunol.* **159:**2318–2326.
77. **Sykes, M.** 1996. Hematopoietic cell transplantation for the induction of allo- and xeno-tolerance. *Clin. Transplant.* **10:**357–363.
78. **Sykes, M., H. Ohdan, J. O. Manilay, T. Wekerle, and Y. G. Yang.** 1998. Hematopoietic chimerism and tolerance of T cells, B cells, and NK cells. *Transplant. Proc.* **30:**4020.
79. **Tay, C. H., E. Szomolanyi-Tsuda, and R. M. Welsh.** 1998. Control of infections by NK cells, p. 193–220. *In* K. Karre and M. Colonna (eds.), *Specificity, Function and Development of NK Cells.* Springer, Berlin, Germany.
80. **Vales-Gomez, M., H. T. Reyburn, M. Mandelboim, and J. L. Strominger.** 1998. Kinetics of interaction of HLA-C ligands with natural killer cell inhibitory receptors. *Immunity* **9:**337–344.
81. **Vance, R. E., J. R. Kraft, J. D. Altman, P. E. Jensen, and D. H. Raulet.** 1998. Mouse CD94/NKG2A is a natural killer cell receptor for the nonclassical major histocompatibility complex (MHC) class I molecule Qa-1(b). *J. Exp. Med.* **188:**1841–1848.
82. **Vance, R. E., D. M. Tanamachi, T. Hanke, and D. H. Raulet.** 1997. Cloning of a mouse homolog of CD94 extends the family of C-type lectins on murine natural killer cells. *Eur. J. Immunol.* **27:**3236–3241.
83. **von Albertini, M., C. Ferran, C. Brostjan, F. H. Bach, and D. J. Goodman.** 1998. Membrane-associated lymphotoxin on natural killer cells activates endothelial cells via an NF-kappaB-dependent pathway. *Transplantation* **66:**1211–1219.
84. **Watier, H., J. M. Guillaumin, I. Vallee, G. Thibault, Y. Gruel, Y. Lebranchu, and P. Bardos.** 1996. Human NK cell-mediated direct and IgG-dependent cytotoxicity against xenogeneic porcine endothelial cells. *Transplant. Immunol.* **4:**293–299.
85. **Whiteside, T. L., N. L. Vujanovic, and R. B. Herberman.** 1998. Natural killer cells and tumor therapy, p. 221–244. *In* K. Karre and M. Colonna (eds.), *Specificity, Function and Development of NK Cells.* Springer, Berlin, Germany.
86. **Winter, C. C., J. E. Gumperz, P. Parham, E. O. Long, and N. Wagmann.** 1998. Direct binding and functional transfer of NK cell inhibitory receptors reveal novel patterns of HLA-C allotype recognition. *J. Immunol.* **151:**571–577.
87. **Wirthmueller, U., T. Kurosaki, M. S. Murakami, and J. V. Ravetch.** 1992. Signal transduction by Fc gamma RIII (CD16) is mediated through the gamma chain. *J. Exp. Med.* **175:**1381–1390.
88. **Yu, Y. Y., T. George, J. R. Dorfman, J. Roland, V. Kumar, and M. Bennett.** 1996. The role of Ly49A and 5E6(Ly49C) molecules in hybrid resistance mediated by murine natural killer cells against normal T cell blasts. *Immunity* **4:**67–76.

Xenotransplantation
Edited by Jeffrey L. Platt

Chapter 5

Cellular Immune Responses to Xenografts

Ronald G. Gill

Discordant xenograft rejection has generally been characterized by the dramatic humoral hyperacute response involving naturally occurring xenoreactive antibodies and complement activation (4, 16, 99). In cases where hyperacute rejection (HAR) can be avoided by complement inhibition, vascularized xenografts still undergo a less-defined delayed hyperacute or acute vascular rejection (AVR), which, as the term implies, results in rapid vascular injury and graft loss within 2 to 3 days after grafting (100). These HAR and AVR reactions form the focus of other contributions in this volume. The dominant participation of the innate immune system, especially complement components, in triggering rapid xenograft rejection has probably limited past concerns over the adaptive or antigen-specific cellular immune response to xenografts. In fact, several early studies indicated that T cells were hyporeactive to xenogeneic antigen-presenting cells (APC), suggesting that cellular responses may only play a limited role in xenograft rejection. Considerable progress has occurred toward inhibiting complement activity, as illustrated by the advent of transgenic pigs bearing human complement regulatory proteins (15, 94). While such exciting advances are tremendously significant, they have resulted in increased attention to cellular xenograft immunity. Contrary to early indications, it has become apparent that xenografts can indeed elicit potent antigen-specific responses that provide an important barrier to the future application of xenotransplantation (5). As such, this review will center on adaptive or antigen-specific cellular responses to xenografts. In particular, much of the following discussion will emphasize the nature of T-lymphocyte–dependent immunity to xenografts.

T-cell–dependent xenograft rejection traditionally has been quite difficult to examine in vivo since it occurs as the backdrop to the humoral HAR and AVR reactions. Thus, the majority of mechanistic studies regarding cellular xenograft immunity have been performed in rodent models where HAR and AVR can be dissociated from classic cellular rejection through the use of defined transgenic and gene-targeted (knockout) animals. To date, most large-animal studies have had to rely on histopathologic evidence to infer mechanisms of cellular rejection (62, 78, 94). Thus, most of the concepts concerning T-cell responses to xenografts developed in this review are derived from rodent studies. However, a major task

Ronald G. Gill • Barbara Davis Center for Childhood Diabetes, University of Colorado Health Sciences Center, Denver, CO 80262.

will be to determine whether these principles generated from small-animal models will translate to large animals and, ultimately, to human application. Another key point is that it can be misleading to make sweeping generalizations regarding the nature of cellular xenograft immunity due to two important variables: (i) Individual species combinations: Although concordant and discordant species combinations were defined according to the absence or presence of natural antibodies, respectively (16), this concept also applies to antigen-specific responses. That is, the magnitude and quality of interspecies T-cell reactivity in particular vary sharply according to the defined responding and stimulating species used (discussed below). (ii) Nature of tissue/organ transplanted: Just as cellular immunity varies according to the type of allograft in question, T-cell–dependent immunity to xenografts also varies strongly, especially in the case of primarily vascularized organs versus cellular (neovascularized) xenografts. Since vascular endothelium is a dominant target of HAR and AVR, there is an especially drastic difference in the rejection seen between organ and cellular xenografts, such as pancreatic islets. Since neovascularized grafts are established by host rather than donor vasculature, it has long been assumed that such cellular grafts are less sensitive to HAR (5). However, this distinction has become less clear in that there is increasing evidence that cellular xenografts may also show sensitivity to rapid humoral injury (48, 64). Overall, these variables should always be considered as important caveats in the following discussion since particular nuances of cellular rejection of defined organs and tissues between specific species combinations will require continuing clarification.

T-LYMPHOCYTE REACTIVITY: REQUIREMENTS FOR ANTIGEN RECOGNITION AND COSTIMULATION

When considering the T-lymphocyte response to non-self antigens, including xenografts, it is imperative to emphasize the two fundamental properties of T-cell reactions. First is the notion that the T-cell receptor recognizes foreign antigens only as a complex with major histocompatibility complex (MHC) molecules (143). Another fundamental paradigm for T-cell activation is that antigen alone is not sufficient for driving the response (13, 73). These restraints on T-cell function can influence the nature of cellular xenograft recognition as discussed below. According to the two-signal model of lymphocyte activation proposed by Lafferty and Cunningham (73), signal one (antigen) is provided by occupancy of the antigen-specific T-cell receptor and signal two is provided by a non–antigen-specific inductive molecule, or *costimulator* (CoS), produced by a metabolically active APC. Although early studies suggested that cytokines could demonstrate CoS activity in vitro (124), later studies provided evidence that accessory molecule interactions between T cells and APC costimulate with antigen to trigger T-cell activation. Primary receptor/ligand surface molecules involved in costimulation are CD28 (54) expressed by T cells interacting with the B7-1 (CD80) and B7-2 (CD86) molecules expressed by APC and activated B cells (18, 111). However, other accessory molecules, such as ICAM-1 and LFA-3 (26), have also been implicated as inducing costimulation of T cells. CD40/CD40L (CD154) interactions between APCs and T cells, respectively, have also emerged as a major costimulatory pathway (45). Notably, the B7/CD28 and CD40/CD40L pathways of costimulation have been used as key targets of therapeutic intervention to prevent allograft (59, 61, 75, 95) and even xenograft rejection (33, 34, 43, 77, 131), indicating the significance of these molecular interactions in triggering cellular immunity. Still other members of the tumor necrosis factor (TNF)/TNF-receptor family, such as 4-1BB, OX-40, and CD30, have likewise been clearly identified as costimulatory molecules (130). Thus, costimulation is actually a complex constellation of receptor–ligand interactions rather than a single signal facilitating T-cell activation. Regardless of the exact nature of costimulatory signals, only those cells providing costimulatory activity will be capable of triggering T-cell responses, whereas other cells will have a nonstimulatory phenotype, such as most tissue parenchymal cells that express the same MHC antigens but do not express costimulatory activity. This idea was very important in transplantation in that it implied that the major source of tissue immunogenicity was derived from the resident hematopoietic APCs, or "passenger leukocytes," rather than in the tissue parenchymal cells themselves (71). The finding that depletion of donor-derived APCs before grafting could result in long-term allograft survival in nonimmunosuppressed recipients provided evidence supporting this concept (71).

Interestingly, our modern concepts of costimulation for T cells are actually derived from early studies of xenoreactivity (73). The notion of costimulation was an attempt to explain the finding that lymphocytes were found to be poor at initiating graft-versus-host disease (GVHD) in xenogeneic recipients despite presumably strong antigenic disparities (70). This finding led to the idea that antigens alone were not sufficient to activate lymphocytes but required an additional inductive signal, or costimulator, that was presumed to be species-specific (70). This principle is actually recapitulated by more recent studies in which immune-deficient mice are repopulated with human cells (scid-hu mice) in order to examine human T-cell function in vivo (86). Although transferred human cells can mediate the rejection of human allografts (58, 105) or porcine xenografts (36, 37) in these animals, they generally fail to initiate vigorous GVHD against the scid mouse host itself. In striking contrast, mature allogeneic mouse T cells trigger acute, lethal GVHD in immunocompromised mice (65). This seemingly paradoxical result is best explained by the relative inability of human T cells to be activated directly by mouse APC (see below).

Direct and Indirect Pathways of Graft Antigen Presentation

A key concept for the following discussion is that two differing pathways of graft antigen presentation can be envisioned that would fulfill the two-signal requirement for T-cell activation described above, each involving APC-dependent processes: (i) donor MHC-restricted responses, whereby host T cells recognize graft antigens *directly* on the surface of donor cells capable of elaborating CoS activity, and (ii) host MHC-restricted responses, whereby host T cells *indirectly* recognize graft antigens, which are processed and presented by host APC (Fig. 1). The direct pathway of antigen presentation would include CD4 and CD8 T cells specific for peptides presented by MHC class II and class I molecules, respectively (123), on donor-derived APCs. Such cells would be capable of directly engaging MHC antigens expressed by transplanted cells. In the indirect pathway, host-type APCs would process and present graft antigens primarily in association with host MHC class II antigens. Such presentation would be expected to activate predominantly CD4 T cells. While indirect antigen presentation has long been assumed to occur through MHC class II presentation, it has become apparent that exogenous antigens can also gain access to the MHC class I processing pathway (10, 14, 68). This pathway, often referred to as "cross-priming," represents an indirect CD8 response that has been shown to contribute to models of autoimmune disease (67). Although there is no clear indication as yet demonstrating a role for this indirect CD8 response in graft rejection, the potential for such reactivity should be considered. A key property of indirect CD4 or CD8 T cells is in their restriction to *host* MHC molecules

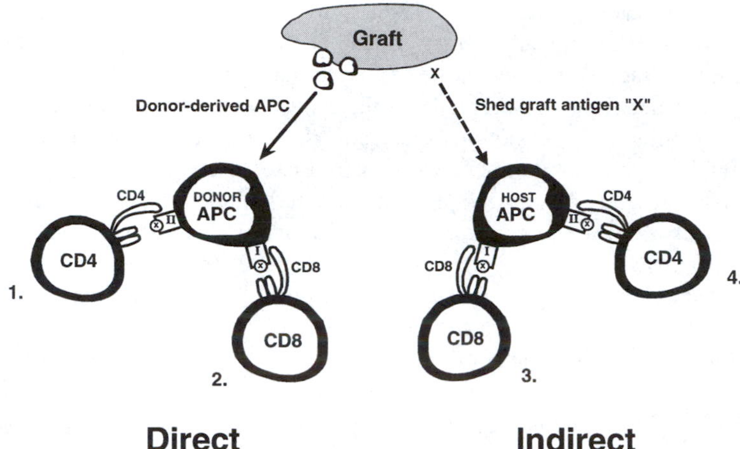

Figure 1. Direct and indirect pathways of graft antigen presentation. Optimal T-lymphocyte activation requires T-cell receptor recognition of processed peptide antigens complexed with MHC molecules plus appropriate secondary costimulatory signals provided by the antigen-presenting cell (APC). Four potential scenarios are depicted whereby CD4 or CD8 T cells can be activated in response to graft-derived antigens: (1) Direct (donor MHC-restricted) CD4 T-cell activation. In this case, the donor-type APC directly presents its own repertoire of peptides associated with MHC class II molecules to specific CD4 T cells. (2) Direct CD8 T-cell activation. Donor APCs directly present MHC class I/peptide complexes to host CD8 T cells. Note that the high alloreactive precursor frequency is attributed largely to the direct CD4 and CD8 T-cell pathways. (3) Indirect (host MHC-restricted) CD8 T-cell activation. In this case, antigens (generically termed "X") derived from donor cells are processed and re-presented in association with MHC class I molecules on host-type APC. This pathway, also referred to as "cross-priming," represents cases in which exogenous antigens enter the MHC class I processing pathway. Although largely disregarded in the past, this pathway may prove to be of greater biological significance than previously considered. (4) Indirect CD4 T-cell activation. This is probably the predominant pathway of responses to most foreign antigens. In this case, graft-derived antigens ("X") are acquired by host-type APCs and re-presented in association with MHC class II molecules. It is generally accepted that exogenous antigens primarily gain access to the MHC class II processing pathway and so primarily induce CD4 T-cell activation.

such that they are not capable of a direct T-cell receptor (TCR)–mediated engagement of transplanted cells. This model of donor MHC-restricted (direct) and host MHC-restricted (indirect) pathways of graft antigen presentation has important implications for the nature of T-cell–dependent immune responses to both allografts and xenografts. Importantly, evidence below will support the idea that cellular xenograft rejection is dominated by indirect, CD4 T-cell–dependent responses in vivo.

T-CELL XENOGENEIC RESPONSES IN VITRO

Example of Deficient Interspecies Direct Activation: Human versus Mouse

Early studies using primarily the human/mouse species combination suggested that the ability of T cells to respond to xenogeneic APC in vitro decreases as the phylogenetic disparity between stimulator and responder cell increases (1, 39, 72, 91, 106). Given that autologous MHC molecules are used as the template for molding the TCR repertoire during positive selection (103), it could be considered that there is a relative paucity of antigen-specific receptors for phylogenetically disparate xenogeneic MHC molecules. However, this proposition appears to be incorrect. Even in the deficient mouse anti-human in vitro response, this hyporeactivity is not due to a low inherent precursor frequency. For example, transgenic studies indicate that genetic restoration of the interspecies CD8/MHC class I interaction restores mouse anti-human CTL responses to levels comparable to allogeneic responses (55). Thus, deficient reactivity is not due simply to a TCR repertoire defect, but rather is due to limitations in other accessory molecule interactions. In species combinations such as human anti-porcine there is already considerable reactivity toward unmodified xenogeneic stimulator cells. Sequence analysis shows that porcine SLA molecules do not differ significantly from human HLA molecule homologs (47). Taken together, such studies indicate that the TCR repertoire can indeed recognize xenogeneic MHC molecules at rather high frequency as seen for allogeneic reactivity.

The relative deficiency of the human/mouse T cell–APC interaction is attributed to species-specific receptor–ligand interactions of accessory molecule and/or cytokines involved in T-cell activation and function (1, 23, 55, 91, 127, 136). For example, the interaction of CD4 and CD8 coreceptors with MHC class II and class I molecules, respectively, can demonstrate species specificity. On one hand, human CD4 is capable of functionally associating with mouse class II (128) and can restore CD4 T-cell development in CD4-deficient mice (76). However, the reciprocal binding of mouse CD4 to human class II is quite weak (7, 22). Similarly, the important association of CD8 with the $\alpha3$ domain of class I MHC molecules also displays species specificity between human and mouse (52, 55). These deficiencies account for the finding that in vitro reactivity between human T cells and mouse APCs is largely dependent on responder-type APCs (82, 90, 141), indicating that the response is due to the indirect pathway and not due to direct stimulation by xenogeneic APCs. These species-specific properties are further illustrated by studies showing that responses to xenogeneic APCs can be restored in vitro by providing appropriate accessory molecule interactions (7, 44, 52, 55) or by the addition of the relevant responder-type cytokines (1, 72). Ironically, some of the costimulatory molecules themselves may not be especially species-specific (46). For example, we found that human B7-1 (CD80) can readily trigger the rejection of mouse islet allografts (24).

Example of Potent Interspecies Direct Activation: Human versus Porcine

The ability of T cells to interact with xenogeneic APCs is dependent on the particular xenogeneic combination studied. The most relevant combination for proposed clinical application is the human anti-porcine response. Unlike the human/mouse combination described above, there appears to be a formidable human anti-porcine direct response (104, 139). That is, porcine APCs are clearly capable of activating human T cells independently of autologous human APCs (104, 139). Such direct reactivity has been demonstrated in responses restricted to both porcine MHC (SLA) class I (114, 138) and class II (12, 139) molecules. Human T cells can even distinguish between particular SLA alleles, as illustrated by the study of human anti-porcine cytotoxic T cells (138, 140). Interestingly, more phylogenetically distant mouse T cells do not appear to readily discriminate between differing SLA alleles (60), suggesting that nonpolymorphic regions of MHC molecules can be recognized by xenoreactive T cells in some cases. What accounts for this vigorous xenogeneic direct reactivity not seen in the human/mouse combination? First, as mentioned above, sequence analysis suggests that porcine SLA molecules are sufficiently similar to their human HLA counterparts to "mimic" human allogeneic MHC molecules (47). Second, many of the accessory molecule interactions found to be deficient in the human anti-mouse response are functional between human and porcine cells (reviewed in reference 120). For example, porcine cells can directly costimulate human T cells via LFA-1 and CD2 interactions (50, 104). Furthermore, binding of human T cells to porcine endothelial cells can be inhibited by antibodies directed toward porcine VCAM, again showing the relevance of this interspecies recognition (92). Thus, human anti-porcine direct reactivity generally appears to be remarkably similar to the human alloreactive counterpart. However, one potentially important distinction from the human allogeneic response in vitro appears to be a more pronounced indirect response to xenogeneic porcine stimulator cells (31, 115, 140). This is a significant and possibly predictable result. It would be assumed that xenogeneic peptides would have increasing sequence divergence from their allogeneic homologs. Thus, the array of non-self epitopes available to be processed and presented by responder-type APCs would be expected to increase for xenogeneic antigens relative to allogeneic antigens (41), increasing the magnitude of the indirect antigen response.

T-CELL XENOGENEIC RESPONSES IN VIVO: DOMINANT INDIRECT CD4 REACTIVITY

A wide range of studies demonstrate that CD4 T cells play an essential role for triggering immunity to both allografts (19, 49, 96, 112, 116, 117, 142) and xenografts (3, 19, 36, 38, 57, 66, 69, 83, 98, 132, 133, 135). However, this does not imply that the role of the CD4 cell is the same in each situation. CD4 T cells can contribute to graft injury in several ways as illustrated in Fig. 2. (i) *CD8 T-cell activation*: CD4 T cells can facilitate the activation and function of CD8 T cells, which in turn mediate graft destruction. This type of T-cell help can be largely attributed to the direct pathway in which CD4 T cells stimulate the donor APC through a CD40-dependent mechanism to facilitate CD8 T-cell activation (9, 102, 110). (ii) *B-cell activation*: CD4 T cells are the classic helper cell for antibody-producing B cells, leading to a graft-specific antibody response. Unlike help for CD8 T cells, this response appears to occur chiefly through indirect CD4 T-cell recognition of antigens presented in the context of MHC class II expressed on B cells. In fact, the pronounced T-cell–dependent antibody response to xenografts that is often observed may be due to enhanced indirect CD4 reactivity. (iii) *Effector cells*: Although CD4 T cells have been traditionally considered to be helper cells, it has become apparent that these cells can act as effector cells either by directly interacting with MHC class II antigens expressed on the graft or through responding to graft antigens displayed by host APCs (39, 129). This multifunctional capacity of the CD4 T-cell subset results in our ambiguity in understanding the precise role of CD4 T cells in different transplant settings. Evidence shown below suggests that indirect CD4 reactivity is the primary pathway of T-cell–dependent xenograft immunity in vivo.

Pancreatic islet transplantation illustrates the contribution of CD4-dependent indirect recognition to xenograft rejection. Both islet allograft and xenograft rejections are dependent on CD4 T cells (38, 57, 66, 69, 83, 119). However, the vigor of CD4-mediated xenograft rejection in vivo does not appear to correlate with the corresponding response in vitro. Many results, including our own, indicate that islet xenograft rejection occurs more rapidly than

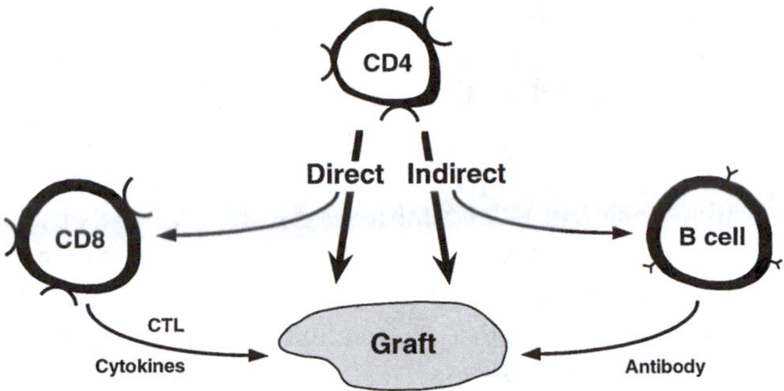

Figure 2. Potential T-cell–dependent pathways of graft destruction. CD4 T cells are considered to be major participants in triggering antigen-specific responses to xenografts (see text). CD4 T cells can respond either directly to donor-type APCs or indirectly to graft-derived antigens presented by host APCs. Both of these responses themselves may participate in tissue injury. Direct CD4 T cells would be capable of TCR engagement of MHC class II antigens expressed by donor APCs and vascular endothelium. Indirect CD4 T cells would interact with graft antigens presented by autologous APCs, possibly producing local inflammatory tissue damage. Alternatively, CD4 T cells may collaborate with other lymphocyte subpopulations that can participate in graft rejection. On one hand, the "direct" type CD4 T cell has been chiefly implicated as helping to activate CD8 lymphocytes, leading to a graft-specific cytotoxic T-cell (CTL) response. Alternatively, "indirect" CD4 T cells are the key helper cells for B cells presenting graft-derived antigens, resulting in a graft-specific antibody response.

the comparable response to allografts (135). Further evidence indicates that this CD4 T-cell–dependent xenograft response is distinct from the allograft response. Unlike islet allograft immunity, xenograft immunity does not appear to require MHC class I–restricted CD8 T cells (28, 29, 38, 40, 66, 135). Also, while MHC class I–deficient islets are accepted as mouse allografts, they are acutely rejected in xenogeneic rat recipients (84). Other studies demonstrate that neither donor MHC class I nor class II expression is necessary for acute xenograft rejection (85). Adoptive transfer studies using scid mice show that while CD4 T cells are both necessary and sufficient to reconstitute these animals for islet xenograft immunity, islet allograft immunity requires both CD4 and CD8 T cells (25, 38). Identical results were found in studying responses to porcine skin xenografts in mice (132). Taken together, in sharp contrast to islet allograft rejection, neither CD8 T cells nor their corresponding class I MHC target antigens are required for islet xenograft rejection. Could the rapid rejection of islet xenografts be due to the contribution of an antibody response that depends on CD4 T-cell help? While antibodies may certainly contribute to xenograft immunity, B cells are not required for the rapid cellular rejection of either rat (38) or porcine (8) islet xenografts in mice. Rather, CD4 T cells appear to be both necessary and sufficient for triggering acute islet xenograft rejection in scid mouse recipients (38).

Our first indication of indirect CD4 reactivity to islet xenografts was the finding that, unlike islet allografts, rat islet xenograft rejection did not require donor-type APCs (135). Furthermore, the rejection of APC-depleted islet xenografts was CD4 T cell–dependent and CD8 T cell–independent. Is this CD4-dependent response really due to indirect antigen presentation? If this is true, then the response will be dependent on host-type and not donor-type MHC class II molecules. The key role of host MHC class II in CD4-dependent xenograft rejection is illustrated by results that show a lack of CD4 T-cell–mediated xenograft rejection in MHC class II–deficient hosts (20, 21). That is, CD4-dependent xenograft rejection depends on host and not on donor MHC class II expression. Our own results using concordant islet xenografts show a similar requirement for host and not donor MHC class II. We find that CD4 T cells trigger rapid rejection of rat islet xenografts established in immunodeficient recombinase-activating gene (*rag*)–deficient hosts. However, none of the islet xenografts are rejected in *rag*-deficient mice that are also MHC class II–deficient (unpublished results). Significant indirect CD4 responses from xenografted animals have also been identified in vitro (93). Taken together, it appears that acute cellular xenograft rejection in small-animal models is largely dependent on host CD4 T cells and MHC class II expression and independent on donor APCs and MHC expression. From such results, it appears that indirect presentation is a predominant form of T-cell–dependent immunity in vivo and is sufficient to account for acute cellular rejection.

The involvement of CD4 indirect reactivity does not preclude a participation for other cellular pathways in xenograft rejection. There are examples of skin and heart xenograft rejection in which CD8 T cells may trigger rejection (66, 79). We have found that predominantly CD8+ xenoreactive (mouse anti-rat) "direct" T-cell lines can mediate xenograft rejection in vivo (134). Also, human CD4 T cells with apparent direct specificity for porcine APCs can trigger xenograft rejection in scid mice, again implicating a role for direct T cells in xenograft rejection (36). The finding that potent direct human anti-porcine T-cell reactivity occurs makes this an important cellular pathway that may strongly contribute to xenograft rejection. However, regardless of the degree of direct reactivity between particular species combinations, we propose that exaggerated CD4-dependent indirect reactivity will be a common feature of virtually all xenograft settings, promoting both antibody and inflammatory responses that exceed typical allograft responses. However, whereas CD8 T cells and B cells may contribute to tissue injury, these cells are not a requisite component of rapid CD4-dependent cellular xenograft rejection.

NATURAL KILLER (NK) CELLS: A POTENTIAL LINK BETWEEN THE INNATE AND ADAPTIVE XENOGRAFT RESPONSES

Xenogeneic organs and tissues may elicit immune reactivity similar to responses triggered by microorganisms that, of course, are xenografts themselves. In particular, the humoral and cellular components of the innate immune response, including complement, granulocytes, and NK cells, are of particular importance for early defense against pathogen intrusion. It would not be surprising if many of these primitive reactions to pathogens influence subsequent antigen-specific cellular immunity to tissue and organ xenografts. It will probably be of key importance to determine how the innate and T-cell–dependent adaptive immune responses interact in order to better understand the cellular rejection of xenografts. As mentioned above, it has been difficult to study cellular xenograft rejection independently from immediate hyperacute rejection and subsequent acute vascular rejection. In particular, the role of NK cells in xenograft cellular immunity has remained rather elusive. On one hand, a number of studies suggest that NK cells are not required for acute cellular xenograft rejection. The finding that xenografts are accepted in severe combined immunodeficient mice provides empirical evidence that the innate immune response is not sufficient for xenograft rejection. Immunodeficient scid and *rag*-deficient mice accept tissue and organ xenografts despite retaining innate immune reactivity, including NK-cell function (88, 126). Also, transplantation of either concordant or discordant xenografts is not prolonged in either NK-deficient or NK-depleted mice (56, 121, 132). Likewise, hamster heart xenografts show only modest prolongation in NK-deficient rats (2). These results emphasize the importance of T cells in cellular xenograft rejection. However, other studies suggest that some xenograft responses can occur with limited involvement of T lymphocytes, as seen in cardiac xenograft rejection in nude rats (17, 79, 80). In our own examination of cellular immunity to concordant islet xenografts (rat-to-mouse), we have not found a requirement for NK cells in the response. For example, we find that purified CD4+ T cells are sufficient for inducing rapid rejection of rat islet xenografts, but not allografts, in scid mice (38). Furthermore, we found that CD4+ T cells transfer equally rapid islet xenograft rejection in either NK-sufficient or NK-deficient scid-*beige* mice (unpublished observations). Conversely, in the absence of T cells, activation of NK activity by poly I:C induction (122) does not trigger destruction of rat islet xenografts established in scid mice (Table 1). That is, intentional activation of systemic NK activity is not sufficient for the rejection of islet xenografts. Taken together, such studies suggest that NK cells are not absolutely required or necessary for rapid cellular xenograft rejection. However, it should be emphasized that these results are for concordant cellular xenografts rather than primarily vascularized transplants.

Despite these findings it should not be construed that NK cells fail to contribute to cellular xenograft immunity. In fact, NK cells are strongly implicated in xenorecognition. NK cells exhibit an interesting dual recognition system in which induction of killing occurs through activating receptors while negative signals are delivered through killer cell–inhibitory receptors (KIRs) (74). Importantly, autologous MHC class I–like molecules play an important role in KIR recognition and subsequent inhibition of NK activity. In the case of xenoreactivity, NK cells have been shown to be capable of interacting with xenogeneic targets through their activating receptors while failing to be inhibited by xenogeneic MHC expression (51, 125), presumably through deficient interspecies KIR recognition. The finding that transfection of porcine cells with human HLA class I molecules can confer resistance to human NK killing supports the concept that xenogeneic cells may lack appropriate inhibitory ligands for NK cells, thus promoting excessive NK activity. A variety of other studies also implicate NK cells as active participants in the response to tissue and organ xenografts. NK cells can form a pronounced component of the early infiltration of xenografts (11, 27, 79). NK cells have also been implicated in the recognition of xenogeneic vascular endothelium (53) and can lead to the activation of discordant endothelial cells (42). Several studies show that human NK cells can lyse porcine target cells, an activity that is enhanced by IL-2 (30, 51, 53, 63,

Table 1. Systemic induction of NK cells does not trigger rejection of rat islet xenografts established in scid mice

Treatment[a]	n	Graft function (days)	NK activity
Saline	3	>50 (×3)	–
Poly I:C	5	>50 (×5)	+++

[a]Chemically induced C.B-17 scid mice were grafted with DA rat islet xenografts. Such grafts uniformly function >100 days in unmanipulated scid recipients. In one group of recipients, NK cells were activated systemically by administration of poly I:C (122). Activation of NK cells was confirmed by in vitro assays of scid spleen cells against NK-sensitive target cells (K562). Despite vigorous NK activation, rat islet xenografts continued functioning >50 days following poly I:C treatment.

113). Importantly, even if NK cells are found to be insufficient for xenograft rejection, they may serve to greatly augment T-cell–dependent reactivity. For example, NK cells have been shown to contribute to the generation of mouse anti-human cytotoxic T-cell immunity in vivo through an interferon-γ–dependent mechanism (121). Alternatively, NK cells have been implicated in triggering rapid cardiac xenograft rejection by mediating antibody-dependent cellular cytotoxicity (79). Thus, NK cells may enhance the consequence of both T-cell and antibody responses in vivo. Taken together, such results suggest that NK cells may help initiate accelerated inflammatory activity against xenogeneic endothelial cells and perhaps other tissue cells and thus exacerbate the cellular response. Thus, NK cells may form an important intermediate innate pathway of reactivity involved in the unusually rapid cellular response to xenografts.

XENOGRAFT CELLULAR RESPONSE: IS THE GRAFT PERCEIVED AS AN EXTRACELLULAR PARASITE?

The cellular xenograft response appears to be quantitatively and qualitatively distinct from the allograft response. Interestingly, the general features of the cellular xenograft response are remarkably similar to those mounted against extracellular parasites (35). T cells cannot directly recognize parasites such as helminths through direct TCR binding, but rather must recognize parasite-derived antigens in the context of self MHC molecules. That is, elimination of the parasite requires indirect antigen recognition, the same pathway proposed to predominate in the cellular response to tissue xenografts. Immunity to intestinal parasites requires CD4 T cells but not CD8 T cells in vivo (35), the same result found in studies of xenograft rejection described above. Also, responses to many extracellular parasites involve a predominant Th2-like cytokine response with concomitant eosinophilia. In fact, elimination of intestinal parasites actually requires Th2 immunity and not Th1 immunity (6, 35), the converse of immune responses to intracellular parasites such as *Leishmania major* (81). This exaggerated Th2-like cytokine production, such as IL-4 and IL-5, and marked eosinophilia are also found in the response to xenografts (87, 89, 137) in contrast to most cases of unmodified allografting, which are predominated by Th1-like cytokines such as IFNγ (97). In rodent models, increasing phylogenetic disparity between the donor and recipient has been correlated with an increased Th2-like humoral response (87). Interestingly, NK cells have also been implicated in the early response to parasite infection (109), contributing to the subsequent response by CD4 T cells. This pronounced NK involvement also is similar to early xenograft reactivity as described above. Thus, it is intriguing to consider that xenografts evoke cellular responses reminiscent of those triggered by more phylogenetically divergent extracellular helminth infections.

How parasitic "xenografts" and organ/cellular xenotransplants elicit such pronounced Th2 immunity remains to be identified. It is possible that prevalent indirect T-cell reactivity and presentation of antigen by B cells help drive Th2 immunity (32). However, the molecular and cellular basis of how differing pathogens elicit different "classes" of responses (e.g., Th1 versus Th2) requires increasing clarification. It should be noted that the general similarity in reactivity to extracellular parasites and xenotransplants does not mean that the elimination of parasites occurs by the same mechanism that produces xenograft rejection. For example, while Th2-deficient mice have impaired nematode immunity (35), IL-4– and IL-5–deficient mice can acutely reject porcine islet xenografts (118). Conversely, animals deficient for the prototypical Th1 cytokine IFNγ can also reject porcine xenografts (108) as well as allografts (101, 107). Clearly, the precise molecular mechanisms of cellular xenograft rejection remain to be identified, especially regarding the role of particular Th1 and Th2 cytokines in triggering tissue injury.

REFERENCES

1. **Alter, B. J., and F. H. Bach.** 1990. Cellular basis of the proliferative response of human T cells to mouse xenoantigens. *J. Exp. Med.* **171:**333–338.
2. **Arakawa, K., T. Akami, M. Okamoto, K. Akioka, P. C. Lee, Y. Sugano, J. Kamei, T. Suzuki, H. Nagase, Y. Tsuchihashi, and T. Oka.** 1994. Prolongation of heart xenograft survival in the NK-deficient rat. *Transplant. Proc.* **26:**1266–1267.
3. **Auchincloss, H., Jr., R. Moses, D. Conti, T. Sundt, C. Smith, D. H. Sachs, and H. J. Winn.** 1990. Rejection of transgenic skin expressing a xeno-class I antigen is CD4-dependent and CD8-independent. *Transplant. Proc.* **22:**1059–1060.
4. **Auchincloss, H. J.** 1998. Xenogeneic transplantation: a review. *Transplantation* **46:**1–20.
5. **Auchincloss, H. J.** 1990. Xenografting: a review. *Transplant. Rev.* **4**:14–27.
6. **Bancroft, A. J., A. N. McKenzie, and R. K. Grencis.** 1998. A critical role for IL-13 in resistance to intestinal nematode infection. *J. Immunol.* **160**:3453–3461.
7. **Barzaga-Gilbert, E., D. Grass, S. Lawrence, P. Peterson, E. Lacy, and V. Engelhard.** 1992. Species specificity and augmentation of responses to class II major histocompatibility complex molecules in human CD4 transgenic mice. *J. Exp. Med.* **175:**1707–1715.
8. **Benda, B., A. Karlsson-Parra, A. Ridderstad, and O. Korsgren.** 1996. Xenograft rejection of porcine islet-like cell clusters in immunoglobulin- or Fc-receptor γ-deficient mice. *Transplantation* **62:**1207–1211.
9. **Bennett, S. R. M., F. R. Carbone, F. Karamalis, R. A. Flavell, J. F. A. P. Miller, and W. R. Heath.** 1998. Help for cytotoxic-T-cell responses is mediated by CD40 signalling. *Nature* **393:**478–480.
10. **Bennett, S. R. M., F. R. Carbone, F. Karamalis, J. F. A. P. Miller, and W. R. Heath.** 1997. Induction of a $CD8^+$ cytotoxic T lymphocyte response by cross-priming requires cognate $CD4^+$ T cell help. *J. Exp. Med.* **186:**65–70.
11. **Blakely, M. L., W. J. Van der Werf, M. C. Berndt, A. P. Dalmasso, F. H. Bach, and W. W. Hancock.** 1994. Activation of intragraft endothelial and mononuclear cells during discordant xenograft rejection. *Transplantation* **58:**1059–1066.
12. **Bravery, C. A., P. Batten, M. H. Yacoub, and M. L. Rose.** 1995. Direct recognition of SLA- and HLA-like class II antigens on porcine endothelium by human T cells results in T cell activation and release of interleukin-2. *Transplantation* **60:**1024–1033.
13. **Bretscher, P., and M. Cohn.** 1970. A theory of self-nonself discrimination. *Science* **169:**1042–1049.
14. **Brossart, P., and M. J. Bevan.** 1997. Presentation of exogenous protein antigens on major histocompatibility complex class I molecules by dendritic cells: pathway of presentation and regulation by cytokines. *Blood* **90:**1594–1599.
15. **Byrne, G. W., K. R. McCurry, M. J. Martin, S. M. McClellan, J. L. Platt, and J. S. Logan.** 1997. Transgenic pigs expressing human CD59 and decay accelerating factor produce an intrinsic barrier to complement-mediated damage. *Transplantation* **63:**149–155.
16. **Calne, R. Y.** 1970. Organ transplantation between widely disparate species. *Transplant. Proc.* **2:**550.
17. **Candinas, D., S. Belliveau, N. Koyamada, T. Miyatake, P. Hechenleitner, W. Mark, F. H. Bach, and W. W. Hancock.** 1996. T cell independence of macrophage and natural killer cell infiltration, cytokine production, and endothelial activation during delayed xenograft rejection. *Transplantation* **62:**1920–1927.
18. **Chen, C., A. Gault, L. Shen, and N. Nabavi.** 1994. Molecular cloning and expression of early T cell costimulatory molecule-1 and its characterization as B7-2 molecule. *J. Immunol.* **152:**4929–4936.
19. **Chen, Z., S. Cobbold, S. Metcalfe, and H. Waldmann.** 1992. Tolerance in the mouse to major histocompatibility complex-mismatched heart allografts, and to rat heart xenografts, using monoclonal antibodies to CD4 and CD8. *Eur. J. Immunol.* **22:**805–810.
20. **Chitilian, H. V., T. M. Laufer, K. Stenger, S. Shea, and H. J. Auchincloss.** 1998. The strength of cell-mediated xenograft rejection in the mouse is due to the CD4+ indirect response. *Xenotransplantation* **5:**93–98.

21. **Chu, G., J. F. Markmann, M. Ahn, E. Chang, R. P. DeMatteo, R. J. Ketchum, K. I. Brayman, S. Deng, and C. F. Barker.** 1997. Xenogeneic but not allogeneic pancreatic islet graft survival in recipients lacking humoral immunity and major histocompatibility complex class II antigens. *Transplant. Proc.* **29:**901–902.
22. **Clayton, L. K., M. Sieh, D. A. Pious, and E. L. Reinherz.** 1989. Identification of residues affecting class II versus HIV-1 gp120 binding. *Nature* **339:**548.
23. **Collins, M. K. L.** 1989. Species specificity of interleukin 2 binding to individual receptor components. *Eur. J. Immunol.* **19:**1517–1520.
24. **Coulombe, M., H. Yang, S. Guerder, R. A. Flavell, K. J. Lafferty, and R. G. Gill.** 1996. Tissue immunogenicity. The role of MHC antigen and the lymphocyte costimulator B7-1. *J. Immunol.* **157:**4790–4795.
25. **Coulombe, M., H. Yang, L. A. Wolf, and R. G. Gill.** 1999. Tolerance to antigen-presenting cell-depleted islet allografts is CD4 T cell dependent. *J. Immunol.* **162:**2503–2510.
26. **Damle, N. K., K. Klussman, P. S. Linsley, and A. Aruffo.** 1992. Differential costimulatory effects of adhesion molecules B7, ICAM-1, LFA-3, and VCAM-1 on resting and antigen-primed CD4+ T lymphocytes. *J. Immunol.* **148:**1985–1992.
27. **Deng, S., R. J. Ketchum, T. Kucher, M. Weber, A. Naji, and K. L. Brayman.** 1997. NK cells, macrophages, and humoral immune responses are dominant in primary nonfunction of islet grafts in the dog-to-rat xenotransplant model. *Transplant. Proc.* **29:**2062–2063.
28. **Desai, N. M., H. Bassiri, J. Kim, B. H. Koller, O. Smithies, C. F. Barker, A. Naji, and J. F. Markman.** 1993. Islet allograft, islet xenograft, and skin allograft survival in $CD8^+$ T lymphocyte-deficient mice. *Transplantation* **55:**718–722.
29. **Desai, N. M., H. Bassiri, J. S. Odorico, B. H. Koller, O. Smithies, A. Naji, C. F. Barker, and J. F. Markmann.** 1993. Pancreatic islet allograft and xenograft survival in CD8+ T-lymphocyte-deficient recipients. *Transplant. Proc.* **25:**961–962.
30. **Donnelly, C. E., C. Yatko, E. W. Johnson, and A. S. Edge.** 1997. Human natural killer cells account for non-MHC class I-restricted cytolysis of porcine cells. *Cell Immunol.* **175:**171–178.
31. **Dorling, A., R. Binns, and R. I. Lechler.** 1996. Significant primary indirect human T-cell anti-pig xenoresponses observed using immature porcine dendritic cells and SLA-class II- negative endothelial cells. *Transplant Proc.* **28:**654.
32. **Duncan, D. D., and S. L. Swain.** 1994. Role of antigen-presenting cells in the polarized development of helper T cell subsets: evidence for differential cytokine production by Th0 cells in response to antigen presentation by B cells and macrophages. *Eur. J. Immunol.* **24:**2506–2514.
33. **Elwood, E. T., C. P. Larsen, H. R. Cho, M. Corbascio, S. C. Ritchie, D. Z. Alexander, C. Tucker-Burden, P. S. Linsley, A. Aruffo, D. Hollenbaugh, K. J. Winn, and T. C. Pearson.** 1998. Prolonged acceptance of concordant and discordant xenografts with combined CD40 and CD28 pathway blockade. *Transplantation* **65:**1422–1428.
34. **Feng, S., R. R. Quickel, J. Hollister-Lock, M. McLeod, S. Bonner-Weir, R. C. Mulligan, and G. C. Weir.** 1999. Prolonged xenograft survival of islets infected with small doses of adenovirus expressing CTLA4Ig. *Transplantation* **67:**1607–1613.
35. **Finkelman, F. D., T. Shea-Donohue, J. Goldhill, C. A. Sullivan, S. C. Morris, K. B. Madden, W. C. Gause, and J. F. Urban, Jr.** 1997. Cytokine regulation of host defense against parasitic gastrointestinal nematodes: lessons from studies with rodent models. *Annu. Rev. Immunol.* **15:**505–533.
36. **Friedman, T., A. Shimizu, R. N. Smith, R. B. Colvin, J. D. Seebach, D. H. Sachs, and J. Iacomini.** 1999. Human CD4+ T cells mediate rejection of porcine xenografts. *J. Immunol.* **162:**5256–5262.
37. **Friedman, T., R. N. Smith, R. B. Colvin, and J. Iacomini.** 1999. A critical role for human CD4+ T-cells in rejection of porcine islet cell xenografts. *Diabetes* **48:**2340–2348.
38. **Gill, R., L. Wolf, D. Daniel, and M. Coulombe.** 1994. CD4 T cells are both necessary and sufficient for islet xenograft rejection. *Transplant. Proc.* **26:**1203.
39. **Gill, R. G.** 1992. The role of direct and indirect antigen presentation in the response to islet xenografts. *Transplant. Proc.* **24:**642–643.
40. **Gill, R. G., and M. Coulombe.** 1992. Rejection of pancreatic islet xenografts does not require CD8+ T-lymphocytes. *Transplant. Proc.* **24:**2877–2878.
41. **Gill, R. G., and L. Wolf.** 1995. Immunobiology of cellular transplantation. *Cell Transplant.* **4:**361–370.
42. **Goodman, D. J., M. von Albertini, A. Willson, M. T. Millan, and F. H. Bach.** 1996. Direct activation of porcine endothelial cells by human natural killer cells. *Transplantation* **61:**763–771.

43. **Gordon, E. J., T. G. Markees, N. E. Phillips, R. J. Noelle, L. D. Shultz, J. P. Mordes, A. A. Rossini, and D. L. Greiner.** 1998. Prolonged survival of rat islet and skin xenografts in mice treated with donor splenocytes and anti-CD154 monoclonal antibody. *Diabetes* **47:**1199–1206.
44. **Greenstein, J. L., J. A. Foran, J. C. Gorga, and S. J. Burakoff.** 1986. The role of T cell accessory molecules in the generation of class II-specific xenogeneic cytolytic T cells. *J. Immunol.* **136:**2358–2363.
45. **Grewal, I. S., H. G. Foellmer, K. D. Grewal, J. Xu, F. Hardardottir, J. L. Baron, C. A. Janeway, Jr., and R. A. Flavell.** 1996. Requirement for CD40 ligand in costimulation induction, T cell activation, and experimental allergic encephalomyelitis. *Science* **273:**1864–1867.
46. **Guerder, S., D. E. Picarella, P. S. Linsley, and R. A. Flavell.** 1994. Costimulator B7-1 confers antigen-presenting-cell function to parenchymal tissue and in conjunction with tumor necrosis factor α leads to autoimmunity in transgenic mice. *Proc. Natl. Acad. Sci. USA* **91:**5138–5142.
47. **Gustafsson, K., S. Germana, F. Hirsch, K. Pratt, C. LeGuern, and D. H. Sachs.** 1990. Structure of miniature swine class II DRB genes: conservation of hypervariable amino acid residues between distantly related mammalian species. *Proc. Natl. Acad. Sci USA* **87:**9798–9802.
48. **Hamelmann, W., D. W. R. Gray, T. D. J. Cairns, T. Ozasa, D. J. P. Ferguson, A. Cahill, K. I. Welsh, and P. J. Morris.** 1994. Immediate destruction of xenogeneic islets in a primate model. *Transplantation* **58:**1109–1114.
49. **Hao, L., Y. Wang, R. G. Gill, and K. J. Lafferty.** 1987. Role of the L3T4+ T cell in allograft rejection. *J. Immunol.* **139:**4022–4026.
50. **Herrlinger, K. R., V. Eckstein, W. Muller-Ruchholtz, and K. Ulrichs.** 1996. Human T-cell activation is mediated predominantly by direct recognition of porcine SLA and involves accessory molecule interaction of ICAM1/LFA1 and CD2/LFA3. *Transplant. Proc.* **28:**650.
51. **Inverardi, L., B. Clissi, A. L. Stolzer, J. R. Bender, M. S. Sandrin, and R. Pardi.** 1997. Human natural killer lymphocytes directly recognize evolutionarily conserved oligosaccharide ligands expressed by xenogeneic tissues. *Transplantation* **63:**1318–1330.
52. **Irwin, M. J., W. R. Heath, and L. A. Sherman.** 1989. Species-restricted interactions between CD8 and the $\alpha 3$ domain of class I influence the magnitude of the xenogeneic response. *J. Exp. Med.* **170:**1091–1101.
53. **Itescu, S., P. Kwiatkowski, S. F. Wang, T. Blood, O. P. Minanov, S. Rose, and R. E. Michler.** 1996. Circulating human mononuclear cells exhibit augmented lysis of pig endothelium after activation with interleukin 2. *Transplantation* **62:**1927–1933.
54. **June, C. H., J. A. Ledbetter, P. S. Linsley, and C. B. Thompson.** 1990. Role of the CD28 receptor in T-cell activation. *Immunol. Today* **11:**211–216.
55. **Kalinke, U., B. Arnold, and G. J. Hammerling.** 1990. Strong xenogeneic HLA response in transgenic mice after introducing an $\alpha 3$ domain into HLA B27. *Nature* **348:**642–644.
56. **Karlsson-Parra, A., A. Ridderstad, A. C. Wallgren, E. Möller, H. G. Ljunggren, and O. Korsgren.** 1996. Xenograft rejection of porcine islet-like cell clusters in normal and natural killer cell-depleted mice. *Transplantation* **61:**1313–1320.
57. **Kaufman, D. S., C. S. Kong, J. A. Shizuru, A. K. Gregory, and C. G. Fathman.** 1988. Use of anti-L3T4 and anti-Ia treatments for prolongation of xenogeneic islet transplants. *Transplantation* **46:**210–215.
58. **Kawamura, T., T. Niguma, J. H. J. Fechner, R. Wolber, M. A. Beeskau, D. A. Hullett, H. W. Sollinger, and W. J. Burlingham.** 1992. Chronic human skin graft rejection in severe combined immunodeficient mice engrafted with human PBL from an HLA-presensitized donor. *Transplantation* **53:**659–665.
59. **Kenyon, N. S., M. Chatzipetrou, M. Masetti, A. Ranuncoli, M. Oliveira, J. L. Wagner, A. D. Kirk, D. M. Harlan, L. C. Burkly, and C. Ricordi.** 1999. Long-term survival and function of intrahepatic islet allografts in rhesus monkeys treated with humanized anti-CD154. *Proc. Natl. Acad. Sci. USA* **96:**8132–8137.
60. **Kievits, F., J. Wijffels, W. Lokhorst, and P. Ivany.** 1988. Recognition of xeno-(HLA, SLA) major histocompatibility complex antigens by mouse cytotoxic T cells is not H-2 restricted: a study with transgenic mice. *Proc. Natl. Acad. Sci. USA* **86:**617–620.
61. **Kirk, A. D., D. M. Harlan, N. N. Armstrong, T. A. Davis, Y. Dong, G. S. Gray, X. Hong, D. Thomas, J. H. Fechner, Jr., and S. J. Knechtle.** CTLA4-Ig and anti-CD40 ligand prevent renal allograft rejection in primates. *Proc. Natl. Acad. Sci. USA* **94:**8789–8794.
62. **Kirk, A. D., J. S. Heinle, J. R. Mault, and F. Sanfilippo.** 1993. Ex vivo characterization of human anti-porcine hyperacute cardiac rejection. *Transplantation* **56:**785–793.

63. **Kirk, A. D., R. A. Li, M. S. Kinch, K. A. Abernethy, C. Doyle, and R. R. Bollinger.** 1993. The human antiporcine cellular repertoire. In vitro studies of acquired and innate cellular responsiveness. *Transplantation* **55:**924–931.

64. **Korbutt, G. S., L. Aspeslet, Z. Ao, G. L. Warnock, J. Ezekowitz, A. Koshal, R. V. Rajotte, and R. W. Yatscoff.** 1996. Porcine islet cell antigens are recognized by xenoreactive natural human antibodies of both IgG and IgM subtypes. *Transplant. Proc.* **28:**837–838.

65. **Korngold, R., and J. Sprent.** 1985. Surface markers of T cells causing lethal graft-vs-host disease to class I vs class II H-2 differences. *J. Immunol.* **135:**3004–3010.

66. **Krieger, N. R., H. Ito, and C. G. Fathman.** 1997. Rat pancreatic islet and skin xenograft survival in CD4 and CD8 knockout mice. *J. Autoimmun.* **10:**309–315.

67. **Kurts, C., F. R. Carbone, M. Barnden, E. Blanas, J. Allison, W. R. Heath, and J. F. A. P. Miller.** 1997. $CD4^+$ T cell help impairs $CD8^+$ T cell deletion induced by cross-presentation of self-antigens and favors autoimmunity. *J. Exp. Med.* **186:**2057–2062.

68. **Kurts, C., W. R. Heath, F. R. Carbone, J. Allison, J. F. A. P. Miller, and H. Kosaka**. 1996. Constitutive class I-restricted exogenous presentation of self antigens in vivo. *J. Exp. Med.* **184:**923–930.

69. **Lacy, P. E., C. Ricordi, and E. H. Finke.** 1989. Effect of transplantation site and αL3T4 treatment on survival of rat, hamster, and rabbit islet xenografts in mice. *Transplantation* **47:**761–766.

70. **Lafferty, K. J., and M. A. S. Jones.** 1969. Reactions of the graft-versus-host (GVH) type. *Aust. J. Exp. Biol. Med. Sci.* **47:**17–54.

71. **Lafferty, K. J., S. J. Prowse, and C. J. Simeonovic.** 1983. Immunobiology of tissue transplantation: a return to the passenger leukocyte concept. *Annu. Rev. Immunol.* **1:**143–173.

72. **Lafferty, K. J., H. S. Warren, J. A. Woolnough, and D. W. Talmage.** 1978. Immunological induction of T lymphocytes: role of antigen and the costimulator. *Blood Cells* **4:**395–404.

73. **Lafferty, K. L., and A. J. Cunningham.** 1975. A new analysis of allogeneic interactions. *Aust. J. Exp. Biol. Med. Sci.* **53:**27–42.

74. **Lanier, L. L.** 1998. NK cell receptors. *Annu. Rev. Immunol.* **16:**359–393.

75. **Larsen, C. P., E. T. Elwood, D. Z. Alexander, S. C. Ritchie, R. Hendrix, C. Tucker-Burden, H. R. Cho, A. Aruffo, D. Hollenbaugh, P. S. Linsley, K. J. Winn, and T. C. Pearson.** 1996. Long-term acceptance of skin and cardiac allografts after blocking CD40 and CD28 pathways. *Nature* **381:**434–438.

76. **Law, Y. M., R. S. M. Yeung, C. Mamalaki, D. Kioussis, T. W. Mak, and R. A. Flavell.** 1994. Human CD4 restores normal T cell development and function in mice deficient in murine CD4. *J. Exp. Med.* **179:**1233–1242.

77. **Lenschow, D. J., Y. Zeng, J. R. Thistlethwaite, A. Montag, W. Brady, M. G. Gibson, P. S. Linsley, and J. A. Bluestone.** 1992. Long-term survival of xenogeneic pancreatic islet grafts induced by CTLA4Ig. *Science* **257:**789–792.

78. **Leventhal, J. R., A. J. Matas, L. H. Sun, S. Reif, R. M. D. Bolman, A. P. Dalmasso, and J. L. Platt.** 1993. The immunopathology of cardiac xenograft rejection in the guinea pig-to-rat model. *Transplantation* **56:**1–8.

79. **Lin, Y., M. P. Soares, K. Sato, K. Takigami, E. Csizmadia, J. Anrather, and F. H. Bach.** 1999. Rejection of cardiac xenografts by CD4+ or CD8+ T cells. *J. Immunol.* **162:**1206–1212.

80. **Lin, Y., M. Vandeputte, and M. Waer.** 1997. Natural killer cell- and macrophage-mediated rejection of concordant xenografts in the absence of T and B cell responses. *J. Immunol.* **158:**5658–5667.

81. **Louis, J., H. Himmelrich, C. Parra-Lopez, F. Tacchini-Cottier, and P. Launois.** 1998. Regulation of protective immunity against *Leishmania major* in mice. *Curr. Opin. Immunol.* **10:**459–464.

82. **Lucas, P. J., G. M. Shearer, S. Neudorf, and R. E. Gress.** 1990. The human anti-murine xenogeneic cytotoxic response. I. Dependence on responder antigen-presenting cells. *J. Immunol.* **144:**4548–4554.

83. **Mandel, T. E., and M. Koulmanda.** 1992. The survival of xeno-, allo- and isografts in NOD mice and xenografts in other strains, after immunosuppression with anti-CD4 monoclonal antibody. *Diab. Nutr. Metab.* **5**(Suppl. 1)**:**91–96.

84. **Markmann, J. F., H. Bassiri, N. M. Desai, J. S. Odorico, J. I. Kim, B. H. Koller, O. Smithies, and C. F. Barker.** 1992. Indefinite survival of MHC class I-deficient murine pancreatic islet allografts. *Transplantation* **54:**1085–1089.

85. **Markmann, J. F., L. Campos, A. Bhandoola, J. I. Kim, N. M. Desai, H. Bassiri, B. R. Claytor, and C. F. Barker.** 1994. Genetically engineered grafts to study xenoimmunity: a role for indirect antigen presentation in the destruction of major histocompatibility complex antigen deficient xenografts. *Surgery* **116:**242–248.

86. **McCune, J. M., R. Namikawa, H. Kaneshima, L. D. Shultz, M. Lieberman, and I. L. Weissman.** 1988. The SCID-hu mouse: murine model for the analysis of human hematolymphoid differentiation and function. *Science* **241:**1632–1639.

87. **Medbury, H. J., M. Hibbins, A. M. Lehnert, W. J. Hawthorne, J. R. Chapman, T. E. Mandel, and P. J. O'Connell.** 1997. The cytokine and histological response in islet xenograft rejection is dependent upon species combination. *Transplantation* **64:**1307–1314.

88. **Mombaerts, P., J. Iacomini, R. S. Johnson, K. Herrup, S. Tonegawa, and V. E. Papaioannou.** 1992. RAG-1-deficient mice have no mature B and T lymphocytes. *Cell* **68:**869–877.

89. **Morris, C. F., C. J. Simeonovic, M.-C. Fung, J. D. Wilson, and A. J. Hapel.** 1995. Intragraft expression of cytokine transcripts during pig proislet xenograft rejection and tolerance in mice. *J. Immunol.* **154:**2470–2482.

90. **Moses, R. D., R. N. Pierson III, H. J. Winn, and J. H. Auchincloss.** 1990. Xenogeneic proliferation and lymphokine production are dependent on CD4+ helper T cells and self antigen-presenting cells in the mouse. *J. Exp. Med.* **172:**567–575.

91. **Moses, R. D., H. J. Winn, and H. J. Auchincloss.** 1992. Evidence that multiple defects in cell-surface molecule interactions across species differences are responsible for diminished xenogeneic T cell responses. *Transplantation* **53:**203–209.

92. **Mueller, J. P., M. A. Giannoni, S. L. Hartman, E. A. Elliott, S. P. Squinto, L. A. Matis, and M. J. Evans.** 1997. Humanized porcine VCAM-specific monoclonal antibodies with chimeric IgG2/G4 constant regions block human leukocyte binding to porcine endothelial cells. *Mol. Immunol.* **34:**441–452.

93. **Murphy, B., H. Auchincloss, Jr., C. B. Carpenter, and M. H. Sayegh.** 1996. T cell recognition of xeno-MHC peptides during concordant xenograft rejection. *Transplantation* **61:**1133–1137.

94. **Pascher, A., C. Poehlein, M. Storck, R. Prestel, J. Mueller-Hoecker, D. J. White, D. Abendroth, and C. Hammer.** 1997. Immunopathological observations after xenogeneic liver perfusions using donor pigs transgenic for human decay-accelerating factor. *Transplantation* **64:**384–391.

95. **Pearson, T. C., D. Z. Alexander, K. J. Winn, P. S. Linsley, R. P. Lowry, and C. P. Larsen.** 1994. Transplantation tolerance induced by CTLA4-Ig. *Transplantation* **57:**1701–1706.

96. **Pearson, T. C., J. C. Madsen, C. P. Larsen, P. J. Morris, and K. J. Wood.** 1992. Induction of transplantation tolerance in adults using donor antigen and anti-CD4 monoclonal antibody. *Transplantation* **54:**475–483.

97. **Piccotti, J. R., S. Y. Chan, A. M. VanBuskirk, E. J. Eichwald, and D. K. Bishop.** 1997. Are Th2 helper T lymphocytes beneficial, deleterious, or irrelevant in promoting allograft survival? *Transplantation* **63:**619–624.

98. **Pierson, R. N., III, H. J. Winn, P. S. Russell, and H. Auchincloss.** 1989. Xenogeneic skin graft rejection is especially dependent on CD4+ T cells. *J. Exp. Med.* **170:**991–996.

99. **Platt, J. L., and F. H. Bach.** 1991. The barrier to xenotransplantation. *Transplantation* **52:**937–947.

100. **Platt, J. L., S. S. Lin, and C. G. McGregor.** 1998. Acute vascular rejection. *Xenotransplantation* **5:**169–175.

101. **Raisanen-Sokolowski, A., P. L. Mottram, T. Glysing-Jensen, A. Satoskar, and M. E. Russell.** 1997. Heart transplants in interferon-γ, interleukin 4, and interleukin 10 knockout mice: recipient environment alters graft rejection. *J. Clin. Invest.* **100:**2449–2456.

102. **Ridge, J. P., F. Di Rosa, and P. Matzinger.** 1998. A conditioned dendritic cell can be a temporal bridge between a CD4+ T-helper and a T-killer cell. *Nature* **393:**474–478.

103. **Rocha, B., and H. von Boehmer.** 1991. Peripheral selection of the T cell repertoire. *Science* **251:**1225–1228.

104. **Rollins, S. A., S. P. Kennedy, A. J. Chodera, E. A. Elliott, G. B. Zavoico, and L. A. Matis.** 1994. Evidence that activation of human T cells by porcine endothelium involves direct recognition of porcine SLA and costimulation by porcine ligands for LFA-1 and CD2. *Transplantation* **57:**1709–1716.

105. **Rouleau, M., R. Namikawa, S. Antonenko, N. Carballido-Perrig, and M. G. Roncarolo.** 1996. Antigen-specific cytotoxic T cells mediate human fetal pancreas allograft rejection in SCID-hu mice. *J. Immunol.* **157:**5710–5720.

106. **Sachs, D. H., and F. H. Bach.** 1990. Immunology of xenograft rejection. *Human Immunol.* **28:**245–251.

107. **Saleem, S., B. T. Konieczny, R. P. Lowry, F. K. Baddoura, and F. G. Lakkis.** 1996. Acute rejection of vascularized heart allografts in the absence of IFNγ. *Transplantation* **62:**1908–1911.

108. **Sandberg, J.-O., B. Benda, N. Lycke, and O. Korsgren.** 1997. Xenograft rejection of porcine islet-like cell clusters in normal, interferon-γ, and interferon-γ receptor deficient mice. *Transplantation* **63:**1446–1452.

109. **Scharton, T. M., and P. Scott.** 1993. Natural killer cells are a source of interferon gamma that drives differentiation of CD4+ T cell subsets and induces early resistance to *Leishmania major* in mice. *J. Exp. Med.* **178:**567–577.
110. **Schoenberger, S. P., R. E. M. Toes, E. I. H. van der Voort, R. Offringa, and C. J. M. Melief.** 1998. T-cell help for cytotoxic T lymphocytes is mediated by CD40-CD40L interactions. *Nature* **393:**480–483.
111. **Schwartz, R. H.** 1992. Costimulation of T lymphocytes: the role of CD28, CTLA-4, and B7/BB1 in interleukin-2 production and immunotherapy. *Cell* **71:**1065–1068.
112. **Scully, R., S. Qin, S. Cobbold, and H. Waldmann.** 1994. Mechanisms in CD4 antibody-mediated transplantation tolerance: kinetics of induction, antigen dependency and role of regulatory T cells. *Eur. J. Immunol.* **24:**2383–2392.
113. **Seebach, J. D., C. Comrack, S. Germana, C. LeGuern, D. H. Sachs, and H. DerSimonian.** 1997. HLA-Cw3 expression on porcine endothelial cells protects against xenogeneic cytotoxicity mediated by a subset of human NK cells. *J. Immunol.* **159:**3655–3661.
114. **Shishido, S., B. Naziruddin, T. Howard, and T. Mohanakumar.** 1997. Recognition of porcine major histocompatibility complex class I antigens by human CD8+ cytolytic T cell clones. *Transplantation* **64:**340–346.
115. **Shishido, S., B. Naziruddin, X. C. Xu, T. Howard, and T. Mohanakumar.** 1998. Indirect recognition of porcine xenoantigens by human CD4+ T cell clones. *Transplantation* **65:**706–712.
116. **Shizuru, J. A., A. K. Gregory, C. T. B. Chao, and C. G. Fathman.** 1987. Islet allograft survival after a single course of treatment of recipient with antibody to L3T4. *Science* **237:**278–280.
117. **Shizuru, J. A., K. B. Seydal, T. F. Flavin, A. P. Wu, C. C. Kong, E. G. Hoyt, N. Fujimoto, M. E. Billingham, V. A. Starnes, and C. G. Fathman.** 1990. Induction of donor specific unresponsiveness to cardiac allografts in rats by pretransplant anti-CD4 monoclonal antibody therapy. *Transplantation* **50:**366–371.
118. **Simeonovic, C. J., M. J. Townsend, J .D. Wilson, K. U. McKenzie, A. J. Ramsay, K. I. Matthaei, D.A. Mann, and I. G. Young.** 1997. Eosinophils are not required for the rejection of neovascularized fetal pig proislet xenografts in mice. *J. Immunol.* **158:**2490–2499.
119. **Simeonovic, C. J., and J. D. Wilson.** 1992. CD4+ T-cell depletion in mice facilitates induction of tolerance to pig proislet xenografts: a comparison of NOD and CBA/H recipient models. *Diab. Nutr. Metab.* **5**(Suppl. 1)**:**133–138.
120. **Simon, A. R., A. N. Warrens, N. P. Yazzie, J. D. Seebach, D. H. Sachs, and M. Sykes.** 1998. Cross-species interaction of porcine and human integrins with their respective ligands: implications for xenogeneic tolerance induction. *Transplantation* **66:**385–394.
121. **Smyth, M. J., and J. M. Kelly.** 1999. Accessory function for NK1.1$^+$ natural killer cells producing interferon-γ in xenospecific cytotoxic T lymphocyte differentiation. *Transplantation* **68:**840–843.
122. **Sobel, D. O., C. H. Ewel, B. Zeligs, V. Abbassi, J. Rossio, and J. A. Bellanti.** 1994. Poly I:C induction of α-interferon in the diabetes-prone BB and normal Wistar rats. Dose-response relationships. *Diabetes* **43:**518–522.
123. **Swain, S. L.** 1983. T cell subsets and the recognition of MHC class. *Immunol. Rev.* **74:**129–142.
124. **Talmage, D., J. Woolnough, H. Hemmingsen, L. Lopez, and K. Lafferty.** 1977. Activation of cytotoxic T cells by nonstimulating tumor cells and spleen cell factor(s). *Proc. Natl. Acad. Sci. USA* **74:**1610–1614.
125. **Torgersen, K. M., M. Salcedo, J. T. Vaage, C. Naper, B. Rolstad, H.-G. Ljunggren, and P. Hoglund.** 1997. Major histocompatibility complex class I-independent killing of xenogeneic targets by rat allospecific natural killer cells. *Transplantation* **63:**119–123.
126. **Tutt, M. M., W. Schuler, W. A. Kuziel, P. W. Tucker, M. Bennett, M. J. Bosma, and V. Kumar.** 1987. T cell receptor genes do not rearrange or express functional transcripts in natural killer cells of scid mice. *J. Immunol.* **138:**2338–2344.
127. **Vignali, D. A. A., J. Moreno, D. Schiller, and G. J. Hammerling.** 1992. Species-specific binding of CD4 to the β2 domain of major histocompatibility complex class II molecules. *J. Exp. Med.* **175:**925–932.
128. **von Hoegen, P., M. C. Miceli, B. Tourvieille, M. Schilham, and J. R. Parnes.** 1989. Equivalence of human and mouse CD4 in enhancing antigen responses by a mouse class II-restricted T cell hybridoma. *J. Exp. Med.* **170:**1879–1886.
129. **Wang, Y., O. Pontesili, R. G. Gill, F. G. LaRosa, and K. J. Lafferty.** The role of CD4$^+$ and CD8$^+$ T cells in the destruction of islet grafts by spontaneously diabetic mice. *Proc. Natl. Acad. Sci. USA* 1991. **88:**527–531.

130. **Watts, T. H., and M. A. DeBenedette.** T cell co-stimulatory molecules other than CD28. *Curr. Opin. Immunol.,* 1999. **11:**286–293.
131. **Weber, C. J., M. K. Hagler, J. T. Chryssochoos, J. A. Kapp, G. S. Korbutt, R. V. Rajotte, and P. S. Linsley.** 1997. CTLA4-Ig prolongs survival of microencapsulated neonatal porcine islet xenografts in diabetic NOD mice. *Cell Transplant.* **6:**505–508.
132. **Wecker, H., H. Winn, and H. J. Auchincloss.** 1994. CD4+ T cells, without CD8+ or B lymphocytes, can reject xenogeneic skin grafts. *Xenotransplantation* **1:**8–16.
133. **Wilson, J. D., C. J. Simeonovic, J. J. L. Ting, and R. Ceredig.** 1989. Role of CD4+ T-lymphocytes in rejection by mice of fetal pig proislet xenografts. *Diabetes* **38**(Supp. 1):217–219.
134. **Wolf, L., and R. G. Gill.** 1993. Xenoreactive T-cell lines initiate pancreatic islet graft destruction in vivo. *Transplant. Proc.* **25:**440–441.
135. **Wolf, L. A., M. Coulombe, and R. G. Gill.** 1995. Donor antigen-presenting cell-independent rejection of islet xenografts. *Transplantation* **60:**1164–1170.
136. **Woolnough, J., I. Misko, and K. J. Lafferty.** 1979. Cytotoxic and proliferative lymphocyte responses to allogeneic and xenogeneic antigens in vitro. *Aust. J. Exp. Bio. Med. Sci.* **57:**467–477.
137. **Wren, S. M., S. C. Wang, N. L. Thai, B. Conrad, R. A. Hoffman, J. J. Fung, R. L. Simmons, and S. T. Ildstad.** 1993. Evidence for early Th2 T cell predominance in xenoreactivity. *Transplantation* **56:**905–911.
138. **Xu, X. C., B. Naziruddin, H. Sasaki, D. M. Smith, and T. Mohanakumar.** 1999. Allele-specific and peptide-dependent recognition of swine leukocyte antigen class I by human cytotoxic T-cell clones. *Transplantation* **68:**473–479.
139. **Yamada, K., D. H. Sachs, and H. DerSimonian.** 1995. Direct and indirect recognition of pig class II antigens by human T cells. *Transplant. Proc.* **27:**258–259.
140. **Yamada, K., D. H. Sachs, and H. DerSimonian.** 1995. Human anti-porcine xenogeneic T cell response. Evidence for allelic specificity of mixed leukocyte reaction and for both direct and indirect pathways of recognition. *J. Immunol.* **155:**5249–5256.
141. **Yoshizawa, K., and A. Yano.** 1984. Mouse T lymphocytes proliferative responses specific for human MHC products in mouse anti-human xenogeneic MLR. *J. Immunol.* **132:**2820–2829.
142. **Zelenika, D., E. Adams, A. Mellor, E. Simpson, P. Chandler, B. Stockinger, H. Waldmann, and S. P. Cobbold.** 1998. Rejection of H-Y disparate skin grafts by monospecific CD4+ Th1 and Th2 cells: no requirement for CD8+ T cells or B cells. *J. Immunol.* **161:**1868–1874.
143. **Zinkernagel, R. M., and P. C. Doherty.** 1974. Restriction of in vitro T cell-mediated cytotoxicity in lymphocytic choriomeningitis within a syngeneic or semiallogeneic system. *Nature* **248:**701–702.

Xenotransplantation
Edited by Jeffrey L. Platt

Chapter 6

Therapeutic Strategies for Xenotransplantation

L. Bühler, M. R. Basker, I. P. J. Alwayn, D. H. Sachs, and D. K. C. Cooper

To achieve successful xenotransplantation, it is necessary to overcome the immunological barriers that evolution has built up between different species. In contrast to allotransplantation, where the cellular response is the main hurdle, in xenotransplantation both humoral and cellular responses have to be overcome (61). However, although the logistics of allotransplantation make it possible to modify only the immune response of the recipient, in xenotransplantation it is also possible to modify the donor in order to facilitate the engraftment of organs or tissues in the recipient. For example, genetic engineering has already been used to create transgenic pigs that express human genes that may protect the porcine organs from the human immune response. Modification of the recipient's immune response includes modulation of the humoral response, i.e., natural antibodies, complement, and induced antibodies, and prevention of the cellular response, which is anticipated to be strong.

In attempts to achieve successful pig-to-human xenotransplantation, several approaches are currently being evaluated. These include (i) the development of inbred and genetically engineered animals as donors and, in the recipient, (ii) depletion or inhibition of xenoreactive natural antibodies (XNA), (iii) depletion or inhibition of complement, (iv) depletion or suppression of B-cell and/or plasma-cell activity, (v) depletion or suppression of T cells, or (vi) the development of immunological tolerance to donor tissues by the creation of mixed hematopoietic cell chimerism or by molecular chimerism. A comprehensive review of the results of some of these approaches obtained in the pig-to-non-human primate model has recently been published by Lambrigts et al. (42).

GENETICALLY INBRED AND/OR ENGINEERED PIGS AS XENOTRANSPLANT DONORS

The establishment of inbred pigs provides major advantages in the development of potential xenograft donors. Furthermore, genetic engineering techniques are being applied to the problems of xenotransplantation. Major efforts are being devoted toward the development

L. Bühler, M. R. Basker, I. P. J. Alwayn, D. H. Sachs, and D. K. C. Cooper • Transplantation Biology Research Center, Massachusetts General Hospital/Harvard Medical School, MGH-East, Building 149-9019, 13th St., Boston, MA 02129.

of pigs whose organs (i) express no or low levels of antigens recognized by XNA and/or (ii) are protected from human complement activation.

Genetically Inbred Pigs of MHC Homozygosity

Over the past 25 years, a herd of miniature swine has been developed in which subgroups of the herd are homozygous for swine leukocyte antigens (SLA) (69) and the coefficient of inbreeding of one subgroup is currently >85% (S. Arn, personal communication). Inbreeding provides several advantages over other pigs as xenograft donors. For example, the exact reproducibility of genetics allows retransplantation of cells or organs with the same immunologic characteristics as the initial donor. In protocols aimed at inducing tolerance by using gene transfer techniques, it is essential to know the precise donor major histocompatibility complex (MHC) (see below). Finally, the size of these miniature swine is similar to that of humans, with maximal weights of approximately 250 lb.

Genetically Engineered Pigs That Express Low Levels of Antigens Recognized by Xenoreactive Antibodies

Current evidence is that nearly all human natural anti-pig antibodies are directed against Galα1-3Gal (αGal) epitopes on the surface of pig vascular endothelium (14, 27). One approach to overcome this problem is to produce a pig that is deficient in αGal epitopes, thus leaving no target for human anti-αGal antibodies (13). In the pig, αGal is produced by the enzyme α1,3galactosyltransferase (α1,3GT) (Fig. 1), which is encoded by a single gene (24). It has been suggested that the α1,3GT gene might be "knocked out" by gene targeting,

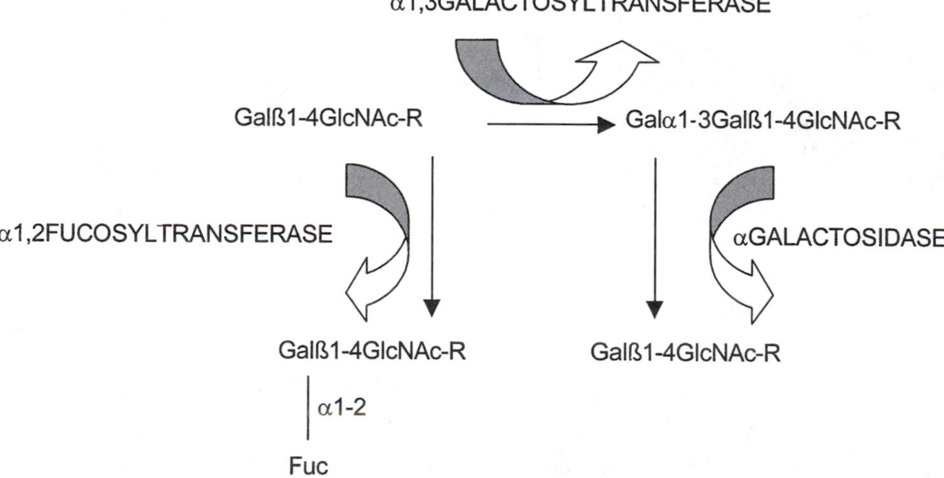

Figure 1. Biosynthetic pathway for synthesis of Galα1-3Gal. The α1,3 galactosyltransferase enzyme adds galactose to *N*-acetyllactosamine (Galβ1-4GlcNAc) to generate Galα1-3Gal. The same substrate can be utilized by transgenically introduced α1,2 fucosyltransferase to produce the H histo-blood group epitope. Galα1-3Gal can also be eliminated by the introduction of α-galactosidase, which enables the N-acetyllactosamine substrate to be available again for further fucosylation. Modified from Sandrin et al. (70).

using a technique such as homologous recombination. This would result in an αGal-deficient pig. However, gene targeting by homologous recombination requires the availability of appropriate pluripotent embryonic stem cells, which are not yet available in pigs.

An alternative approach is to introduce a gene for an enzyme that would compete with the α1,3GT for the underlying substrate, *N*-acetyllactosamine (Fig. 1). Initially, suggested candidates were the genes for sialic acid (α2,3 or α2,6 neuraminic acid) or for the H (O) histo-blood group antigen, α1,2fucosyltransferase (α1,2FT) (13, 14). More recently, other candidate genes have been suggested (reviewed in reference 10). This method, involving the microinjection of a gene for the enzyme that will produce the required oligosaccharide, is possible in the pig. Pigs do, in fact, have the gene for α1,2FT and express H oligosaccharide epitopes, not on vascular endothelium, but in certain other tissues (58). It is, therefore, essential to ensure that the α1,2FT produced as a result of the introduction of α1,2FT cDNA functions at the correct site, and this may prove to be more difficult than is immediately obvious.

Nevertheless, good progress has been made by Sandrin et al. (70, 71), who have demonstrated in vitro that competition between α1,2FT and α1,3GT takes place for *N*-acetyllactosamine. For various reasons, α1,2FT is significantly more successful and the H epitope predominates, reducing the presence of αGal to approximately 10 to 20% of its original expression. Unless H epitopes replace the αGal epitopes completely, however, the number of αGal epitopes remaining on the vascular endothelium would still make such a pig organ susceptible to hyperacute rejection (HAR) or acute vascular rejection (AVR). Galili et al. (24) have estimated that each pig endothelial cell expresses approximately $10^7$$\alpha$Gal epitopes per cell. The ultimate solution, therefore, may be to combine expression of α1,2FT with that of αgalactosidase (15, 71) (Fig. 1). αGalactosidase is an enzyme that has the opposite effect to that of α1,3GT—it removes the terminal αGal molecule rather than adds it. Cell culture studies by Sandrin et al. indicate that insertion of the gene for αgalactosidase alone results in an approximately 70% downregulation of αGal expression. The combined presence of the genes for both αgalactosidase and α1,2FT results in a complete absence of αGal expression. It would appear that wherever α1,2FT is not successful in competing for substrate with α1,3GT, any αGal epitopes that remain are removed by the αgalactosidase. It will be more difficult, however, to replace or remove the αGal epitopes in a pig than from cells in culture.

Transgenic Pigs That Express Human Complement-Regulatory Proteins

A major advance has come from efforts to genetically engineer a pig that expresses one or more of the human complement-regulatory proteins. Under most circumstances, complement-regulatory proteins are largely species-specific, i.e., they block activation of autologous complement but not that of other species (28, 30). For example, pig organs express complement-regulatory proteins that block activation of pig complement but do not adequately block that of human complement. The development of pigs that express a human complement-regulatory protein on their vascular endothelium has been demonstrated to successfully block human (or non-human primate) complement activation in vitro and prevent HAR when a pig organ is transplanted into a primate (17, 48, 72, 92).

The human complement-regulatory system includes several different proteins, e.g., CD46 (membrane cofactor protein, MCP), CD55 (decay-accelerating factor, DAF), and CD59.

Pigs have been bred by transgenesis that express one or more of these proteins (16, 17, 52, 84). The best results published to date have been by the Cambridge, U.K., group of White and his colleagues, who have reported survival of transplanted transgenic (for hDAF) pig kidneys or heterotopic hearts for >2 months in a small number of non-human primates that were also intensively immunosuppressed. The most successful therapy has consisted of 3 to 4 induction doses of cyclophosphamide (20 to 40 mg/kg intravenously on each occasion) and maintenance therapy with cyclosporine (25 mg/kg/day intramuscularly or 200 mg/kg/day orally), prednisolone (1 mg/kg/day, reduced to 0.2 mg/kg/day by day 18), and another agent, such as a rapamycin or mycophenolate mofetil analog (59, 72, 81, 92). The pig-to-cynomolgus monkey model used frequently by this group, however, is unusual in that some of the control (nontransgenic) pig organs survive up to 30 days, suggesting that HAR is not uniform in this combination (17). Nevertheless, the almost consistent prevention of HAR when hDAF organs have been transplanted demonstrates the therapeutic benefit of this approach.

Lin et al. (48) reported the use of transgenic pigs expressing two human complement-regulatory proteins, hDAF and CD59, in a pig-to-baboon heterotopic heart transplant model. In unmanipulated recipient baboons, the transgenic pig hearts were not hyperacutely rejected but underwent AVR within 5 days, demonstrating that the use of transgenic pigs as donors can overcome the problem of HAR. When the recipients were treated by extracorporeal immunoadsorption of XNA and pharmacologic immunosuppression, AVR was delayed and the pig hearts survived up to 29 days. Although it is likely that the combination of transgenic donors, extracorporeal immunoadsorption, and pharmacologic immunosuppression will allow progressive prolongation of survival of xenotransplanted tissues into primates, the limitations of the current immunosuppressive agents are becoming obvious (59, 72, 81, 92).

Nuclear Transfer

With the recent development of nuclear transfer in large mammals (85), the genetic manipulation of embryonic or even adult cells has significantly advanced. It may soon be possible to delete or add a gene or genes in a cultured pig cell, which can then be cloned selectively and used to provide a nucleus, which, after nuclear transfer into an embryonic cell, can produce a herd of animals that incorporates the genetic change. The ability to genetically modify animals in this way should prove a great advantage for the economic production of genetically modified pigs.

IMMUNE MODULATION OF THE RECIPIENT

Depletion or Inhibition of Xenoreactive Antibodies

Initial experiments in the 1960s and 1970s directed at removing xenoreactive antibodies were performed by perfusion of the recipient's blood or plasma through a donor-specific organ, such as a pig kidney or liver (54, 75, 77, 79). Antibodies were adsorbed onto the perfused organ's vascular endothelium, thus temporarily depleting the subject's anti-species antibody and enabling modestly prolonged survival of a subsequently transplanted organ. Initial experiments in the pig-to-non-human primate model (12, 47) showed the pig liver to be a better immunoadsorbent than the kidney, a finding confirmed recently by Azimzadeh et al. (4). The pig liver was used extensively as an immunoadsorbent by Sablinski et al.

(68). Evidence has also been presented that perfusion of human blood through pig lungs is more effective in removing anti-pig antibody than perfusion through pig liver or spleen (49). Other methods for depleting anti-αGal include (i) plasma exchange, (ii) plasma perfusion through nonspecific immunoadsorbants (e.g., protein columns), and (iii) plasma perfusion through specific antibody sorbents (e.g., synthetic αGal immunoaffinity columns).

Plasma Exchange

Plasma exchange—the complete removal of the subject's plasma with replacement of volume by other fluids—is utilized as a treatment for numerous conditions, such as myasthenia gravis, thrombotic microangiopathies, and cryoglobulinemias. All or most circulating antibodies, including anti-αGal, are removed. Because of this temporary state of agammaglobulinemia, the patient is at risk for infection. Furthermore, the patient may be depleted of plasma proteins important to the coagulation cascade. Alexandre and coworkers were successful in using repeated plasma exchange to remove circulating anti-A and anti-B blood group antibodies from potential kidney allograft recipients (1), and demonstrated that the phenomenon of accommodation could result. This technique was also moderately successful in depleting xenoreactive natural antibodies from baboons in a pig-to-baboon kidney transplant model (2), but, although the porcine grafts functioned for up to 22 days, accommodation did not occur, and the grafts were lost to AVR.

Nonspecific Antibody Sorbents

Nonspecific antibody adsorption differs from plasma exchange in that the plasma is passed through an immunoaffinity column containing proteins that remove immunoglobulins from the plasma. The remaining plasma is then returned to the patient, reducing the need for replacement fluids. The proteins (such as staphylococcal protein A or G) are efficient in removing mainly IgG by binding to the Fc portion of the antibody. Since the proteins are nonspecific, all antibodies are removed, resulting in hypogammaglobulinemia and transient predisposition for infectious complications. Several groups reported success in the use of protein A columns to deplete anti-HLA antibodies in potential renal transplant recipients (60, 62), and this technique has been used in xenotransplantation studies.

Specific Antibody Sorbents

Specific antibody sorbents utilize immunoaffinity columns that remove anti-αGal antibodies from plasma by binding them to natural or synthetic αGal oligosaccharides conjugated to a matrix. Significant hypogammaglobulinemia does not occur. Initial studies performed by Ye et al. (91) demonstrated that extracorporeal immunoadsorption (EIA) of baboon plasma, utilizing immunoaffinity columns of melibiose on 4 consecutive days, could reduce cytotoxicity to pig kidney epithelial cells (PK15), which express abundant αGal, by 80%. When highly specific synthetic αGal oligosaccharides became available, a course of EIA resulted in successful depletion of anti-αGal antibodies for 4 to 5 days after which anti-αGal antibodies returned and led to rejection of a transplanted porcine organ (11, 68, 78, 87). Kozlowski et al. (39) provided evidence indicating that EIAs should be carried out approximately 2 to 4 days apart in order to enable equilibration of anti-αGal antibody between the intra- and extravascular spaces to occur, and that four extracorporeal immunoadsorptions were optimal. Although αGal immunoaffinity columns are efficient in depleting anti-αGal, in order to maintain depletion, other therapeutic modalities need to be employed, such as inhibiting the production of antibody. This has proved much more difficult, and is perhaps the major barrier to successful xenotransplantation facing us at the present time (see below).

Neutralization of Xenoreactive Antibodies

A simple approach to prevent HAR is the in vivo neutralization of the recipient's XNA by the intravenous infusion of oligosaccharides terminating in αGal. In vitro experiments demonstrated that many αGal oligosaccharides (e.g., disaccharide [Galα1-3Gal] or trisaccharide [Galα1-3Galβ1-4Glc]) are bound by anti-αGal antibodies, temporarily preventing the binding of the antibodies to pig cells. Simon et al. (76) and Romano et al. (66) perfused synthetic αGal oligosaccharides into baboons without complication. During the period when blood concentrations of the oligosaccharide were above 1 mmol/liter, serum cytotoxicity to pig endothelial cell lines was abolished. Porcine hearts were transplanted heterotopically into two baboons treated without other therapy. HAR was delayed for several hours, but early features of antibody-mediated rejection could not be totally prevented, suggesting that this approach would not be successful if used alone. However, if combined with other approaches (e.g., complement depletion), it might play a useful role. Furthermore, if the oligosaccharide could be bound to a suitable polymer, it might lead to tolerization of the B and/or plasma cells that produce anti-αGal antibody.

An alternative approach to the use of synthetic oligosaccharides is the use of anti-idiotypic antibodies (AIA) directed against idiotypic epitopes expressed on anti-αGal antibodies and B cells. AIAs recognize specific idiotypes that are antigenic determinants within the hypervariable regions of immunoglobulins. AIAs are also directed against the B lymphocyte subpopulations that bear the same idiotypes as surface receptors. Koren et al. (38) produced AIAs by injection into mice of human anti-pig antibodies (eluted from pig organs after repeated perfusion with human plasma) and by the subsequent creation of hybridomas. Several of these AIAs, when incubated with human serum, had a major inhibitory effect on serum cytotoxicity toward pig PK15 cells in vitro. Furthermore, when two selected AIAs were infused intravenously in combination into baboons, serum cytotoxicity was markedly reduced (from 100% to approximately 10%). As not all AIAs had this effect, nonspecific factors, such as anticomplementarity, were not thought to play a role.

Recently, we have produced a polyclonal AIA by immunizing a pig with human anti-αGal antibodies (L. Bühler et al., unpublished data). The purified final preparation contained 1 to 2% AIA. When this was injected repeatedly into a baboon (combined with extracorporeal immunoadsorption of anti-αGal antibodies), a temporary delayed return of anti-αGal antibodies and cytotoxicity to pig cells was observed. Furthermore, the baboon serum was able to partially inhibit cytotoxicity of other highly cytotoxic sera, which was not due to residual AIA. The effect was mediated by the IgG fraction, since removal of the IgM fraction of this inhibitory serum completely abolished its cytotoxicity but did not change its inhibitory effect. This suggests that AIA therapy might have induced the production of noncytotoxic IgG.

Depletion or Inhibition of Complement

Complement is a major factor in the HAR of xenografts. Depletion or inhibition of complement was one of the first therapies explored in an effort to prevent HAR and to prolong discordant organ survival (reviewed in reference 35). Purified cobra venom factor (CVF) is a modified form of C3. CVF binds mammalian factor B and induces the activation of the alternative pathway. However, as it has a modified structure, it cannot be inhibited by a physiological negative feedback (e.g., factor H) and escapes regulation, which results in rapid depletion of C3. CVF alone can clearly protect a discordant organ from HAR (46). However, even when complement is completely inhibited, histopathological features of AVR begin to develop within several days, most probably mediated by the combined action of antibodies and macrophages (37). The addition of concomitant pharmacologic immunosuppressive therapy, by suppressing both B- and T-cell activity, delays rejection further for <27 days (37), but AVR still occurs.

Human complement receptor 1 is a single-chain cell-surface glycoprotein found on erythrocytes, some T lymphocytes, all mature B lymphocytes, neutrophils, eosinophils, basophils, monocytes/macrophages, and certain other cells (51). It is also found circulating in a soluble form in plasma at low concentrations. The interaction of complement receptor 1 with some fractions of the complement cascade regulates complement activation through its convertase decay-accelerating activity and its factor 1 cofactor activity. Fearon and colleagues constructed a soluble form of complement receptor 1 (sCR1), which lacked the transmembrane and cytoplasmic protein domains (82). This sCR1 retains all the known activities of the native cell surface receptor and has been demonstrated to be a potent and selective inhibitor of both the classical and alternative complement pathways. Discordant xenografts have survived for <6 weeks when protected by recombinant sCR1 (9, 63, 64, 86).

Other agents that inhibit complement have been explored, such as FUT and K76 (36), but have been found to be less successful than either CVF or sCR1. However, it is clear that complement depletion or inhibition alone, although a valuable therapeutic approach to assist in overcoming HAR, is not sufficient to prolong discordant xenograft survival indefinitely. The potential risk of infection prevents the long-term administration of any agent that depletes or inhibits complement. In any case, the presence of antibody, even in the absence of complement, appears to lead to the development of AVR by mechanisms that are independent of complement, such as antibody-dependent cellular cytotoxicity (5, 48).

The intravenous administration of concentrated human immunoglobulin (IVIG) has been used clinically in the treatment of certain autoimmune disorders, e.g., thrombotic thrombocytopenic purpura (19, 20, 31), and more recently as therapy to reduce anti-HLA antibodies in highly sensitized patients awaiting organ transplantation (18, 26, 53, 80). Different hypotheses have been proposed to explain the mechanism of action of IVIG, including anti-idiotypic antibodies (65, 67) or complement inhibition (25). In the field of xenotransplantation, IVIG has been shown to prevent the HAR of discordant xenografts. In a guinea pig-to-rat model, human IVIG therapy significantly prolonged the survival of transplanted hearts (25). Furthermore, in pig-to-cynomolgus monkey and pig-to-baboon heart transplantation models, human IVIG delayed HAR in 4 of 6 animals for periods of 18 h, 7.5, 7.5, and 10 days, respectively (50). In these models of xenotransplantation, it was suggested that the possible mechanism of action might be anticomplementarity (50), but other mechanisms are also possible.

B-Cell and Plasma-Cell Suppression

To achieve a reduction of synthesis of XNA, several pharmacologic agents, monoclonal antibodies, and immunotoxins have been investigated.

Pharmacologic Suppression

In the pig-to-primate model, immunosuppressive drugs have been tested in combination with EIA in an attempt to maintain low levels of XNA. Lambrigts et al. (43) used various pharmacologic treatments in baboons and showed that cyclosporin, administered as a single agent, is inefficient in suppressing return of XNA after EIA, indicating that XNA production is not influenced greatly by T-cell–dependent mechanisms. Other pharmacologic agents that have some action on B or plasma cells, e.g., cyclophosphamide, melphalan, mycophenolate mofetil, and brequinar sodium, reduced the rate of return of XNA after EIA. However, no agent alone or in combination was successful in completely preventing production of antibody, although the level could be maintained at approximately 20 to 45% of pretreatment level during EIA therapy. Once EIA was discontinued, however, XNA rose to 50 to 70% of baseline despite continuing drug therapy. These lower levels of XNA remained cytotoxic to pig cells (PK15), suggesting that the remaining XNA would be sufficient to induce HAR of a transplanted pig organ. Furthermore, these modest suppressions of XNA production were only obtained at doses of immunosuppressive drugs that were associated with significant side effects, such as thrombocytopenia (brequinar, cyclophosphamide) or leukopenia (cyclophosphamide).

More recently, our laboratory has begun to investigate other agents that may be more specifically toxic to B or plasma cells. These include cladribine (leustatin) and zidovudine (AZT). Cladribine (2-chloro-2′-deoxy-β-D-adenosine) is an antineoplastic drug used for therapy of lymphoproliferative malignancies that is being explored for use in transplantation as an immunosuppressive agent. Unlike other chemotherapeutic agents affecting purine metabolism, it is not only toxic to actively dividing lymphocytes but also to quiescent lymphocytes. We have tested the efficacy of this drug to suppress B cells and thereby to reduce anti-αGal antibody production following EIA. Little effect on total white blood cell count was seen, and flow cytometry analysis indicated few changes in the B- or T-cell populations in the blood or bone marrow. However, following EIA, XNA was maintained at levels between 50 and 80% of the baseline level for 1 to 3 weeks. In contrast, return of XNA occurs within 48 h in untreated baboons undergoing EIA (39).

Zidovudine is a purine analog used primarily in the treatment of HIV infection. It inhibits mammalian DNA polymerase-alpha and gamma, enzymes that are responsible for mitochondrial DNA synthesis. As antibody production by the B cells/plasma cells is a highly energy-dependent process, interference with the function of mitochondria could reduce the amplitude of antibody rebound following EIA by impairing B-cell/plasma-cell proliferation and antibody production. Baboons have been administered zidovudine in high dosage for <50 days without evidence of toxicity (M. Basker et al., unpublished data). One week after a course of EIA, anti-αGal IgG and IgM levels showed a fall of 55 to 95% (mean 75%) and 50 to 90% (mean 70%), respectively, compared to baseline levels. Low levels were maintained for about 2 weeks. However, neither zidovudine nor cladribine suppressed B-cell and/or plasma-cell function sufficiently to be of clinical potential.

Anti–B-Cell and Plasma-Cell Monoclonal Antibodies and Immunotoxins

Several monoclonal antibodies (MAbs) directed against B cells or plasma cells have become available or are being developed for the treatment of B-cell or plasma-cell malignancies. The efficacy of some of these agents in suppressing B-cell and/or plasma-cell function, and thereby preventing the synthesis of XNA, is under investigation at our center. For example, anti-human CD20 MAb is a chimeric mouse–human MAb specific for CD20 receptors on B cells. Baboons have been treated with this MAb at weekly intervals for 4 weeks. Following this therapy, no B cells were detected in the blood or bone marrow for over 3 months, while lymph nodes showed a maximum 80% reduction, although recovery began within 6 weeks. However, XNA production was largely unaffected. Two weeks after a course of EIA, anti-αGal IgM and IgG levels had recovered to approximately 70% of pretreatment levels, and further recovery of both IgM and IgG occurred relatively rapidly (Fig. 2).

Anti-CD22 MAb is directed against human CD22, which is present on primate B cells. We have used this antibody conjugated to ricin A to make it directly cytotoxic without requiring complement or cell-mediated lysis. Its administration into a baboon resulted in an 80% depletion of B cells in blood and bone marrow, and of 60% in lymph nodes. However, in this baboon the rapid development of anti-ricin antibodies reduced the efficacy of subsequent doses and there was a rapid recovery of anti-αGal antibody levels.

From these preliminary studies it would seem that B cells are not the major cell population of XNA production. Plasma cells may have to be depleted if XNA production is to be significantly reduced.

Prevention of Induced (or T-Cell–Dependent) Antibodies

Induced high-affinity anti-αGal IgG (22) and possibly antibody directed against new porcine (non-αGal) antigenic determinants are considered to play a major role in AVR.

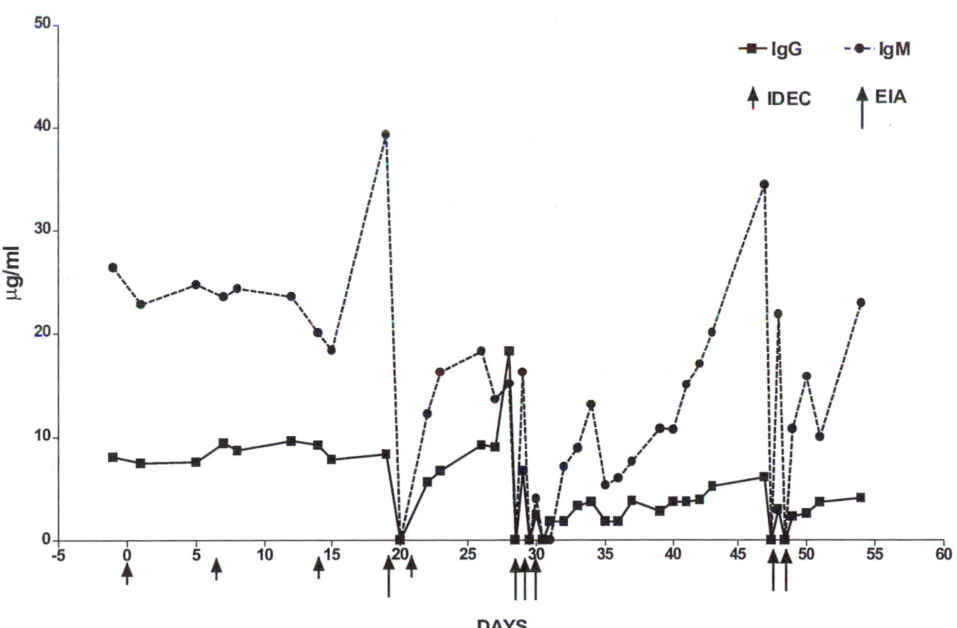

Figure 2. Anti-αGal IgG and IgM levels during treatment with anti-CD20 MAb (short arrows) and adsorption with EIA (long arrows). After four injections of anti-CD20 MAb and four of EIA, the level of anti-αGal IgM returned to pretreatment values within 2 weeks, whereas IgG remained below baseline.

Production of these induced antibodies is generally considered to be T cell–dependent. In animal models, transplantation of porcine cartilage (23), kidneys (41), hearts (11, 41), or bone marrow cells (40) has resulted in a marked increase (of 100- to 300-fold) in anti-pig or anti-αGal IgG and, to a lesser extent, IgM. Transgenic porcine hDAF organs transplanted into non-human primates have survived longer than organs from nontransgenic pigs but, because of the development of AVR, have not shown truly long-term survival despite intensive immunosuppressive therapy (70, 92).

The costimulatory pathway of CD40, which is present on the antigen-presenting cell, and the T-cell ligand, CD40L (or CD154), is crucial for effective activation of T cells to antigen (3) and plays an important role in establishing T-cell–dependent B-cell activity (57). Blockade of this pathway alone or in combination with blockade of the B7/CD28 pathway effectively prolongs survival of skin and organ allografts in rodents (44) and of kidney allografts in monkeys (33, 34). At our center, costimulatory blockade has been shown to facilitate the establishment of mixed chimerism and tolerance to skin allografts in mice when combined with a nonmyeloablative regimen (83). In xenotransplantation, costimulatory blockade has allowed prolonged survival of rat-to-mouse skin and heart grafts, as well as of pig-to-mouse skin grafts (21).

Recently, we have incorporated murine anti-human CD40L MAb therapy in baboons pretreated with a nonmyeloablative regimen and transplanted with high doses of porcine hematopoietic cells (7). This regimen prevented sensitization to all pig antigens, including αGal. Although there was a return of αGal-reactive IgM and IgG to pretransplant levels, there was no increase of either immunoglobulin above those levels. Furthermore, the development of antibody to other pig antigens (anti–non-αGal antibody) was prevented (Fig. 3b and d). This is in contrast to baboons that received porcine hematopoietic cells under the same regimen, but without anti-CD40L MAb, in which sensitization to both αGal and new porcine non-αGal determinants occurred (Fig. 3a and c). By preventing sensitization, therapy with anti-CD40L MAb may have considerable potential in allowing the development of mixed chimerism following porcine hematopoietic cell transplantation, which may lead to immunological tolerance to transplanted pig tissues. Furthermore, in the absence of tolerance, anti-CD40L MAb may enable pig organ survival in primates to be achieved without the need for high doses of pharmacologic immunosuppressive therapy to suppress induced immunoglobulin production. These results support the hypothesis that the induced anti-pig antibody response is T cell–dependent, as anti-CD40L MAb therapy, which is directed against T cells but not B cells, prevented a humoral response. The preexisting natural anti-pig antibody production would seem to be T cell–independent, as baseline synthesis of anti-αGal Ab was not inhibited. We believe this finding will make a significant contribution to achieving successful discordant xenotransplantation.

T-Cell Suppression

Experimental data on the cellular immune response of humans and non-human primates to discordant xenografts are scarce, mainly because early graft destruction from HAR or AVR prevents evaluation of the subsequent cellular response. Most of the information that is thought to be predictive of the human cellular immune response to a discordant xenograft comes from in vitro experiments (55). In pig-to-primate xenotransplantation it would appear that both $CD4^+$ and $CD8^+$ T lymphocytes have the potential to recognize

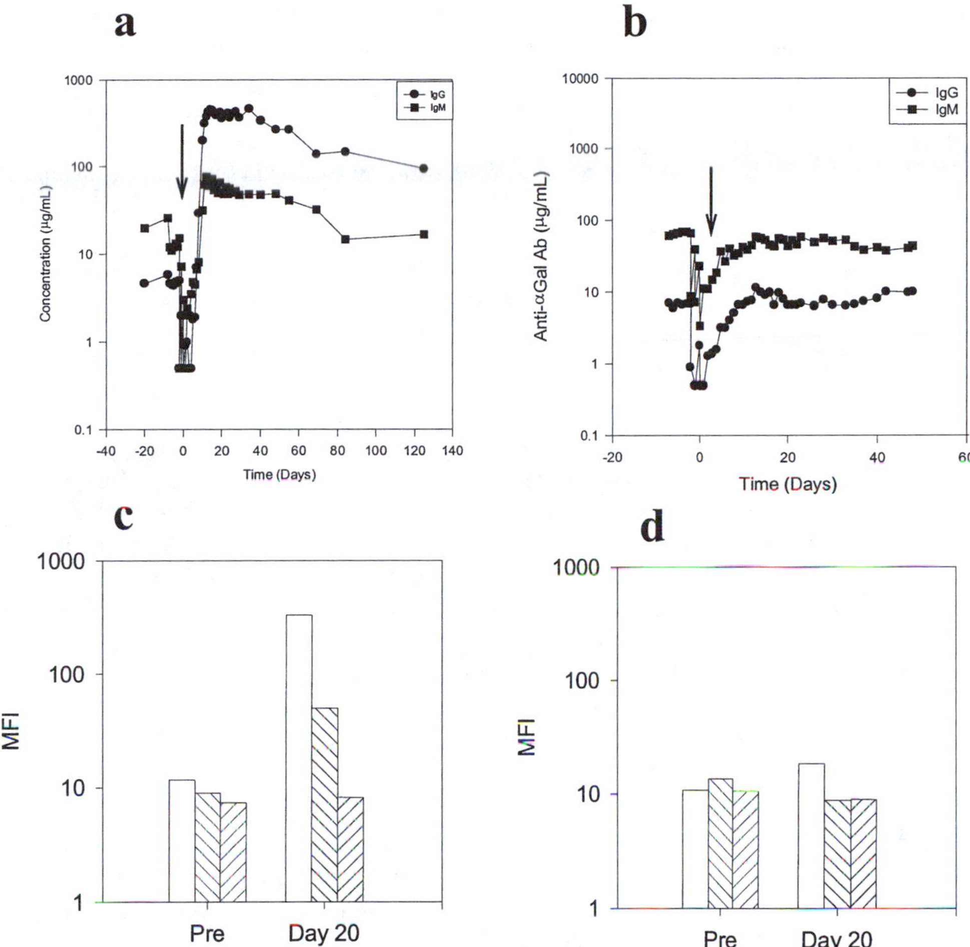

Figure 3. Anti-αGal IgG and IgM responses following porcine peripheral blood mobilized progenitor cell (PBPC) transplantation in representative baboons receiving a tolerance-inducing regimen without (a) and with (b) anti-CD40L MAb. The arrows indicate the first day of porcine PBPC transplantation, which was administered after the extracorporeal immunoadsorption of anti-αGal antibodies. (a) A rise in both anti-αGal IgG and IgM occurred by day 10, indicating sensitization to the Gal determinants on the PBPC. (b) No rise in αGal-reactive IgG or IgM occurred, indicating that sensitization to Gal did not develop when anti-CD40L MAb was administered. The non–αGal-reactive anti-pig antibody response is shown expressed as median fluorescence intensity (MFI), in the same representative baboons treated without (c) and with (d) anti-CD40L MAb. The first column represents the total anti-pig antibody level, column 2 represents the same serum after immunoadsorption of anti-αGal antibody over an αGal matrix, and column 3 represents this serum after further depletion over a pig cell matrix. The difference between columns 1 and 2 therefore indicates the amount of anti-αGal antibody, and the difference between columns 2 and 3 indicates the amount of non-αGal anti-pig antibody. (c) Antibody directed to porcine non-αGal determinants on the PBPC developed within 20 days. (d) No antibody against porcine non-αGal determinants developed.

porcine xenoantigens and do not require the presence of antigen-presenting cells. Vigorous $CD4^+$ proliferation and cytotoxic activity have been documented to be important, and the cellular response is at least equivalent or stronger than that to an allograft (56, 88). This apparent critical role for $CD4^+$ cells in xenotransplantation indicates that strategies to prevent cellular rejection of porcine xenografts should be particularly directed against the $CD4^+$ population. Human anti-porcine cell-mediated cytotoxicity is furthermore mediated in vitro by natural killer (NK) cells (8, 89). This contrasts markedly with allogeneic cellular cytotoxicity, in which NK cells rarely play a role. These differences between T-cell allo- and xenorecognition probably explain why conventional immunosuppressive agents, such as cyclosporin, have to date been shown to be insufficient to block the xenoreactive cellular response. Apart from pharmacologic interventions, potential strategies include the induction of T-cell tolerance in the recipient (see below).

The Induction of Immunological Tolerance

As it seems likely that conventional immunosuppressive therapy will prevent neither the development of AVR nor of acute cellular rejection of a xenograft, we believe alternative approaches will be required to achieve long-term xenograft survival. The induction of donor-specific tolerance would eliminate the development of acute and chronic rejection. The elimination of chronic rejection (e.g., graft atherosclerosis or bronchiolitis obliterans) is possibly even more important than that of acute rejection as there is no effective treatment for chronic rejection, even in allografts. If tolerance could be achieved to some or all xenogeneic antigens, pharmacologic immunosuppressive therapy could be minimized and therefore the accompanying risks of opportunistic infection, malignancy, and drug toxicity would be decreased. Strategies that aim to induce donor-specific tolerance are largely based on the induction of mixed hematopoietic cell chimerism or of molecular chimerism, both of which are major fields of interest at our center.

Tolerance to Donor Species by Mixed Hematopoietic Cell Chimerism

The successful transplantation of donor bone marrow cells has been shown to induce tolerance in allogeneic rodent and non-human primate models (32, 73). In these models, the main mechanism of tolerance induction is intrathymic clonal deletion of preexisting alloreactive T cells. This requires (prior to the bone marrow transplantation) a conditioning regimen that depletes the recipient T cells and creates bone marrow and thymic "space." This is achieved by whole-body and thymic irradiation combined with the administration of polyclonal antibodies or MAbs directed against T cells. In some models, whole-body irradiation can be avoided by increasing the number of bone marrow cells transplanted or by the use of agents that block a costimulatory pathway, such as anti-CD40L MAb or CTLA4-Ig (83).

Cosimi and his colleagues at our center have successfully achieved tolerance to allografts in non-human primates, with some kidney allografts currently surviving for several years without maintenance immunosuppressive therapy (32). This approach has been extended to concordant xenogeneic rodent (rat-to-mouse) (74) and non-human primate (baboon-to-cynomolgus monkey) models (45). Long-term tolerance was achieved in the rodent model, and prolonged organ survival (over 6 months) has been obtained in the primate models.

Although the allograft model requires only the induction of T-cell tolerance, B-cell tolerance can also be achieved by hematopoietic cell chimerism. Sykes' group has demonstrated that transplantation of bone marrow from wild-type (αGal-positive) mice into irradiated αGal-knockout (αGal-negative) mice, which produce anti-αGal antibodies, leads to αGal-reactive B-cell tolerance once engraftment takes place (90). The presence of the αGal-positive bone marrow cells leads to suppression of production of anti-αGal antibody, probably through clonal deletion of the specific B cells.

We have attempted to extend this approach toward achieving mixed chimerism in the discordant pig-to-primate combination (41, 68). The conditioning regimen is based on the experience gained in allotransplantation (32). The major addition to the protocol is the need to remove XNA from the recipient's circulation to avoid HAR. This has been attempted by EIA of the primate's plasma through specific synthetic oligosaccharide (αGal) columns (as discussed above), and has been carried out immediately prior to porcine bone marrow and organ transplantation. Using this regimen, pig kidney and heart grafts have functioned for <15 days in cynomolgus monkeys and baboons but, in the absence of the development of B-cell tolerance, have failed from the development of AVR after return of antibody. In contrast to the allograft model, until recently there has been generally only transient or intermittent evidence for pig cell chimerism, with a low level of pig cells detectable in the blood by polymerase chain reaction. In more recent studies, high doses of pig peripheral blood mobilized progenitor cells (1 to 3×10^{10} cells/kg) have been transplanted and have resulted in higher levels of chimerism (detectable by FACS) for up to 3 weeks (Fig. 4). MLR demonstrates donor-specific hyporesponsiveness for 2 to 3 months. However, return of anti-αGal antibody has prevented complete success to date.

Tolerance to Donor Species by Molecular Chimerism

One approach explored at our center has been the development of what has been termed "molecular chimerism" through the expression in the recipient bone marrow of a swine (SLA) class II antigen or of the αGal epitope.

One approach has been to transfer (ex vivo) into baboon bone marrow cells an SLA class II gene of a specific MHC-inbred miniature swine genotype (29). After infusion of the transduced cells into the baboon from which the cells were originally obtained (as an

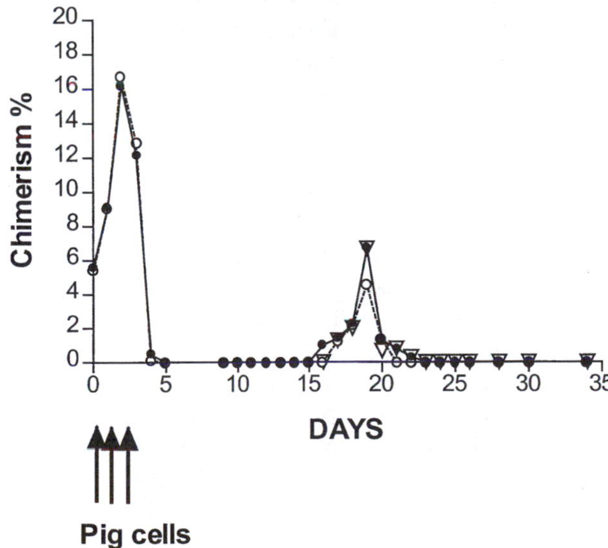

Figure 4. Detection by flow cytometry of pig cell chimerism in the blood of a baboon pretreated with a nonmyeloablative regimen and anti-CD40L MAb. The pig cells were injected on days 0 to 2, with detection of pig cells constituting up to 16% of the white blood cells in the baboon. These cells stained positive for a pig marker (pan pig) and for pig CD9 and pig MAC (monocyte and granulocyte markers). After day 5, no pig cells were detectable until day 16, when a pig monocyte population could be detected until day 22, indicating pig cell engraftment in the baboon.

autologous transplant), the class II transgene was detected long-term in blood and bone marrow, but the transcription of the transgene was transient. Pig organ or skin transplants were rejected within 8 to 22 days. However, long-term follow-up demonstrated that the induction of IgG directed to porcine non-αGal antigenic targets was prevented. This was in contrast to the results obtained in control baboons, where bone marrow cells were transduced with the neomycin gene, in which there was a strong response to porcine non-αGal determinants after pig organ or skin transplants. These results strongly suggest that the presence of the pig class II gene in the baboon's own bone marrow cells prevented the T-cell–dependent response to the xenograft. For this approach to be successful, the availability of inbred pigs with a known SLA genotype is essential.

In studies by Bracy et al. (6), the gene for α1,3GT was introduced into the bone marrow of αGal-knockout mice. The transduced bone marrow was returned to the mouse after a myeloablative regimen of irradiation. The autologous bone marrow graft, including cells transduced with the α1,3GT gene, reconstituted the bone marrow and led to the production of αGal in these αGal-knockout mice. The presence of αGal expressed on cells resulted in suppression of production of anti-αGal antibodies by the mouse. αGal-reactive B-cell tolerance was therefore achieved. This successful study has been followed by preliminary studies in baboons. After transduction of bone marrow cells with the porcine α1,3GT gene, expression of αGal was detected by flow cytometry in the baboon bone marrow. After autologous bone marrow transplantation, however, expression was transient for a few weeks only, and B-cell tolerance was not achieved. Further studies are planned using improved vectors.

COMMENT

Methods that allow successful discordant xenotransplantation will clearly open up new areas of surgical therapy. Patients with organ failure who are in need of a transplant will be able to undergo the procedure electively or immediately when the need arises. Patients with borderline contraindications to allotransplantation will be given the opportunity of organ transplantation as there will no longer be a restriction on the number of donor organs. Transplantation will become a common procedure in countries such as Japan, where to date there have been cultural barriers to cadaveric allotransplantation. The ethical problem of whether retransplantation should be offered to a patient will be overcome by the abundance of donor organs. There will, therefore, be a great expansion in organ transplantation worldwide, and it is likely that both patients and physicians will not wish to persist with inadequate medical therapy, including dialysis, if successful organ xenotransplantation is readily available.

To achieve successful xenotransplantation, it will probably be necessary to combine several therapeutic techniques and/or agents, as is the case with allotransplantation today. There will almost certainly be several steps of development, but the ultimate goal is to develop tolerance in the human recipient to the transplanted pig organ.

Xenotransplantation offers the first opportunity for modifying the donor as opposed to the recipient, which opens up new possibilities in this era of rapidly developing techniques such as genetic engineering, gene transfer, and cloning. The breeding of a pig with a vascular endothelial structure against which humans have no preformed antibodies would be a major advance. In the recipient, however, it will still be necessary to inhibit the production of induced antibodies, as well as the strong cellular response, either by some form of immunosuppressive therapy or by the induction of tolerance.

Acknowledgments. We thank our many collaborators at the Massachusetts General Hospital and at BioTransplant, Inc., who have contributed to the studies reviewed in this chapter, many of which were supported by a Sponsored Research Agreement between the Massachusetts General Hospital and BioTransplant, Inc.

REFERENCES

1. **Alexandre, G. P., J. P. Squifflet, M. De Bruyere, D. Latinne, R. Reding, P. Gianello, M. Carlier, and Y. Pirson.** 1987. Present experiences in a series of 26 ABO-incompatible living donor renal allografts. *Transplant. Proc.* **19:**4538–4542.
2. **Alexandre, G. P., P. Gianello, and D. Latinne.** 1989. Plasmapheresis and splenectomy in experimental renal xenotransplantation, p. 28. *In* M. A. Hardy (ed.), *Xenograft 25*. Elsevier, New York, N.Y.
3. **Armitage, R. J., W. C. Fanslow, L. Strockbine, T. A. Sato, K. N. Clifford, B. M. Macduff, D. M. Anderson, S. D. Gimpel, T. Davis-Smith, C. R. Maliszewski, E. A. Clark, C. A. Smith, K. H. Grabstein, D. Cosman, and M. K. Spriggs.** 1992. Molecular and biological characterization of a murine ligand for CD40. *Nature* **357:** 80–82.
4. **Azimzadeh, A., C. Meyer, H. Watier, J. P. Beller, M. P. Chenard-Neu, R. Kieny, K. Boudjema, D. Jaeck, J. Cinqalbre, and P. Wolf.** 1998. Removal of primate xenoreactive natural antibodies by extracorporeal perfusion of pig kidneys and livers. *Transplant. Immunol.* **1:**13–22.
5. **Bach, F. H., H. Winkler, C. Ferran, W. W. Hancock, and S. C. Robson. 1996.** Delayed xenograft rejection. *Immunol. Today* **17:**379–384.
6. **Bracy, J. L., D. H. Sachs, and J. Iacomini.** 1998. Inhibition of xenoreactive natural antibody production by retroviral gene therapy. *Science* **281:**1845–1847.
7. **Bühler, L., M. Awwad, M. Basker, S. Gojo, A. Watts, S. Treter, K. Nash, G. Oravec, Q. Chang, A. Thall, J. Down, M. Sykes, D. Andrews, R. Sackstein, M. White-Scharf, D. H. Sachs, and D. K. C. Cooper.** 2000. High-dose porcine hematopoietic cell transplantation combined with CD40 ligand blockade in baboons prevents an induced anti-pig humoral response. *Transplantation* **69:**2296–2304.
8. **Chan, D. V., and H. Auchincloss, Jr.** 1996. Human anti-pig cell-mediated cytotoxicity in vitro involves non-T as well as T cell components. *Xenotransplantation* **3:**158–165.
9. **Chrupcala, M., S. Pomer, G. Staehler, R. Waldherr, and C. Kirschfink.** 1994. Prolongation of discordant renal xenograft survival by depletion of complement. Comparative effects of systemically administered cobra venom factor and soluble complement receptor type 1 in a guinea pig to rat model. *Transplant. Int.* **7:**S650.
10. **Cooper, D. K. C.** 1998. Xenoantigens and xenoantibodies. *Xenotransplantation* **5:**6–17.
11. **Cooper, D. K. C., T. D. H. Cairns, and D. H. Taube.** 1996. Extracorporeal immunoadsorption of anti-pig antibody in baboons using αGal oligosaccharide immunoaffinity columns. *Xeno* **4:**27–29.
12. **Cooper, D. K. C., P. A. Human, G. Lexer, A. G. Rose, J. Rees, M. Keraan, and E. Dutoit.** 1988. Effects of cyclosporine and antibody adsorption on pig cardiac xenograft survival in the baboon. *J. Heart Lung Transplant.* **7:**238–246.
13. **Cooper, D. K. C., E. Koren, and R. Oriol.** 1993. Genetically-engineered pigs. *Lancet* **342:**682–683.
14. **Cooper, D. K. C., E. Koren, and R. Oriol.** 1994. Oligosaccharides and discordant xenotransplantation. *Immunol. Rev.* **141:** 31–58.
15. **Cooper, D. K. C., E. Koren, and R. Oriol.** 1996. Manipulation of the anti-αGal antibody-αGal epitope system in experimental discordant xenotransplantation. *Xenotransplantation* **3:**102–111.
16. **Cozzi, E., and D. J. G. White.** 1995. The generation of transgenic pigs as potential organ donors for humans. *Nature Med.* **1:**964–966.
17. **Cozzi, E., N. Yannoutsos, G. A. Langford, G. Pino-Chavez, J. Wallwork, and D. J. G. White.** 1997. Effect of transgenic expression of human decay-accelerating factor on the inhibition of hyperacute rejection of pig organs, p. 665–682. *In* D. K. C. Cooper, E. Kemp, J. L. Platt, and D. J. G. White (ed.), *Xenotransplantation*, 2nd ed. Springer, Heidelberg, Germany.
18. **DeMarco, T., L. Damon, B. Colombe, F. Keigh, K. Chatterjee, and M. Garovoy.** 1997. Successful immunomodulation with intravenous gamma globulin and cyclophosphamide in an alloimmunized heart transplant recipient. *J. Heart Lung Transplant.* **16:**360–365.
19. **Dwyer, J. M.** 1987. Intravenous therapy with gamma globulin. *Adv. Intern. Med.* **32:**111–135.
20. **Dwyer, J. M.** 1992. Manipulating the immune system with immune globulin. *N. Engl. J. Med.* **326:**107–116.

21. **Elwood, E. T., C. P. Larsen, H. R. Cho, M. Corbascio, S. C. Ritchie, D. Z. Alexander, C. Tucker-Burden, P. S. Linsley, A. Aruffo, D. Hollenbaugh, K. J. Winn, and T. C. Pearson**. 1998. Prolonged acceptance of concordant and discordant xenografts with combined CD40 and CD28 pathway blockade. *Transplantation* **65:**1422–1428.
22. **Galili, U.** 1997. Anti-αgalactosyl (anti-Gal) damage beyond hyperacute rejection, p. 95–103. *In* D. K. C. Cooper, E. Kemp, J. L. Platt, and D. J. G. White (ed.), *Xenotransplantation*, 2nd ed. Springer, Heidelberg, Germany.
23. **Galili, U., D. C. Latemple, A. W. Walgenbach, and K. R. Stone**. 1997. Porcine and bovine cartilage transplants in cynomolgus monkeys: II. Changes in anti-gal response during chronic rejection. *Transplantation* **63:**646–651.
24. **Galili, U., S. B. Shohet, E. Kobrin, C. L. M. Stults, and B. A. Macher.** 1988. Man, apes and Old World monkeys differ from other mammals in the expression of αgalactosyl epitopes on nucleated cells. *J. Biol. Chem.* **263:**17755–17762.
25. **Gautreau, C., T. Kojima, G. Woimant, J. Cardoso, P. H. Devillier, and D. Houssin.** 1995. Use of intravenous immunoglobulin to delay xenogeneic hyperacute rejection. An in vivo and in vitro evaluation. *Transplantation* **60:**903–907.
26. **Glotz, D., J. Haymann, N. Sansonetti, A. Francois, V. Menoyo-Calonge, J. Bariety, and P. Druet.** 1993. Suppression of HLA-specific alloantibodies by high-dose intravenous immunoglobulins (IVIG). *Transplantation* **56:**335–337.
27. **Good, A. H., D. K. C. Cooper, A. J. Malcolm, R. M. Ippolito, E. Koren, F. A. Neethling, Y. Ye, N. Zuhdi, and L. R. Lamontagne.** 1992. Identification of carbohydrate structures which bind human anti-porcine antibodies: implications for discordant xenografting in man. *Transplant. Proc.* **24:**559–562.
28. **Hansch, G., C. H. Hammer, P. Vanguri, and M. L. Shin.** 1981. Homologous species restriction in lysis of erythrocytes by terminal complement proteins. *Proc. Natl. Acad. Sci. USA* **78:**5118–5121.
29. **Ierino, F. L., S. Gojo, P. T. Bajerjee, M. Giovino, Y. Xu, J. Gere, C. Kaynor, M. Awwad, R. Monroy, J. Rembert, T. Hatch, A. Foley, T. Kozlowski, K. Yamada, F. A. Neethling, J. Fishman, M. Bailin, R. R. Spitzer, D. K. C. Cooper, A. B. Cosimi, C. LeGuern, and D. H. Sachs.** 1999. Transfer of swine major histocompatibility complex class II genes into autologous bone marrow cells of baboons for the induction of tolerance across xenogeneic barriers. *Transplantation* **67:**1119–1128.
30. **Ish, C., G. L. Ong, N. Desai, and M. J. Mattes.** 1993. The specificity of alternative complement pathway-mediated lysis of erythrocytes: the survey of complement and target cells from 25 species. *Scand. J. Immunol.* **38:**113–122.
31. **Kaveri, S. V., G. Dietrich, V. Hurez, and M. D. Kazatchkine.** 1991. Intravenous immunoglobulins (IVIG) in the treatment of autoimmune diseases. *Clin. Exp. Immunol.* **86:**192.
32. **Kawai, T., A. B. Cosimi, R. B. Colvin, J. Powelson, J. Eason, T. Kozlowski, M. Sykes, R. Monroy, M. Tanaka, and D. S. Sachs.** 1995. Mixed allogeneic chimerism and renal allograft tolerance in cynomolgus monkeys. *Transplantation* **59:**256–262.
33. **Kirk, A. D., L. C. Burkly, D. S. Batty, R. E. Baumgartner, J. D. Berning, K. Buchanan, J. H. Fechner, R. L. Germond, R. L. Kampen, N. B. Patterson, S. J. Swanson, D. K. Tadaki, C. N. TenHor, L. White, S. J. Knechtle, and D. M. Harlan.** 1999. Treatment with humanized monoclonal antibody against CD154 prevents acute renal allograft rejection in nonhuman primates. *Nature Med.* **5:**686–693.
34. **Kirk, A. D., D. M. Harlan, N. N. Armstrong, T. A. Davis, Y. Dong, G. S. Gray, X. Hong, D. Thomas, J. H. Fechner, Jr., and S. J. Knechtle.** 1997. CTLA4-Ig and anti-CD40 ligand prevent renal allograft rejection in primates. *Proc. Natl. Acad. Sci. USA* **94:**8789–8794.
35. **Kobayashi, T., E. Kemp, and D. K. C. Cooper.** 1997. Prolongation of discordant xenograft survival by cobra venom factor, p. 425–436. *In* D. K. C. Cooper, E. Kemp, J. L. Platt, and D. J. G. White (ed.), *Xenotransplantation*, 2nd ed. Springer, Heidelberg, Germany.
36. **Kobayashi, T., F. A. Neethling, S. Taniguchi, Y. Ye, M. Niekrasz, E. Koren, W. W. Hancock, H. Takagi, and D. K. C. Cooper.** 1996. Investigation of the anti-complement agents, FUT-175 and K76COOH, in discordant xenotransplantation. *Xenotransplantation* **3:**237–245.
37. **Kobayashi, T., S. Taniguchi, F. A. Neethling, A. G. Rose, W. W. Hancock, Y. Ye, M. Niekrasz, S. Kosanke, L. J. Wright, D. J. G. White, and D. K. C. Cooper.** 1997. Delayed xenograft rejection of pig-to-baboon cardiac transplants after cobra venom factor therapy. *Transplantation* **64:**1255–1261.
38. **Koren, E., F. Milotec, F. A. Neethling, M. Koscec, D. Fei, T. Kobayashi, S. Taniguchi, and D. K. C. Cooper.** 1996. Monoclonal anti-idiotypic antibodies neutralize cytotoxic effects of anti-αGal antibodies. *Transplantation* **62:**837–843.

39. **Kozlowski, T., F. L. Ierino, D. Lambrigts, A. Foley, D. Andrews, M. Awwad, R. Monroy, A. B. Cosimi, D. K. C. Cooper, and D. H. Sachs.** 1998. Depletion of anti-αGal1-3Gal antibody in baboons by specific immunoaffinity columns. *Xenotransplantation* **5:**122–131.

40. **Kozlowski, T., R. Monroy, Y. Xu, T. Glaser, M. Awwad, D. K. C. Cooper, and D. H. Sachs.** 1998. Anti-αGal antibody response to porcine bone marrow in unmodified baboons and baboons conditioned for tolerance induction. *Transplantation* **66:**176–182.

41. **Kozlowski, T., A. Shimizu, D. Lambrigts, K. Yamada, Y. Fuchimoto, R. Glaser, R. Monroy, Y. Xu, M. Awwad, R. B. Colvin, A. B. Cosimi, S. C. Robson, J. Fishman, T. R. Spitzer, D. K. C Cooper, and D. H. Sachs.** 1999. Porcine kidney and heart transplantation in baboons undergoing a tolerance induction regimen and antibody adsorption. *Transplantation* **67:**18–30.

42. **Lambrigts, D., D. H. Sachs, and D. K. C. Cooper.** 1998. Discordant organ xenotransplantation in primates—world experience and current status. *Transplantation* **66:**547–561.

43. **Lambrigts, D., P. Van Calster, X. Xu, M. Awwad, F. A. Neethling, T. Kozlowski, A. Foley, A. Watts, S. J. Chae, J. Fishman, A. D. Thall, M. E. White-Scharf, D. H. Sachs, and D. K. C. Cooper.** 1998. Pharmacologic immunosuppressive therapy and extracorporeal immunoadsorption in the suppression of anti-αGal antibody in the baboon. *Xenotransplantation* **5:**274–283.

44. **Larsen, C. P., E. T. Elwood, D. Z. Alexander, S. C. Ritchie, R. Hendrix, C. Tucker-Burden, H. R. Cho, A. Aruffo, D. Hollenbaugh, P. S. Linsley, K. J. Winn, and T. C. Pearson.** 1996. Long-term acceptance of skin and cardiac allografts after blocking CD40 ligand. *Nature* **381:**434–438.

45. **Latinne, D., P. Gianello, C. V. Smith, V. Nickeleit, T. Kawai, M. Beadle, C. Haug, M. Sykes, E. Lebowitz, H. Bazin, R. Colvin, A. B. Cosimi, and D. H. Sachs.** 1993. Xenotransplantation from pig to cynomolgus monkey: an approach toward tolerance induction. *Transplant. Proc.* **250:**336–338.

46. **Leventhal, J. R., A. P. Dalmasso, J. W. Cromwell, J. L. Platt, C. J. Manivel, R. M. Bolman III, and A. J. Matas.** 1993. Prolongation of cardiac xenograft survival by depletion of complement. *Transplantation* **55:**857–865.

47. **Lexer, G., D. K. C. Cooper, A. G. Rose, W. N. Wicomb, J. Rees, M. Keraan, and E. Du Toit.** 1986. Hyperacute rejection in a discordant (pig-to-baboon) cardiac xenograft model. *J. Heart Transplant.* **5:**411–418.

48. **Lin, S. S., B. C. Weidner, G. W. Byrne, L. E. Diamond, J. H. Lawson, C. W. Hoopes, L. J. Daniels, C. W. Daggett, W. Parker, R. C. Harland, R. D. Davis, R. R. Bollinger, J. S. Logan, and J. L. Platt.** 1998. The role of antibodies in acute vascular rejection of pig-to-baboon cardiac transplants. *J. Clin. Invest.* **101:**1745–1756.

49. **Macchiarini, P., R. Oriol, A. Azimzadeh, V. De Montpreville, R. Rieben, N. Bovin, M. Mazmanian, and P. Dartevelle.** 1998. Evidence of human non-alpha-galactosyl antibodies involved in the hyperacute rejection of pig lungs and their removal by pig organ perfusion. *J. Thorac. Cardiovasc. Surg.* **5:**831–843.

50. **Magee, J. C., B. H. Collins, R. C. Harland, B. J. Lindman, R. R. Bollinger, M. M. Frank, and J. L. Platt.** 1995. Immunoglobulin prevents complement-mediated hyperacute rejection in swine-to-primate xenotransplantation. *J. Clin. Invest.* **96:**2404–2412.

51. **Marsh, H. C., and U. S. Ryan.** 1997. The therapeutic effect of soluble complement receptor type I (sCR1) in xenotransplantation, p. 437–455. *In* D. K. C. Cooper, E. Kemp, J. L. Platt, and D. J. G. White (ed.), *Xenotransplantation*, 2nd ed. Springer, Heidelberg, Germany.

52. **McCurry, K. R., D. L. Kooyman, C. G. Alvarado, A. H. Cotterell, M. J. Martin, J. S. Logan, and J. L. Platt.** 1995. Human complement regulatory proteins protect swine-to-primate cardiac xenografts from humoral injury. *Nature Med.* **1:**423–427.

53. **McIntyre, J., N. Higgins, R. Britton, S. Faucett, S. Johnson, D. Beckman, D. Hormuth, J. Fehrenbacher, and H. Halbrook.** 1996. Utilization of intravenous immunoglobulin to ameliorate alloantibodies in a highly sensitized patient with a cardiac assist device awaiting heart transplantation. *Transplantation* **62:**691–693.

54. **Moberg, A. W., A. R. Shons, H. Gerwurz, M. Mozes, and J. S. Najarian.** 1971. Prolongation of renal xenografts by the simultaneous sequestration of preformed antibody, inhibition of complement, coagulation, and antibody synthesis. *Transplant. Proc.* **3:**538–541.

55. **Moses, R. D., and H. Auchincloss.** 1997. Mechanism of cellular xenograft rejection, p. 140–174. *In* D. K. C. Cooper, E. Kemp, J. L. Platt, and D. J. G. White (ed.), *Xenotransplantation*, 2nd ed. Springer, Heidelberg, Germany.

56. **Murray, A. G., M. M. Khodadoust, J. S. Pober, and A. L. Rothwell.** 1994. Porcine aortic endothelial cells activate human T cells: direct presentation of MHC antigens and costimulation by ligands for human CD2 and CD28. *Immunity* **1:**57–63.

57. **Noelle, R., M. Roy, D. Shepherd, I. Stamenkovic, J. Ledbetter, and A. Aruffo.** 1992. A 39-kDa protein on activated helper T cells binds CD40 and transduces the signal for cognate activation of B cells. *Proc. Natl. Acad. Sci. USA* **89:**6550–6554.
58. **Oriol, R., Y. Ye, E. Koren, and D. K. C. Cooper.** 1993. Carbohydrate antigens of pig tissues reacting with human natural antibodies as potential targets for hyperacute vascular rejection in pig-to-man organ xenotransplantation. *Transplantation* **56:**1433–1442.
59. **Ostlie, D. J., E. Cozzi, C. M. Vial, F. N. K. Bhatti, G. Pino-Chavez, S. Thiru, B. Soin, D. J. G. White, and P. J. Friend.** 1999. Improved renal function and fewer rejection episodes using SDZ RAD in life-supporting hDAF pig-to-primate renal xenotransplantation. *Abstr. Am. Soc. Transplant.*
60. **Palmer, A., D. Taube, K. Welsh, M. Bewick, P. Gjorstrup, and M. Thick.** 1989. Removal of HLA antibodies by extracorporeal immunoadsorption to enable renal transplantation. *Lancet* **i:**10–12.
61. **Perper R. J., and J. S. Najarian.** 1966. Experimental renal heterotransplantation. I. In widely divergent species. *Transplantation* **4:**377–388.
62. **Pretagostini, R., P. Berloco, L. Poli, P. Cinti, A. Di Nicuolo, P. De Simone, M. Colonnello, A. Salerno, D. Alfani, and R. Cortesini.** 1996. Immunoadsorption with protein A in humoral rejection of kidney transplants. *ASAIO Journal* **42:**M645–M648.
63. **Pruitt, S. K., W. M. Baldwin, H. C. Marsh, Jr., S. S. Lin, C. G. Yeh, and R. R. Bollinger.** 1991. The effect of soluble complement receptor type 1 on hyperacute xenograft rejection. *Transplantation* **52:**868–873.
64. **Pruitt, S. K., A. D. Kirk, R. R. Bollinger, H. C. Marsh, Jr., B. H. Collins, J. L. Levin, J. R. Mault, J. S. Heinle, S. Ibrahim, and A. R. Rudolph.** 1994. The effect of soluble complement receptor type 1 on hyperacute rejection of porcine xenografts. *Transplantation* **57:**363–370.
65. **Reed, E., M. Hardy, A. Benvenisty, C. Lattes, J. Brensilver, R. McCabe, K. Reemstma, D. W. King, and N. Suciu-Foca.** 1987. Effect of antiidiotypic antibody to HLA on graft survival in renal allograft recipients. *N. Engl. J. Med.* **316:**1450–1455.
66. **Romano, E., F. A. Neethling, K. Nilsson, S. Kosanke, A. Shimizu, S. Magnusson, L. Svensson, B. Samuelsson, and D. K. C. Cooper.** 1999. Intravenous synthetic αGal saccharides delay hyperacute rejection of a pig-to-baboon heart transplant. *Xenotransplantation* **6:**36–42.
67. **Rossi, F., G. Dietrich, and M. D. Kazatchkine.** 1989. Antiidiotypic suppression of autoantibodies with normal polyspecific immunoglobulins. *Res. Immunol.* **140:**19–31.
68. **Sablinski, T., D. Latinne, P. Gianello, M. Bailin, K. Bergen, R. B. Colvin, A. Foley, H. Z. Hong, S. Meehan, R. Monroy, J. A. Powelson, M. Sykes, M. Tanaka, A. B. Cosimi, and D. H. Sachs.** 1995. Xenotransplantation of pig kidneys to nonhuman primates: I. Development of the model. *Xenotransplantation* **2:**264–270.
69. **Sachs, S. H., G. Leight, J. Cone, S. Schwarz, L. Stuart, and S. Rosenberg.** 1976. Transplantation in miniature swine. I. Fixation of the major histocompatibility complex. *Transplantation* **22:**559–567.
70. **Sandrin, M. S., S. Cohney, N. Osman, and I. F. C. McKenzie.** 1997. Overcoming the anti-Galα1-3Gal reaction to avoid hyperacute rejection: molecular genetic approaches, p. 683–700. *In* D. K. C. Cooper, E. Kemp, J. L. Platt, and D. J. G. White (ed.), *Xenotransplantation*, 2nd ed. Springer, Heidelberg, Germany.
71. **Sandrin, M. S., W. L. Fodor, E. Mouhtouris, N. Osman, S. Cohney, S. A. Rollins, E. R. Guilmette, E. Setter, S. P. Squinto, and I. F. C. McKenzie.** 1995. Enzymatic remodeling of the carbohydrate surface of a xenogenic cell substantially reduces human antibody binding and complement-mediated cytolysis. *Nature Med.* **1:**1261–1267.
72. **Schmoeckel, M., F. N. K. Bhatti, A. Zaidi, E. Cozzi, P. D. Waterworth, M. J. Tolan, M. Goddard, R. G. Warner, G. A. Langford, J. J. Dunning, J. Wallwork, and D. J. G. White.** 1998. Orthotopic heart transplantation in a transgenic pig-to-primate model. *Transplantation* **65:**1570–1577.
73. **Sharabi, Y., V. S. Abraham, M. Sykes, and D. H. Sachs.** 1992. Mixed allogeneic chimeras prepared by a non-myeloablative regimen: requirement for chimerism to maintain tolerance. *Bone Marrow Transplant.* **9:**191–197.
74. **Sharabi, Y., I. Aksentijevich, T. M. Sundt III, D. H. Sachs, and M. Sykes.** 1990. Specific tolerance induction across a xenogeneic barrier: production of mixed rat/mouse lymphohematopoietic chimeras using a nonlethal preparative regimen. *J. Exp. Med.* **172:**195–202.
75. **Shons, A. R., M. Beir, J. Jetzer, and J. S. Najarian.** 1973. Techniques of in vivo plasma modification for the treatment of hyperacute rejection. *Surgery* **73:**28–37.
76. **Simon, P., F. A. Neethling, S. Taniguchi, P. L. Good, D. Zopf, W. W. Hancock, and D. K. C. Cooper.** 1998. Intravenous infusion of αGal oligosaccharides in baboons delays hyperacute rejection of porcine heart xenografts. *Transplantation* **65:**346–353.

77. **Slapak, M., M. Greenbaum, W. Bardawil, C. Saravis, J. Joison, and W. V. McDermott, Jr.** 1971. Effect of heparin, arvin, liver perfusion, and heterologous antiplatelet serum on rejection of pig kidney to dog. *Transplant. Proc.* **3:**558–561.
78. **Taniguchi, S., F. A. Neethling, E. Y. Korchagina, N. Bovin, Y. Ye, T. Kobayashi, M. Niekrasz, S. Li, E. Koren, R. Oriol, and D. K. C. Cooper.** 1996. In vivo immunoadsorption of antipig antibodies in baboons using a specific Galα1-3Gal column. *Transplantation* **10:**1379–1384.
79. **Terman, D. S., R. Garcia-Rinaldi, R. McCalmon, C. C. Crumb, C. Mattioli, G. Cook, and R. Poser.** 1979. Modification of hyperacute renal xenograft rejection after extracorporeal immunoadsorption of heterospecific antibody. *Int. J. Artif. Organs* **2:**35–41.
80. **Tyan, D., V. A. Li, L. Czer, A. Trento, and S. Jordan.** 1994. Intravenous immunoglobulin suppression of HLA alloantibody in highly sensitized transplant candidates and transplantation with a histoincompatible organ. *Transplantation* **57:**553–562.
81. **Vial, C. M., D. H. Ostlie, E. Cozzi, G. Pino-Chavez, S. Thiru, D. J. G. White, and P. J. Friend.** 1999. Mycophenolic acid-sodium (ERL080) permits prolonged function in hDAF pig-to-primate renal xenotransplantation. *Abstr. Am. Soc. Transplant Surgeons.*
82. **Weisman, H. F., T. Bartow, M. K. Leppo, H. C. Marsh, Jr., G. R. Carson, M. F. Concino, M. P. Boyle, K. H. Roux, M. L. Weisfeldt, and D. T. Fearon.** 1990. Soluble human complement receptor type 1: in vivo inhibitor of complement suppressing post-ischemic myocardial inflammation and necrosis. *Science* **249:**146–151.
83. **Wekerle, T., M. H. Sayegh, J. Hill, Y. Zhao, A. Chandraker, K. G. Swenson, G. Zhao, and M. Sykes.** 1998. Extrathymic T cell deletion and allogeneic stem cell engraftment induced with costimulatory blockade is followed by central T cell tolerance. *J. Exp. Med.* **187:**2037–2044.
84. **White, D. J. G., G. A. Langford, E. Cozzi, and V. J. Young.** 1995. Production of pigs transgenic for human DAF. A strategy for xenotransplantation. *Xenotransplantation* **2:**213–217.
85. **Wilmut, I., A. E. Schnieke, J. McWhir, A. J. Kind, and K. H. Campbell.** 1997. Viable offspring derived from fetal and adult mammalian cells. *Nature* **385:**810–813.
86. **Xia, W., D. T. Fearon, and R. L. Kirkman.** 1993. Effect of repetitive doses of soluble human complement receptor type 1 on survival of discordant cardiac xenografts. *Transplant. Proc.* **25:**410–411.
87. **Xu, Y., T. Lorf, T. Sablinski, P. Gianello, M. Bailin, R. Monroy, T. Kozlowski, M. Awwad, D. K. C. Cooper, and D. H. Sachs.** 1998. Removal of anti-porcine natural antibodies from human and nonhuman primate plasma in vitro and in vivo by a Galα1-3Galβ1-4Glc-X immunoaffinity column. *Transplantation* **65:**172–179.
88. **Yamada, K., D. H. Sachs, and H. DerSimonian.** 1995. The human anti-porcine xenogeneic T-cell response: evidence for allelic specificity of MLR and for both direct and indirect pathways of recognition. *J. Immunol.* **155:**5249–5256.
89. **Yamada, K., J. D. Seebach, H. DerSimonian, and D. H. Sachs.** 1996. Human anti-pig T-cell mediated cytotoxicity. *Xenotransplantation* **3:**179–187.
90. **Yang, Y. G., E. DeGoma, H. Ohdan, J. L. Bracy, Y. Xu, J. Iacomini, A. D. Thall, and M. Sykes.** 1998. Tolerization of anti-Galα1-3Gal natural antibody-forming B cells by induction of mixed chimerism. *J. Exp. Med.* **187:**1335–1342.
91. **Ye, Y., F. A. Neethling. M. Niekrasz, E. Koren, S. V. Richards, M. Martin, S. Kosanke, R. Oriol, and D. K. C. Cooper.** 1994. Evidence that intravenously administered alpha-galactosyl carbohydrates reduce baboon serum cytotoxicity to pig kidney cells (PK15) and transplanted pig hearts. *Transplantation* **58:**330–337.
92. **Zaidi, A., M. Schmoeckel, F. N. K. Bhatti, P. D. Watterworth, M. J. Tolan, E. Cozzi, G. Chavez, G. A. Langford, S. Thiru, J. Wallwork, D. J. G. White, and P. Friend.** 1998. Life-supporting pig-to-primate renal xenotransplantation using genetically modified donors. *Transplantation* **65:**1584–1590.

Section III

IMPACT OF THERAPEUTIC MANIPULATIONS ON THE HOST RESPONSE TO INFECTION

Xenotransplantation
Edited by Jeffrey L. Platt

Chapter 7

Manipulation of the Humoral Immune System and the Host Immune Response to Infection

Eric Wagner and Michael M. Frank

The humoral immune system comprises elements that, in part, provide protection against invading organisms. Indeed, the early years of immunology focused on the bactericidal activity of human and animal sera (117). Factors in serum were soon identified that interacted with bacterial strains and prevented their infectivity (93). These factors were characterized and ultimately named antibody and complement. Cellular mechanisms were also identified as important in the host defense against infectious agents. It was assumed in these early studies that a decrease or inhibition of antibodies or complement function would affect natural protection against infection.

As discussed in detail elsewhere, discordant xenotransplantation using porcine organs in human transplant recipients is viewed by many as the most promising alternative to allotransplantation. In the latter case, a dramatic organ shortage is a barrier to successful transplantation for disease that cannot be overcome (58, 95). However, the success of transplantation procedures that involve vascularized pig organs currently is extremely limited because of the efficiency of immune rejection. The first barrier to xenotransplantation, termed hyperacute rejection, appears within minutes after reperfusion of the grafted organ and consists of an intense inflammatory reaction with clotting of vessels that involves natural antibodies and complement activation (58, 95, 110). To avoid hyperacute rejection, it is tempting to lower or inhibit the amount of xenoreactive natural antibodies that react with porcine antigens and/or interfere with the complement system function (96).

Here we discuss the effects of manipulating the humoral immune system on the risk of developing microbial infections. Manipulations aimed at lowering the concentration of circulating antibodies and inhibiting fluid-phase complement activation will be reviewed in their relation to potential infectious risk.

Eric Wagner • Departments of Pediatrics and Surgery, Duke University Medical Center, Durham, NC 27710.
Michael M. Frank • Departments of Pediatrics and Immunology, Duke University Medical Center, Durham, NC 27710.

NATURAL ANTIBODIES

For many years, it has been known that a large fraction of circulating antibody in humans and animals appears not to be synthesized as a response to a sensitizing event but is the product of normally circulating cells (13, 75). One characteristic of a fraction of these natural antibodies is that they react with multiple unrelated antigens. They can react with antigens of bacterial, viral, fungal, protozoan, and self origin (6, 24). These antibodies, because of their ability to bind many different antigens, are termed polyreactive. Natural antibodies can be of IgM, IgG, or IgA isotype; the IgM isotype apparently represents the majority of natural antibodies (24). Antigens recognized by natural antibodies include proteins, polysaccharides, phospholipids, and nucleic acids. The affinity with which natural antibodies bind varies according to the antigen that is recognized and with the antibody itself (48). In humans, the source of most natural antibody is a subset of B cells termed the B-1 cells (6, 23, 24, 55, 69). Both B-1a cells ($CD5^{+}$) and B-1b cells ($CD5^{-}$, $CD45RA^{lo}$) are responsible for the synthesis of these antibodies. These B cells possess immunoglobulin genes that remain in the germline configuration (24). Although there is clear evidence for a preferential V_H gene usage by B-1a and B-1b cells that may correlate with polyreactivity of the synthesized antibodies, isotype class switch upon proper activation can occur (24).

The function of natural antibodies in humoral immunity is still not understood. Because of their ability to interact with a wide variety of infectious agents, many investigators believe that they play a role in primary defense against invasion of microorganisms (13, 23, 24). Numerous reports have documented the binding of natural antibodies to microorganisms. For example, natural antibodies are reported to react with bacteria such as anaerobic bacteria (119), *Haemophilus influenzae* (130), *Streptococcus mutans* (25), and bacterial products such as alkaline phosphatase (106) and β-galactosidase (48). Furthermore, natural antibodies exist that react with viruses such as HIV-1 (48), vesicular stomatitis virus (10), primate type C RNA viruses (4), and oncoviruses (118) among other viruses. Natural antibodies to parasites have been documented that neutralize these agents by enhancing phagocytosis (61). This natural antibody in theory can function to protect individuals in a number of ways. It may coat organisms directly and, by then interacting with phagocytes via Fc receptors, promote phagocytosis. It may activate complement, facilitating complement-mediated lysis or opsonization. It may facilitate clearance of the organism from the circulation by interacting with Fc receptors of the cells of the mononuclear phagocyte system or facilitate complement deposition with interaction with phagocyte complement receptors. Interestingly, one example of natural antibody function in protection against bacterial infection has been demonstrated in a murine model of X-linked immunodeficiency (15). Reconstitution of natural antiphosphatidylcholine antibodies found in normal mouse serum provided protection against type 3 *Streptococcus pneumoniae* in the immunoglobulin-deficient mice. Furthermore, using RAG-2−/− mice that lack serum immunoglobulin or Btk−/− mice that have reduced levels of IgG3 and IgM, Reid et al. demonstrated that these animals are more sensitive to endotoxic shock than normal mice and that introduction of purified normal mouse IgM as a source of natural antibody enhanced the ability of immunoglobulin-deficient mice to clear endotoxin (105).

A certain proportion of natural antibodies bind self antigens. To explain this phenomenon, it has been proposed that maintenance of homeostasis is an additional function of these antibodies. For example, recognition of exposed antigens on senescent cells and cellular debris by natural antibodies might allow for their proper clearance (94). Furthermore, it has been suggested recently that some natural antibodies have regulatory effects on various metabolic processes and cellular activities, thus protecting from critical physiologic errors (107).

There exist xenoreactive natural antibodies in humans and Old World primates that recognize the galα1-3gal epitope at the surface of porcine vascular endothelial cells and mediate hyperacute rejection of porcine xenografts. These antibodies belong to the family of natural antibodies that comprise isohemagglutinins and antibodies to blood group substances (92). These antibodies are clearly polyreactive and can recognize determinants expressed at the surface of enteric bacteria (45). A protective role of these antibodies against infection caused by the normal gut bacterial flora and parasites such as *Trypanosoma cruzi* and *Leishmania* sp. has been proposed (45), but clear physiological relevance of these potential properties of human xenoreactive natural antibodies has not been established. Nevertheless, it is interesting to note that Kearns-Jonker et al. recently demonstrated that rat monoclonal antibodies that react against porcine endothelial cells and partially block the binding of human xenoreactive natural antibodies to these cells are encoded by genes in germline configuration and share structural homologies with natural antibodies to infectious agents (57). Therefore, they proposed that xenoreactive natural antibodies are natural antibodies recognizing microbial antigens with cross-reactivity to other molecular structures that bear the galα1-3gal epitope. Whether the same is true with human xenoreactive natural antibodies remains to be studied.

It is clear that patients with severe immunoglobulin deficiency with associated deficiency of natural antibody are at increased risk of developing serious infections (121). Infectious agents associated with disease in antibody-deficient patients include gram-positive bacteria, viruses (139), and protozoa. Thus far, no patient has been described with a specific deficiency in the cell lines that produce natural antibody but with a normal adaptive immune response.

PLASMAPHERESIS

Methods that have been used to reduce the level of pathogenic antibodies from the circulation in a variety of immunologically mediated diseases include plasmapheresis and immunoadsorption (47, 114). These methods have been used to remove xenoreactive antibody as well. Details of the different techniques employed have been reviewed (47, 114) and will not be addressed here. Plasmapheresis (also called plasma exchange) has been utilized as a therapy for a limited number of immunological diseases that are caused by autoantibodies, including thrombocytic thrombocytopenia/hemolytic uremic syndrome, cryoglobulinemia, Goodpasture's syndrome, Guillain-Barré syndrome, and myasthenia gravis (122). Plasma is exchanged with a physiologic salt solution, allowing a reduction of circulating immunoglobulin. It has been estimated that 60% of intravascular immunoglobulin levels can be removed; however, only about 20% of total immunoglobulin is depleted during a 4-liter plasma exchange procedure (26). Therefore, repeated plasma exchanges are necessary to significantly lower the total immunoglobulin pool. Because immune complexes may be tissue-associated and usually are efficiently removed from the circulation by the mononuclear phagocyte system, plasmapheresis is more likely to be of use in diseases where circulating autoantibodies are present and often is not useful in immune complex–mediated diseases. As reviewed by Griffin et al. (47), plasmapheresis has several possible benefits. First, plasma exchange may remove a portion of pathogenic autoantibodies. Second, removal of some circulating immune complexes may be achieved by plasmapheresis, although it has almost no effect on tissue-bound immune complexes that may be formed in situ (87, 112). Third, in some instances, plasmapheresis may improve the clearance of immune complexes in patients in whom the function of the reticuloendothelial system is impaired. Removal of pathogenic autoantibodies in patients by means of plasmapheresis is often accompanied by immunosuppression with cyclophosphamide or other immunosuppressive agent in an attempt to inhibit de novo synthesis of antibody by autoantibody-secreting B cells. Therefore, comparative studies of the beneficial effect of plasmapheresis as a single therapy are difficult to perform and often not available.

IMMUNOADSORPTION

Plasmapheresis, in addition to depleting antibodies and immune complexes from the circulation, also depletes other plasma proteins such as coagulation factors and complement proteins. In some situations, this may be harmful, although the possibility is more theoretical than real. Although it may have an advantage in some inflammatory diseases (47), plasmapheresis is nonselective. Important protective antibodies may be removed at the same time as the antibody of interest. Therefore, more specific methods, such as specific immunoadsorption methods, have been developed to remove specific pathogenic antibodies. As reviewed recently (47, 114), immunoadsorbents have been developed that remove immunoglobulins nonspecifically or that remove specific antibodies selectively. Immunoadsorbent columns can absorb immunoglobulin nonspecifically via biochemical interaction (protein A, tryptophan, phenylalanine, C1q, IG-Therasorb) (114) or can remove specific antibody via interaction with a specific ligand (67). Immunoadsorption, in addition to being more selective than plasmapheresis, induces less hemodynamic alteration with less need for replacement fluid such as fresh frozen plasma or colloid (5% albumin). If the immunoadsorbent is specific for a pathogenic antibody, it is far more likely to leave essential protective antibodies in the circulation (47). Although immunoadsorption is often considered safe, it is important to note that many immunoadsorbants activate complement during the absorption procedure. There is evidence that immunoadsorption is often followed by a reduction of antibody levels to many antigens, and some have suggested that regulatory complement peptides like C3dg are released that downregulate antibody synthesis (2). In addition, the generation of anaphylatoxins such as C3a and C5a theoretically could induce a harmful inflammatory response. So far, there have been a few limited clinical trials of this type of therapy in cases of systemic lupus erythematosus, primary vasculitis, antiglomerular basement membrane-autoantibody syndromes (114), and transplant recipients with high levels of pre- and posttransplant antibodies (47). Its widespread application awaits controlled clinical trials.

Plasmapheresis and Immunoadsorption in Transplantation

Plasmapheresis and immunoadsorption have been used to remove natural and specific antibody in organ transplantation. It is known that vascularized organ allografting cannot be performed when the donor and recipient are ABO blood group-incompatible. Crossing the ABO barrier leads to hyperacute rejection. Furthermore, patients with prior history of sensitization to human antigens (previous grafts, blood transfusions, multiple pregnancies) often cannot receive transplants because of high levels of antibodies that may cross-react with donor antigens. Acute rejection of allografts is known to depend on the presence of anti-donor antibodies. Therefore, it is tempting to remove the pathogenic antibodies in these patients either nonspecifically by plasmapheresis or specifically to allow the transplanted graft to survive. Plasmapheresis has been used to remove isohemagglutinins from patients, allowing transplantation across the ABO blood group barrier of kidneys (52) and livers (36, 82), and to allow for kidney transplantation in highly sensitized patients (3). In addition, plasmapheresis has shown benefits in treating humoral rejection of kidney (86, 111) and heart (11, 90) allografts.

Immunoadsorption has been proposed to lower the level of donor-specific antibodies prior to transplantation in sensitized recipients or to treat antibody-mediated rejection of organ allografts. Adsorption of plasma IgG using protein A columns in presensitized recipients of both renal and cardiac allografts has been reported to be beneficial (49, 89, 101). Nevertheless, since immunosuppressive treatments with cyclophosphamide are often included to prevent the re-synthesis of harmful antibodies, it is difficult to assign a specific role to the immunoadsorption in the posttransplant period. It is also noteworthy that this approach to treatment has not yet reached widespread application in the clinical arena.

Because of the crucial role xenoreactive natural antibodies play in discordant vascularized xenograft rejection, their removal from the circulation by either plasmapheresis or immunoadsorption has been employed to better study their role and to prolong graft survival in animal models (30, 65, 67, 113, 127). In general, using these methods, investigators have proven the essential role of natural antibodies in inducing hyperacute xenograft rejection and have succeeded in significantly prolonging survival of the graft.

Infectious Risk of Plasmapheresis and Immunoadsorption

Both naturally occurring and elicited antibodies have an important role to play in the control of infectious agents. Therefore, removal of such antibodies from the circulation by means of plasmapheresis or even immunoadsorption might pose a risk for a patient. However, as with studies of graft survival, it is very difficult to assess the impact of plasmapheresis or immunoadsorption in patients who receive these therapies since they are often treated concomitantly with immunosuppressive drugs, such as cyclophosphamide, which themselves increase the risk of infection (47). The incidence of infection in patients treated with plasmapheresis alone has been reported to be very low, and it is considered an extremely safe procedure without serious side effects (47, 79, 97, 141). Nevertheless, a recent report has suggested that plasmapheresis added to immunosuppressive therapy increases the risk of serious bacterial and viral infections as compared to immunosuppression alone (5). Although there is general agreement that plasmapheresis alone does not increase the infectious risk per se, the addition of antibiotics following plasmapheresis has been recommended in certain cases, such as plasmapheresis in septic shock to avoid multiorgan failure (120).

COMPLEMENT

The complement system is one element of innate immunity comprising more than 20 proteins that interact to mediate or regulate its biological effects. It appears that a principal function of the complement system is to mediate destruction of invading organisms, but it clearly functions in many different aspects of natural and acquired immunity. A detailed description of the system is beyond the scope of this chapter, and the reader is referred to excellent reviews (42, 83, 133). The importance of the system in host defense against microorganisms has been recognized since the early days of immunology, and activation in response to microbial infection has been shown to have several effects. (i) The triggering of complement activation can lead to direct lysis of the target. (ii) Often, complement binding by microorganisms leads to opsonization, a process in which fragments of complement components bound to the target can interact with specific receptors on phagocytes, thus inducing phagocytosis. (iii) Complement activation leads to the release of small peptides that have proinflammatory properties. Among these are the "anaphylatoxins," molecules that induce an anaphylactic response. Therefore, complement activation is not only limited to the direct killing of invading organisms but also induces a potent inflammatory response to increase the efficiency of microbe elimination.

Complement can be activated via three main pathways: the classical pathway, the lectin pathway, and the alternative pathway (Fig. 1). The classical pathway usually requires the presence of an antibody–antigen complex for activation. The lectin pathway is activated by the binding of mannan-binding lectin to the appropriate carbohydrate moiety on a target organism. The binding of mannan-binding lectin recruits two circulating proteases, mannan-binding lectin-associated serine proteases 1 and 2, that in turn activate the classical and alternative complement pathways. The alternative pathway can be activated directly on molecular structures that allow interaction with the hydrolyzed form of the third component of complement (C3) or can be activated by antibodies binding to a microbial target. Complement can be activated by other "nonclassical" means that appear to be important in host defense against microorganisms. We will review briefly the mechanisms by which microorganisms can be eliminated by products of the complement cascade.

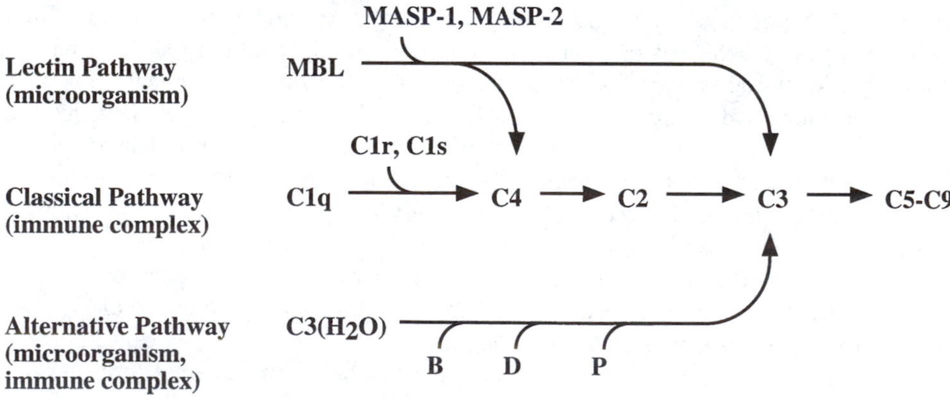

Figure 1. Pathways of complement activation. Activators of complement such as microorganisms and antigen–antibody complexes bind the first component of each pathway to initiate activation of the entire cascade. Reactions beyond C3 activation are common to all three pathways and result in the formation of the C5–9 complex known as the membrane attack complex. C, complement component; MBL, mannan-binding lectin; MASP, mannan-binding lectin-associated serine protease; C3(H_2O), C3 that underwent spontaneous hydrolysis of its thiolester group; B, factor B; D, factor D; P, properdin.

Interaction of Complement with Microorganisms

In the absence of antibody, the alternative pathway can be directly activated on the surface of a variety of bacteria, viruses, fungi, parasites, and virally infected cells (91). Activation of the alternative pathway usually proceeds without any initiating factor. However, its activation can be augmented by IgG (81) or triggered by IgA (142) or mannan-binding lectin (116, 123). On microbial surfaces, alternative pathway activation is triggered by the interaction of amino or hydroxyl groups present on proteins or carbohydrates and the thiolester present in the α chain of the two-chain molecule of C3, when the thiolester group undergoes spontaneous hydrolysis (91). This interaction favors the formation and amplification of the alternative pathway C3 convertase, an enzymatic complex that leads to efficient alternative pathway complement activation. As stated above, many microorganisms activate the alternative pathway. In general, most gram-positive and gram-negative bacteria activate this pathway (43). Whereas teichoic acid of gram-positive bacterial cell walls is the main target for alternative pathway activation, lipopolysaccharide plays this role in gram-negative bacteria. The assembly of the membrane attack complex upon completion of complement activation generates lesions that induce cell death via membrane pore formation and osmotic imbalance in several model systems studied. However, cell death is not the end result for a number of bacteria on which complement is activated. Indeed, the thickness of the peptidoglycan layer of gram-positive bacteria ($\sim$20 nm) interferes with the lytic activity of the membrane attack complex. Therefore, gram-positive bacteria are generally not susceptible to bacteriolysis induced by direct complement activation (43). In addition, the long chain of the O-polysaccharide linked to lipid A in lipopolysaccharide confers resistance to complement-mediated bacterial killing by allowing sites of complement activation far from the bacterial cell membrane (93). Encapsulation of both gram-positive and gram-negative bacteria may provide additional protection against the bactericidal activity of complement. Even in susceptible organisms, the precise mechanism of complement-mediated killing is unknown. To be killed, the organisms must be in log phase growth, and in the case of bacteria, it is not clear that organisms die because of osmotic disequilibrium.

If bacterial lysis does not occur, bacteria can still be eliminated by phagocytes of the reticuloendothelial system via interaction of complement cleavage peptides such as C3b or iC3b with specific complement receptors on phagocytic cells. It is believed that this opsonic function of complement is far more important than direct lysis. A wide variety of viral particles, either enveloped or nonenveloped, can activate the alternative pathway, leading to deposition of huge amounts of C3 on the viral surface. In addition, it has been shown that the binding of complement proteins to the viral surface may in some instances cause direct viral neutralization (27). In addition to bacteria and viruses, many pathogenic fungi such as *Cryptococcus neoformans* and *Candida albicans* have the capacity to activate the alternative pathway (62).

Some microorganisms activate the classical pathway directly, even in the absence of specific antibody. C1q appears to bind directly to lipopolysaccharide of many bacteria. In addition, binding of C1q occurs on outer membrane proteins of some bacterial strains such as *Salmonella minnesota*, *Legionella pneumophila*, and *Klebsiella pneumoniae* (93). A number of viruses have also been shown to activate complement via the classical pathway without antibody requirement (27). Although specific antibody may not be required for complement activation on a number of microorganisms, its presence greatly amplifies the efficiency of complement activation. Interestingly, many microorganisms have evolved means to evade direct complement attack (39). The ability to form antibody is particularly valuable in the elimination of these infectious agents. It has been shown that the fine specificity of the antibody dictates the exact location of complement activation and its lytic activity. Indeed, even if different antibodies react efficiently with the same bacterium and induce the binding of the same numbers of complement molecules, some may lead to bacteriolysis whereas others may confer protection (44).

Two acute-phase proteins have the potential to activate complement on the surface of microorganisms, namely C-reactive protein and mannan-binding lectin. C-reactive protein was initially shown to bind to phosphorylcholine present in type C polysaccharide of the cell wall and membrane of *S. pneumoniae* and activate complement upon binding (56). Activation of components of the classical pathway results from the binding of C-reactive protein to its substrate. The importance of C-reactive protein-mediated complement activation in protection against *S. pneumoniae* infection has been shown in a mouse model (51, 125). Mannan-binding lectin is an acute-phase protein that appears to be a crucial initiator of complement activation during the first years of life, before adaptive immunity and immunological memory are established. Mannan-binding lectin is a calcium-dependent lectin that reacts with terminal carbohydrates as they are expressed on microbial surfaces such as mannose, fucose, glucose, and N-acetyl-glucosamine (34). It is structurally related to C1q and reacts with a variety of gram-negative bacteria, gram-positive bacteria, viruses, yeasts, mycobacteria, parasites, and protozoa (34, 131). As stated above, it can activate the alternative pathway but also activates the classical pathway via an interaction with C1r and C1s or specific C1-like serine proteases termed mannan-binding lectin-associated serine proteases 1 and 2 (73, 128).

Role of Complement in Infectious Diseases

The role complement plays in the control of various infections has been investigated using two main approaches. First, animals genetically deficient in one complement protein have been examined for defects in control of infectious agents (12, 41). The second approach uses complement-activating agents such as cobra venom factor to deplete components of the classical and alternative pathways. Cobra venom factor is a human C3 analog that activates the alternative pathway and depletes serum of many of the late-acting complement components (132). Treated animals have circulating complement activation peptides. Nevertheless, they have been used widely to study the effect of complement on the control of infectious agents. Several animal models in which cobra venom factor was employed demonstrate the importance of complement activation in resistance against infections. These include models of resistance to bacteria (1, 17, 18, 77, 115), viruses (50, 88), parasites (20, 46, 66), and fungi (62). C4-deficient guinea pigs have also been used in studies of resistance to microbial infection. Discrimination between the alternative pathway and the classical pathway is possible since these animals have a block in the classical pathway and an intact alternative pathway. Using C4-deficient guinea pigs, it was shown that the alternative pathway is crucial in protection against some bacterial (19) and fungal infectious agents (62). The use of these animals demonstrates the importance of the classical pathway in optimal clearance of bacteria from the bloodstream (19), but the alternative pathway was able to allow for survival of the animal. Recently, C3 and C4 knockout mice have been generated. Both types of complement-deficient mice showed increased sensitivity to endotoxic shock as compared to normal mice (40), further demonstrating the importance of the complement system in the clearance of bacteria and bacterial products. This observation was also reported some years ago using C4-deficient guinea pigs (74).

Perhaps the most striking evidence of a role of complement in defense against microbial agents comes from following the clinical course of individuals genetically deficient in one complement component. Patients deficient in one of the early classical pathway components (C1, C4, C2) usually have relatively low rates of recurrent bacterial infections. However, patients with deficiencies of components of the alternative pathway (factor D, properdin), C3, components of the membrane attack complex (C5, C6, C7, C8, C9), or proteins that regulate complement activation by cleaving C3 (factor H, factor I) show a high incidence of infections (32, 38). A very high prevalence of infections of the sinopulmonary tree prevails in these individuals. *Neisseria meningitidis* infection occurs frequently in complement-deficient patients, particularly patients with deficiency of C5–C8, further demonstrating the sensitivity of this bacterial strain to the lytic action of complement. This also demonstrates that opsonization alone is not sufficient to eliminate some bacterial strains. *S. pneumoniae* infection develops frequently in patients lacking one of the early classical pathway components or C3.

Role of Complement in Transplantation

One major hurdle to successful pig-to-human or pig-to-non-human primate vascularized organ transplantation is hyperacute rejection, which depends on classical complement pathway activation (28, 95). The classical complement pathway may as well be involved in acute vascular rejection of xenografts (96). The importance of this system was clearly demonstrated using agents that deplete complement or control complement activation. For example, blockade of complement activation using such agents as cobra venom factor (64), soluble complement receptor type 1 (22, 102), synthetic inhibitors (78), C1 inhibitor (29), or antibodies to complement components (109) prolongs xenograft survival in animal models and prevents cellular damage in in vitro systems. The use of C6-deficient rats further demonstrates the importance of the complement system in the initiation of hyperacute rejection of cardiac xenografts (53).

Except in presensitized patients (donor-recipient ABO blood group incompatibility, or sensitizing events preceding transplantation in the recipient, both leading to hyperacute allograft rejection), the precise role that complement plays in the rejection of allografts has been unclear. Prolonged cardiac allograft survival in C6-deficient rats when compared to normal animals has been reported (14, 104). Furthermore, using soluble complement receptor type 1 in rat renal allotransplantation experiments, Sacks' group showed prolonged graft survival as well as impaired alloantibody responses in recipients, suggesting a role for complement in the rejection of allografts (99, 100). In addition, C3 and C4 knockout mice have prolonged skin allograft survival as compared to normal animals (72). Alloantibody production is also significantly impaired in these complement-deficient mice. Even though these reports suggest that complement is important in allograft rejection, the focus of attention has been on cell-mediated immunity and the role of complement remains controversial.

Agents That Control Complement Activation

Although the complement system is crucial for protection against microorganisms, its activation can also lead to pathologic consequences. A major function of complement activation is to promote inflammation, thereby destroying invading pathogens, tumor cells, etc. There are many diseases in humans associated with uncontrolled complement activation leading to untoward organ damage (71). These range from autoimmune diseases like systemic lupus erythematosus to diseases that might not be expected to be complement-related like ischemia-reperfusion injury in myocardial infarcts. Therefore, control of complement activation using an appropriate agent would be beneficial to patients with a variety of disorders. Until recently, there have been few agents available for clinical application. Nevertheless, new complement inhibitors are being produced and tested for their efficiency in controlling complement activation in various disease models and in man. We will focus on the agents that have proven efficient in various models and show promise in clinical situations. For a complete description of all the potential agents that could be used to block complement activation, the reader is referred to recent reviews on the subject (59, 71, 134).

One promising agent for controlling complement activation in various pathological states is soluble complement receptor type 1. The most common form of complement receptor type 1 (CR1) is a 205-kDa protein that acts as a receptor for C3b and C4b (60). It possesses decay-accelerating activity toward both the C3 and C5 convertases, enzymes that are crucial for the function of the classical and alternative complement pathways (37). As such, it binds to the convertases and accelerates their decay. In addition, CR1 serves as a cofactor for factor I-mediated cleavage of two important complement peptides, C3b and C4b (84). Because it is an extended rod-like molecule, CR1 not only protects the cell it is expressed on but also is capable of protecting neighboring cells from complement attack. Through genetic engineering, a soluble form of this complement receptor (sCR1) has been generated that lacks the transmembrane and cytoplasmic domains of the molecule (140). This agent has been used in a wide range of animal models where complement activation is a key element of the pathological state. It showed high potency in reducing myocardial infarct size in a rat model of ischemia-reperfusion injury (140). Furthermore, sCR1 was shown to significantly reduce complement-mediated tissue injury in models of xenograft and allograft rejection; vasculitis; lung injury; multiple sclerosis; myasthenia gravis; reperfusion injury of the heart, intestine, and liver; thermal injury; brain trauma; glomerulonephritis; anaphylaxis; and immune pleuritic reactions (71, 134). Therefore, this agent is an excellent candidate for clinical trials in patients in whom complement activation leads to severe pathological conditions. Nevertheless, sCR1, because of its high molecular weight, has a short half-life in vivo and has to be given parenterally, thus limiting its long-term use (83). Work is being conducted to improve its bioavailability (54).

One important natural complement inhibitor that acts principally on the classical complement pathway is C1 inhibitor. It inhibits classical pathway activation by interacting with activated C1r and C1s, the active enzymatic sites on C1 (42). In doing so, it slows C1 activation and destroys C1 activity once C1 is activated. A high concentration of C1 inhibitor was shown to efficiently block classical complement pathway activation in an in vitro model of hyperacute xenograft rejection (29) and reduce tissue damage in a feline model of myocardium reperfusion injury (21). In patients with hereditary angioedema, a concentrated vapor-heated C1 inhibitor preparation prevented acute attacks (138). The major limitation to its use is the difficulty of purifying adequate amounts for widespread therapy. However, methods are being developed to alleviate this problem (98).

Another promising agent for blocking complement activation in a variety of complement-dependent diseases is a monoclonal antibody that recognizes C5. The rationale for its use is that C5 is common to both the classical and alternative pathways, and the blockade of its activation would interfere with the potent proinflammatory properties of C5a. Blocking C5 activation would also inhibit the formation of the membrane attack complex. In this way, it would limit tissue injury but allow deposition of complement fragments such as C3b on microorganisms. Thus, it should not interfere with proper clearance of bacteria via phagocytosis. Monoclonal antibody reacting with mouse C5 was shown to prevent collagen-induced arthritis in a mouse model (137). It also reduced glomerulonephritis and increased the survival of mice with a lupus-like disease (136). Anti-human C5 monoclonal antibodies have also been produced that proved potent in inhibiting complement-mediated injury to xenografts in in vitro cell culture and ex vivo perfusion systems (63, 109). To increase the compatibility and efficiency of anti-C5 use in humans, humanized monoclonal antibodies to human C5 and recombinant single-chain antibody (scFv) have been produced and shown to efficiently block C5 activation (35, 129). Such a humanized anti-C5 recombinant single-chain antibody is currently in clinical trials in humans and has recently been reported to significantly reduce inflammation and myocardial tissue injury in patients undergoing cardiopulmonary bypass surgery (108).

Another natural molecule that has been used in the control of complement-mediated disease is human IgG injected intravenously (IVIg). IVIg is prepared from pooled plasma of thousands of donors. It is used for replacement therapy in primary and secondary immunodeficiencies as well as in patients with autoimmune and inflammatory diseases such as idiopathic thrombocytopenic purpura, Kawasaki's disease, Guillain-Barré syndrome, and myasthenia gravis (33). The mode of action of IVIg is still not fully understood, and investigators have postulated effects that include idiotype–anti-idiotype interactions, blockade of Fc receptors on phagocytic cells, modulation of T- and B-cell functions, selection of immune repertoires, and modulation of cytokine production (85). From the observation that as much as 30% of C3 deposited to a bacterial surface is bound to IgG and not to the target, we postulated that one function of IgG is to serve as a preferential acceptor of activated C3 (16). It was further demonstrated that high-dose IVIg was effective in interfering with complement-dependent in vivo reactions such as Forssman shock in guinea pigs (9) and hyperacute rejection of pig hearts implanted in primates (70). In humans, IVIg is reported to inhibit C3b and C5b-9 deposits on endomysial capillaries in patients with dermatomyositis (8) and reduce C3 binding to erythrocytes in patients with paroxysmal nocturnal hemoglobinuria (7). It would appear that the way high-dose IVIg blocks complement activation is by inhibiting C4 binding to the sensitized target surface (76). Other proposed mechanisms of action include interference with C1 binding to the target cell (80, 103) and degradation of C3b by factors H and I by the formation of C3b-IgG complexes (68).

Other agents that might prove useful in controlling complement activation in various clinical settings have been produced and are listed in detail in recent reviews (59, 71, 134). Examples include complement regulatory molecules naturally present on cells, which are prepared by recombinant technology and genetically modified for clinical use. Some examples include soluble complement receptor type 2, soluble decay-accelerating factor, soluble membrane cofactor protein, soluble CD59, and hybrids of decay-accelerating factor and CD59. Also, various natural products with inherent anticomplementary activity and peptides that serve as C5a or C3a receptor antagonists are being developed as potent anti-inflammatory agents.

Infectious Risk Associated with the Use of Agents That Control Complement Activation

Though the complement system is recognized as crucial for the control of microbial infection, very little is known about the potential infectious risk of using pharmacologic agents that control its activation. As mentioned in a previous section of this chapter, complement depletion induced by injection of cobra venom factor has permitted the assessment of the importance of complement in the resistance to various infectious agents. However, because of its nature, cobra venom factor has no clinical utility since it induces massive complement activation (134). Only one study has focused on the infectious risk of using soluble complement receptor type 1 (sCR1) as a complement inhibitor. Swift and coworkers used a rat model to demonstrate that sCR1 treatment inhibits the phagocytosis of *S. pneumoniae*, even when the organism is preopsonized (124). Resistance to both *S. pneumoniae* and *Pseudomonas aeruginosa* was greatly reduced in this model when animals were administered sCR1. Nevertheless, clinical trials of sCR1 in myocardial infarction and burn-induced adult respiratory distress syndrome that are as yet unpublished have not suggested that bacterial infections will be a common clinical problem (71). In two limited xenotransplantation studies, infectious complications were reported with the use of either sCR1 (31) or K76COOH (a fungal metabolite isolated from *Stachybotrys complementi* that inhibits C5 activation) (126). However, investigators in both of these studies used immunosuppressive agents such as cyclophosphamide, cyclosporine A, steroids, and tacrolimus. Therefore, it is difficult to determine the role of complement blockade on infectious complications. Studies on the long-term use of complement-inhibiting agents will prove necessary to assess the potential risk of infectious complications associated with their use.

As detailed previously in this chapter, it is known that IVIg interferes with classical pathway-mediated complement binding to sensitized targets. We have studied the effect of IVIg on complement–bacteria interactions in vitro (135). Unlike sCR1, even at high concentrations, IVIg does not interfere with the amount of C3 that binds to bacteria that activate the alternative or the classical pathways directly. Furthermore, IVIg has no effect on complement-mediated lysis of complement-sensitive bacteria. Only when sensitizing antibodies were needed for proper complement activation did IVIg have an effect on C3 deposition. Using serum samples from patients treated with high-dose IVIg, no effect on C3 deposition nor bacterial killing of a complement-sensitive strain was observed, suggesting lack of interference in direct complement–bacteria interactions in vivo.

CONCLUDING REMARKS

Elements of innate immunity such as natural antibodies and complement have clearly been shown to play an important role in host resistance against microorganisms. Therefore, removal of such antibodies from the circulation or pharmacologic blockade of the complement system may lead to infectious complications in a graft recipient. Although well-controlled studies are lacking, there is general belief that methods that lower plasma protein concentrations (plasmapheresis, immunoadsorption) may place the treated animal or recipient at an increased risk of developing infections. Agents that lower complement activity have not been examined in detail. Experimental and clinical studies are needed to fully appreciate the beneficial and harmful effects of methods that interfere with unwanted pathologic effects of elements of the humoral immune system.

REFERENCES

1. **Ahlstedt, S.** 1981. Experimental *Escherichia coli* 06 infection in mice. *Acta Pathol. Microbiol. Scand.* **89**(C)**:**23–28.
2. **Alarabi, A. A., B. Nilsson, U. Nilsson, B. Wikström, and B. G. Danielson.** 1993. Complement activation during tryptophan immunoadsorption treatment. *Artif. Organs* **17:**782–786.
3. **Alarabi, A., U. Backman, O. Wikstrom Sjoberg, and G. Tufveson.** 1997. Plasmapheresis in HLA-immunosensitized patients prior to kidney transplantation. *Int. J. Artif. Organs* **20:**51–56.
4. **Aoki, T., M. J. Walling, G. S. Bushar, M. Liu, and K. C. Hsu.** 1976. Natural antibodies in sera from healthy humans to antigens on surfaces of type C RNS viruses and cells from primates. *Proc. Natl. Acad. Sci. USA* **73:**2491–2495.
5. **Aringer, M., J. S. Smolen, and W. B. Graninger.** 1998. Severe infections in plasmapheresis-treated systemic lupus erythematosus. *Arthritis Rheum.* **41:**414–420.
6. **Avrameas, S.** 1991. Natural antibodies: from "horror autotoxicus" to "gnothi seauton." *Immunol. Today* **12:**154–159.
7. **Basta, M.** 1996. Modulation of complement-mediated immune damage by intravenous immune globulin. *Clin. Exp. Immunol.* **104**(Suppl. 1)**:**21–25.
8. **Basta, M., and M. C. Dalakas.** 1994. High-dose intravenous immunoglobulin exerts its beneficial effect in patients with dermatomyositis by blocking endomysial deposition of activated complement fragments. *J. Clin. Invest.* **94:**1729–1735.
9. **Basta, M., P. Kirshbom, M. M. Frank, and L. F. Fries.** 1989. Mechanism of therapeutic effect of high-dose intravenous immunoglobulin. Attenuation of acute, complement-dependent immune damage in a guinea pig model. *J. Clin. Invest.* **84:**1974–1981.
10. **Beebe, D. P., and N. R. Cooper.** 1981. Neutralization of vesicular stomatitis virus (VSV) by human complement requires a natural IgM antibody present in human serum. *J. Immunol.* **126:**1562–1568.
11. **Berglin E., C. Kjellstrom, V. Mantovani, G. Stelin, C. Svalander, and L. Wiklund.** 1995. Plasmapheresis as a rescue therapy to resolve cardiac rejection with vasculitis and severe heart failure. A report of five cases. *Transplant Int.* **8:**382–387.
12. **Bitter-Suermann D., and R. Burger.** 1986. Guinea pigs deficient in C2, C4, C3 or the C3a receptor. *Prog. Allergy* **39:**134–158.
13. **Boyden, S.** 1964. Natural antibodies and the immune response. *Adv. Immunol.* **5:**1–28.
14. **Brauer, R. B., W. M. Baldwin III, S. Ibrahim, and F. Sanfilippo.** 1995. The contribution of the terminal complement components to acute and hyperacute allograft rejection in the rat. *Transplantation* **59:**288–293.
15. **Briles, D., M. Nahm, K. Schroer, J. Davie, P. Baker, J. Kearney, and R. Barlettas.** 1981. Antiphosphocholine antibodies found in normal mouse serum are protective against intravenous infection with type 3 *Streptococcus pneumoniae. J. Exp. Med.* **153:**694–705.
16. **Brown, E. J., M. Berger, K. A. Joiner, and M. M. Frank.** 1983. Classical pathway activation by antipneumococcal antibodies leads to covalent binding of C3b to antibody molecules. *Infect. Immun.* **42:**594–598.
17. **Brown, E. J., S. W. Hosea, and M. M. Frank.** 1981. Reticuloendothelial clearance of radiolabeled pneumococci in experimental bacteremia: correlation of changes in clearance rates, sequestration patterns, and opsonization requirements at different phases of the bacterial growth cycle. *J. Reticuloendothelial Soc.* **30:** 23–31.
18. **Brown, E. J., S. W. Hosea, and M. M. Frank.** 1981. The role of the spleen in experimental pneumococcal bacteremia. *J. Clin. Invest.* **67:**975–982.
19. **Brown, E. J., S. W. Hosea, C. H. Hammer, C. G. Burch, and M. M. Frank.** 1982. A quantitative analysis of the interactions of antipneumococcal antibody and complement in experimental pneumococcal bacteremia. *J. Clin. Invest.* **69:**85–98.
20. **Budzko, D. B., M. C. Pizzimenti, and F. Kierszenbaum.** 1975. Effects of complement depletion in experimental Chagas disease: immune lysis of virulent blood forms of *Trypanosoma cruzi. Infect. Immun.* **11:**86–91.

21. **Buerke, M., T. Morohara, and A. M. Lefer.** 1995. Cardioprotective effects of a C1 esterase inhibitor in myocardial ischemia and reperfusion. *Circulation* **91:**393–402.
22. **Candinas, D., B.-A. Lesnikoski, S. C. Robson, T. Miyatake, S. M. Scesney, H. C. Marsh, Jr., U. S. Ryan, A. P. Dalmasso, W. W. Hancock, and F. H. Bach.** 1996. Effect of repetitive high-dose treatment with soluble complement receptor type 1 and cobra venom factor on discordant xenograft survival. *Transplantation* **62:**336–342.
23. **Casali, P., and A. L. Notkins.** 1989. CD5+ B lymphocytes, polyreactive antibodies and the human B cell repertoire. *Immunol. Today* **10:**364–368.
24. **Casali, P., and E. W. Schettino.** 1996. Structure and function of natural antibodies. *Curr. Top. Microbiol. Immunol.* **210:**167–179.
25. **Challacombe, S. J., L. A. Bergmeier, C. Czerkinsky, and A. S. Rees.** 1984. Natural antibodies in man to *Streptococcus mutans*: specificity and quantification. *Immunology* **52:**143–150.
26. **Chopek, M., and J. McCullogh.** 1980. Protein and biochemical changes during plasma exchange, p. 13–52. *In* J. Ulmas and B. Berkman (ed.), *Therapeutic Haemapheresis: A Technical Workshop*. American Association of Blood Banks, Washington, D.C.
27. **Cooper, N. R.** 1998. Complement and viruses, p. 393–407. *In* J. E. Volanakis and M. M. Frank (ed.), *The Human Complement System in Health and Disease*. Marcel Dekker, Inc., New York, N.Y.
28. **Dalmasso, A. P.** 1992. The complement system in xenotransplantation. *Immunopharmacology* **24:**149–160.
29. **Dalmasso, A. P., and J. L. Platt.** 1993. Prevention of complement-mediated activation of xenogeneic endothelial cells in an in vitro model of xenograft hyperacute rejection by C1 inhibitor. *Transplantation* **56:**1171–1176.
30. **Dalmasso, A. P., G. M. Vercellotti, R. J. Fischel, R. M. Bolman, F. H. Bach, and J. L. Platt.** 1992. Mechanism of complement activation in the hyperacute rejection of porcine organs transplanted into primate recipients. *Am. J. Pathol.* **140:**1157–1166.
31. **Davis, E. A., S. K. Pruitt, P. S. Greene, S. Ibrahim, T. T. Lam, J. L. Levin, W. M. Baldwin III, and F. Sanfilippo.** 1996. Inhibition of complement, evoked antibody, and cellular response prevents rejection of pig-to-primate cardiac xenografts. *Transplantation* **62:**1018–1023.
32. **Densen, P.** 1998. Complement deficiencies and infection, p. 409–421. *In* J. E. Volanakis and M. M. Frank (ed.), *The Human Complement System in Health and Disease*. Marcel Dekker, Inc., New York, N.Y.
33. **Dwyer, J. M.** 1992. Manipulating the immune system with immune globulin. *N. Engl. J. Med.* **326:**107–116.
34. **Epstein, J., Q. Eichbaum, S. Sheriff, and R. A. B. Ezekowitz.** 1996. The collectins in innate immunity. *Curr. Opin. Immunol.* **8:**29–35.
35. **Evans, M. J., S. A. Rollins, D. W. Wolff, R. P. Rother, A. J. Norin, D. M. Therrien, G. A. Grijalva, J. P. Mueller, S. H. Nye, S. P. Squinto, and J. A. Wilkins.** 1995. In vitro and in vivo inhibition of complement activity by a single-chain Fv fragment recognizing human C5. *Mol. Immunol.* **32:**1183–1195.
36. **Farges, O., A. N. Kalil, D. Samuel, F. Saliba, J. L. Arulnaden, P. Debat, A. Bismuth, D. Castaing, and H. Bismuth.** 1995. The use of ABO-incompatible grafts in liver transplantation: a life-saving procedure in highly selected patients. *Transplantation* **59:**1124–1133.
37. **Fearon, D. T.** 1984. Cellular receptors for fragments of the third component of complement. *Immunol. Today* **5:**105–110.
38. **Figueroa, J. E., and P. Densen.** 1991. Infectious diseases associated with complement deficiencies. *Clin. Microbiol. Rev.* **4:**359–395.
39. **Fishelson, Z.** 1994. Complement-related proteins in pathogenic organisms. *Springer Semin. Immunopathol.* **15:**345–368.
40. **Fisher, M. B., A. P. Prodeus, A. Nicholson-Weller, M. Ma, J. Murrow, R. R. Reid, H. B. Warren, L. Lage, F. D. Moore, Jr., F. S. Rosen, and M. C. Carroll.** 1997. Increased susceptibility to endotoxin shock in complement C3- and C4-deficient mice is corrected by C1 inhibitor replacement. *J. Immunol.* **159:**976–982.
41. **Frank, M. M.** 1995. Animal models for complement deficiencies. *J. Clin. Immunol.* **15:**113S–121S.
42. **Frank, M. M., and L. F. Fries.** 1989. Complement, p. 679–701. *In* W. E. Paul (ed.), *Fundamental Immunology*, 2nd ed. Raven Press, Ltd., New York, N.Y.
43. **Frank, M. M., and L. F. Fries.** 1998. The role of complement in defence against bacterial disease. *Bailliere's Clin. Immunol. Allergy* **2:**335–361.
44. **Frank, M. M., K. A. Joiner, and C. H. Hammer.** 1987. The function of antibody and complement in the lysis of bacteria. *Rev. Infect. Dis.* **9:**S537–S545.

45. **Galili, U.** 1993. Evolution and pathophysiology of the human natural anti-galactosyl IgG (anti-Gal) antibody. *Springer Semin. Immunopathol.* **15:**155–171.
46. **Goes, A. M., and F. J. Ramalho-Pinto.** 1991. Protective immunity to *Schistosoma mansoni* in mice is dependent on antibody and complement but not on radiosensitive leukocytes. *Immunol. Lett.* **28:**57–64.
47. **Griffin, S. V., C. M. Lockwood, and C. D. Pusey.** 1996. Plasmapheresis and immunoadsorption, p. 636–651. *In* K. F. Austen, S. J. Burakoff, F. S. Rosen, and T. B. Strom (ed.), *Therapeutic Immunology*. Blackwell Science, Inc., Cambridge, Mass.
48. **Harindranath, N., H. Ikematsu, A. L. Notkins, and P. Casali.** 1993. Structure of the V_H and V_L segments of polyreactive and monoreactive human natural antibodies to HIV-1 and *Escherichia coli* β-galactosidase. *Int. Immunol.* **5:**1523–1533.
49. **Higgins, R. M., D. J. Bevan, B. S. Carey, C. K. Lea, M. Fallon, R. Buhler, R. W. Vaughan, P. J. O'Donnell, S. A. Snowden, M. Bewick, and B. M. Hendry.** 1996. Prevention of hyperacute rejection by removal of antibodies to HLA immediately before renal transplantation. *Lancet* **348:**1208–1211.
50. **Hirsh, R. L., D. E. Griffin, and J. A. Winkelstein.** 1978. The effect of complement depletion on the course of sindbis virus infection in mice. *J. Immunol.* **121:**1276–1278.
51. **Horowitz, J., J. E. Volanakis, and D. E. Briles.** 1987. Blood clearance of *Streptococcus pneumoniae* by C-reactive protein. *J. Immunol.* **138:**2598–2603.
52. **Ishiwaka, A., M. Itoh, T. Ushlyama, K. Suzuki, and K. Fujita.** 1998. Experience of ABO-incompatible living kidney transplantation after double filtration plasmapheresis. *Clin. Transplant.* **12:**80–83.
53. **Jakobs, F. M., E. A. Davis, T. White, F. Sanfilippo, and W. M. Baldwin III.** 1998. Prolonged discordant xenograft survival by inhibition of the intrinsic coagulation pathway in complement C6-deficient recipients. *J. Heart Lung Transplant.* **17:**306–311.
54. **Kalli, K. R., P. Hsu, and D. T. Fearon.** 1994. Therapeutic uses of recombinant complement protein inhibitors. *Semin. Immunopathol.* **15:**417–431.
55. **Kantor, A. B.** 1991. The development and repertoire of B-1 cells (CD5 B cells). *Immunol. Today* **12:**389–391.
56. **Kaplan, M. H., and J. E. Volanakis.** 1974. Interaction of C-reactive protein complexes with the complement system. I. Consumption of human complement associated with the reaction of C-reactive protein with pneumococcal C-polysaccharide and with the choline phosphatides, lecithin and sphingomyelin. *J. Immunol.* **112:**2135–2147.
57. **Kearns-Jonker, M., M. Fraiman, W. Chu, E. Gochi, J. Michel, G.-D. Wu, and D. V. Cramer.** 1998. Xenoantibodies to pig endothelium are expressed in germline configuration and share a conserved immunoglobulin V_H gene structure with antibodies to common infectious agents. *Transplantation* **65:**1515–1519.
58. **Kemp, E.** 1996. Xenotransplantation. *J. Intern. Med.* **239:**287–297.
59. **Kirschfink, M.** 1997. Controlling the complement system in inflammation. *Immunopharmacology* **38:**51–62.
60. **Klickstein, L. B., T. J. Bartow, V. Miletic, L. D. Rabson, J. A. Smith, and D. T. Fearon.** 1988. Identification of distinct C3b and C4b recognition sites in the human C3b/C4b receptor (CR1, CD35) by deletion mutagenesis. *J. Exp. Med.* **168:**1699–1717.
61. **Konishi, E., and M. Nakao.** 1992. Naturally occurring immunoglobulin M antibodies: enhancement of phagocytic and microbicidal activities of human neutrophils against *Toxoplasma gondii*. *Parasitology* **104:**427–432.
62. **Kozel, T. R.** 1996. Activation of the complement system by pathogenic fungi. *Clin. Microbiol. Rev.* **9:**34–46.
63. **Kroshus, T. J., S. A. Rollins, A. P. Dalmasso, E. A. Elliott, L. A. Matis, S. P. Squinto, and R. M. Bolman III.** 1995. Complement inhibition with an anti-C5 monoclonal antibody prevents acute cardiac tissue injury in an ex vivo model of pig-to-human xenotransplantation. *Transplantation* **60:**1194–1202.
64. **Leventhal, J. R., A. P. Dalmasso, J. W. Cromwell, J. L. Platt, C. J. Manivel, R. M. Bolman III, and A. J. Matas.** 1993. Prolongation of cardiac xenograft survival by depletion of complement. *Transplantation* **55:**857–866.
65. **Leventhal, J. R., R. John, J. P. Fryer, J. C. Witson, J.-M. Derlich, J. Remiszewski, A. P. Dalmasso, A. J. Matas, and R. M. Bolman III.** 1995. Removal of baboon and human antiporcine IgG and IgM natural antibodies by immunoadsorption. Results of in vitro and in vivo studies. *Transplantation* **59:**294–300.
66. **Leventhal, R., H. Bonner, E. J. L. Soulsby, and A. D. Schreiber.** 1978. The role of complement in *Ascaris suum* induced histopathology. *Clin. Exp. Immunol.* **32:**69–76.

67. **Lin, S. S., D. L. Kooyman, L. J. Daniels, C. W. Daggett, W. Parker, J. H. Lawson, C. W. Hoopes, C. Gullotto, L. Li, P. Birch, R. D. Davis, L. E. Diamond, J. S. Logan, and J. L. Platt.** 1997. The role of natural anti-galα1-3gal antibodies in hyperacute rejection of pig-to-baboon cardiac transplants. *Transplant. Immunol.* **5:**212–218.
68. **Lutz, H. U., P. Stammler, E. Jelezarova, M. Nater, and P. J. Spath.** 1996. High doses of immunoglobulin G attenuate immune aggregate-mediated complement activation by enhancing physiologic cleavage of C3b in (C3b)n-IgG complexes. *Blood* **88:**184–193.
69. **Lydyard, P. M., A. Lamour, L. E. MacKenzie, C. Jamin, R. A. Mageed, and P. Youinou.** 1993. CD5+ B cells and the immune system. *Immunol. Lett.* **38:**159–166.
70. **Magee, J. C., B. H. Collins, R. C. Harland, B. J. Lindman, R. R. Bollinger, M. M. Frank, and J. L. Platt.** 1995. Immunoglobulin prevents complement-mediated hyperacute rejection in swine-to-primate xenotransplantation. *J. Clin. Invest.* **96:**2404–2412.
71. **Makrides, S. C.** 1998. Therapeutic inhibition of the complement system. *Pharmacol. Rev.* **50:**59–87.
72. **Marsh, J. E., M. C. Carroll, and S. H. Sacks.** 1998. The classic pathway augments production of alloantibodies. *Mol. Immunol.* **35:**393.
73. **Matsushita, M., and T. Fujita.** 1996. The lectin pathway. *Res. Immunol.* **147:**115–118.
74. **May, J. E., M. A. Kane, and M. M. Frank.** 1972. Host defense against bacterial endotoxemia. Contribution of the early and late components of complement to detoxification. *J. Immunol.* **109:**893–895.
75. **Michael, J. G.** 1969. Natural antibodies. *Curr. Top. Microbiol. Immunol.* **48:**43–62.
76. **Miletic, V. D., C. G. Hester, and M. M. Frank.** 1996. Regulation of complement activity by immunoglobulin. I. Effect of immunoglobulin isotype on C4 uptake on antibody-sensitized sheep erythrocytes and solid phase immune complexes. *J. Immunol.* **156:**749–757.
77. **Miller, T. E., S. Phillips, and T. J. Simpson.** 1978. Complement-mediated immune mechanisms in renal infection. II. Effect of decomplementation. *Clin. Exp. Immunol.* **33:**115–121.
78. **Miyagawa, S., R. Shirakura, G. Matsumiya, N. Fukushima, S. Nakata, H. Matsuda, M. Matsumoto, H. Kitamura, and T. Seya.** 1993. Prolonging discordant xenograft survival with anticomplement reagents K76COOH and FUT-175. *Transplantation* **55:**709–713.
79. **Mokrzycki, M. H., and A. A. Kaplan.** 1994. Therapeutic plasma exchange: complications and management. *Am. J. Kidney Dis.* **23:**817–827.
80. **Mollnes, T. E., K. Hogasen, B. F. Hoaas, T. E. Michaelsen, P. Garred, and M. Harboe.** 1995. Inhibition of complement-mediated red cell lysis by immunoglobulins is dependent on the Ig isotype and its C1 binding preperties. *Scand. J. Immunol.* **41:**449–456.
81. **Moore, F. D., Jr., D. T. Fearon, and K. F. Austen.** 1981. IgG on mouse erythrocytes augments activation of the human alternative complement pathway by enhancing deposition of C3b. *J. Immunol.* **126:**1805–1809.
82. **Mor, E., D. Skerrett, C. Manzarbeitia, P. A. Sheiner, M. E. Schwartz, S. Emre, S. N. Thung, and C. M. Miller.** 1995. Successful use of an enhanced immunosuppressive protocol with plasmapheresis for ABO-incompatible mismatched grafts in liver transplant recipients. *Transplantation* **59:**986–990.
83. **Morgan, B. P.** 1995. Physiology and pathophysiology of complement: progress and trends. *Crit. Rev. Clin. Lab. Sci.* **32:**265–298.
84. **Morgan, B. P., and S. Meri.** 1994. Membrane proteins that protect against complement lysis. *Semin. Immunopathol.* **15:**369–396.
85. **Mouthon, L., S. V. Kaveri, S. H. Spalter, S. Lacroix-Desmazes, C. Lefranc, R. Desai, and M. D. Kazatchkine.** 1996. Mechanism of action of intravenous immune globulin in immune-mediated diseases. *Clin. Exp. Immunol.* **104**(Suppl. 1):3–9.
86. **Naik, R. B., R. Ashlin, C. Wilson, D. S. Smith, H. A. Lee, and M. Slapak.** 1979. The role of plasmapheresis in renal transplantation. *Clin. Nephrol.* **11:**245–250.
87. **Norrgren, K., S. E. Strand, and C. Ingvar.** 1992. Contrast enhancement in RII and modification of the therapeutic ratio in RIT: a theoretical evaluation of simulated extracorporeal immunoadsorption. *Antibody Immunoconj. Radiopharmaceut.* **5:**61–73.
88. **Ohta, H., Y. Yoshikawa, C. Kai, K. Yamanouchi, H. Taniguchi, K.-I. Komine, Y. Ishijima, and H. Okada.** 1986. Effect of complement depletion by cobra venom factor on fowlpox virus infection in chickens and chicken embryos. *J. Virol.* **57:**670–673.
89. **Olivari, M.-T., C. B. May, N. A. Johnson, W. S. Ring, and M. K. Stephens.** 1994. Treatment of acute vascular rejection with immunoadsorption. *Circulation* **90:**II70–II73.

90. **Olsen, S. L., L. E. Wagoner, E. H. Hammond, D. O. Taylor, R. L. Yowell, R. D. Ensley, M. R. Bristow, J. B. O'Connell, and D. G. Renlund.** 1993. Vascular rejection in heart transplantation: clinical correlation, treatment options, and future considerations. *J. Heart Lung Transplant.* **12:**S135–S142.
91. **Pangburn, M. K., and H. J. Müller-Eberhard.** 1984. The alternative pathway of complement. *Semin. Immunopathol.* **7:**163–192.
92. **Parker, W., D. Bruno, and J. L. Platt.** 1995. Xenoreactive antibodies in the world of natural antibodies: typical or unique? *Transplant. Immunol.* **3:**181–191.
93. **Petry, F., and M. Loos.** 1998. Bacteria and complement, p. 375–391. *In* J. E. Volanakis and M. M. Frank (ed.), *The Human Complement System in Health and Disease*. Marcel Dekker, Inc., New York, N.Y.
94. **Platt, J. L.** 1995. Natural antibodies, p. 55–80. *In* J. L. Platt (ed.), *Hyperacute Xenograft Rejection*. R.G. Landes Co., Georgetown, Tex.
95. **Platt, J. L.** 1998. New directions for organ transplantation. *Nature* **392:**11–17.
96. **Platt, J. L., S. S. Lin, and C. G. A. McGregor.** 1998. Acute vascular rejection. *Xenotransplantation* **5:**169–175.
97. **Pohl, M. A., S.-P. Lan, T. Berl, and the Lupus Nephritis Collaborative Study Group.** 1991. Plasmapheresis does not increase the risk for infection in immunosuppressed patients with severe lupus nephritis. *Ann. Intern. Med.* **114:**924–929.
98. **Poulle, M., M. Burnouf-Radosevich, and T. Burnouf.** 1994. Large-scale preparation of highly purified human C1 inhibitor for therapeutic use. *Blood Coagul. Fibrinolysis* **5:**543–549.
99. **Pratt, J. R., A. W. Harmer, J. Levin, and S. H. Sacks.** 1997. Influence of complement on the allospecific antibody response to a primary vascularized organ graft. *Eur. J. Immunol.* **27:**2848–2853.
100. **Pratt, J. R., M. J. Hibbs, A. J. Laver, A. G. Smith, and S. H. Sacks.** 1996. Effects of complement inhibition with soluble complement receptor-1 on vascular injury and inflammation during renal allograft rejection in the rat. *Am. J. Pathol.* **149:**2055–2066.
101. **Pretagostini, R., P. Berloco, L. Poli, P. Cinti, A. Di Nicuolo, P. De Simone, M. Colonnello, A. Salerno, D. Alfani, and R. Cortesini.** 1996. Immunoadsorption with protein A in humoral rejection of kidney transplants. *ASAIO J.* **42:**M645–M648.
102. **Pruitt, S. K., A. D. Kirk, R. R. Bollinger, H. C. Marsh, Jr., B. H. Collins, J. L. Levin, J. R. Mault, J. S. Heinle, S. Ibrahim, A. R. Rudolph, V. M. Baldwin III, and F. Sanfilippo.** 1994. The effect of soluble complement receptor type 1 on hyperacute rejection of porcine xenografts. *Transplantation* **57:**363–370.
103. **Qi, M., and J. A. Shifferli.** 1995. Inhibition of complement activation by intravenous immunoglobulins. *Arthritis Rheum.* **38:**146.
104. **Qian, Z., F. M. Jakobs, T. Pfaff-Amesse, F. Sanfilippo, and W. M. Baldwin III.** 1998. Complement contributes to the rejection of complete and class I major histocompatibility complex-incompatible cardiac allografts. *J. Heart Lung Transplant.* **17:**470–478.
105. **Reid, R. R., A. P. Prodeus, W. Khan, T. Hsu, F. S. Rosen, and M. C. Carroll.** 1997. Endotoxin shock in antibody-deficient mice. Unraveling the role of natural antibody and complement in the clearance of lipopolysaccharide. *J. Immunol.* **159:**970–975.
106. **Ritter, K., A. Fudickar, N. Heine, and R. Thomssen. 1997.** Autoantibodies with a protective function: polyreactive antibodies against alkaline phosphatase in bacterial infections. *Med. Microbiol. Immunol.* **186:**109–113.
107. **Rodman, T. C., S. E. To, J. J. Sullivan, and R. Winston.** 1997. Innate natural antibodies. Primary roles indicated by specific epitopes. *Hum. Immunol.* **55:**87–95.
108. **Rollins, S. A., J. C. K. Fitch, S. Sherman, C. S. Rinder, H. M. Rinder, B. R. Smith, C. D. Collard, G. L. Stahl, B. L. Alford, L. Li, and L. A. Matis.** 1998. Anti-C5 single chain antibody therapy blocks complement and leukocyte activation and reduces myocardial tissue damage in CPB patients. *Mol. Immunol.* **35:**397.
109. **Rollins, S. A., L. A. Matis, J. P. Springhorn, E. Setter, and D. W. Wolff.** 1995. Monoclonal antibodies directed against human C5 and C8 block complement-mediated damage of xenogeneic cells and organs. *Transplantation* **60:**1284–1292.
110. **Saadi, S., and J. L. Platt.** 1998. Immunology of xenotransplantation. *Life Sci.* **62:**365–387.
111. **Salmela, K. T., E. O. von Willebrand, L. E. Kyllonen, B. H. Eklund, K. A. Hockerstedt, H. M. Isoniemi, L. Krogerus, E. Taskinen, and P. J. Ahonen.** 1992. Acute vascular rejection in renal transplantation: diagnosis and outcome. *Transplantation* **54:**858–862.

112. **Sanaka, T., S. Wakai, S. Teraoka, T. Takuma, N. Sugino, and T. Agishi.** 1990. Effect of therapeutic plasma exchange on immunological and renal pathological findings in patients with lupus nephritis, p. 351–353. *In* G. Rock (ed.), *Apharesis*. Alan R. Liss, Inc., New York, N.Y.
113. **Sato, Y., M. Kimikawa, H. Suga, Y. Hayasaka, S. Teraoka, T. Agishi, and K. Ota.** 1992. Prolongation of cardiac xenograft survival by double filtration plasmapheresis and ex vivo immunoadsorption. *ASAIO J.* **38:**M673–M675.
114. **Schneider, K. M.** 1998. Plasmapheresis and immunoadsorption: different techniques and their current role in medical therapy. *Kidney Int.* **53:**S61–S65.
115. **Schreiber, J. R., C. Basker, and G. R. Siber.** 1987. Effect of complement depletion on anticapsular-antibody-mediated immunity to experimental infection with *Haemophilus influenzae* type b. *Infect. Immun.* **55:**2830–2833.
116. **Schweinle, J. E., R. A. B. Ezekowitz, A. J. Tenner, M. Kuhlman, and K. A. Joiner.** 1989. Human mannose-binding protein activates the alternative complement pathway and enhances serum bactericidal activity on a mannose-rich isolate of *Salmonella*. *J. Clin. Invest.* **84:**1821–1829.
117. **Silverstein, A. M.** 1993. The history of immunology, p. 21–41. *In* W. E. Paul (ed.), *Fundamental Immunology*, 3rd ed. Raven Press, Ltd., New York, N.Y.
118. **Snyder, H. W., and E. Fleissner.** 1980. Specificity of human antibodies to oncovirus glycoproteins: recognition of antigen by natural antibodies directed against carbohydrate structures. *Proc. Natl. Acad. Sci. USA* **77:**1622–1626.
119. **Sonnenwirth, A. C.** 1979. Antibody response to anaerobic bacteria. *Rev. Infect. Dis.* **1:**337–341.
120. **Stegmayr, B. G.** 1996. Plasmapheresis in severe sepsis or septic shock. *Blood Purif.* **14:**94–101.
121. **Stiehm, E. R., T. W. Chin, A. Haas, and A. G. Peerless.** 1986. Infectious complications of the primary immunodeficiencies. *Clin. Immunol. Immunopathol.* **40:**69–86.
122. **Strauss, R. G., D. Clavarella, R. O. Gilcher, D. O. Kasprisin, D. D. Kiprov, H. G. Klein, and B. C. McLoed.** 1993. An overview of current management. *J. Clin. Apharesis* **8:**189–194.
123. **Suankratay, C., X.-H. Zhang, Y. Zhang, T. F. Lint, and H. Gewurz.** 1998. Requirement for the alternative pathway as well as C4 and C2 in complement-dependent hemolysis via the lectin pathway. *J. Immunol.* **160:**3006–3013.
124. **Swift, A. J., T. S. Collins, P. Bugelski, and J. A. Winkelstein.** 1994. Soluble complement receptor type 1 inhibits complement-mediated host defense. *Clin. Diagn. Lab. Immunol.* **1:**585–589.
125. **Szalai, A. J., D. E. Briles, and J. E. Volanakis.** 1996. Role of complement in C-reactive-protein-mediated protection of mice from *Streptococcus pneumoniae*. *Infect. Immun.* **64:**4850–4853.
126. **Tanaka, M., N. Murase, Q. Ye, W. Miyazaki, M. Nomoto, H. Miyazawa, R. Manez, Y. Toyama, A. J. Demetris, S. Todo, and T. E. Starzl.** 1996. Effect of anticomplement agent K76 COOH on hamster-to-rat and guinea pig-to-rat heart xenotransplantation. *Transplantation* **62:**681–688.
127. **Taniguchi, S., S. Kitamura, K. Kawachi, M. Fukutomi, Y. Yoshida, and Y. Kondo.** 1992. Effects of double-filtration plasmapheresis and a platelet-activating factor antagonist on the prolongation of xenograft survival. *J. Heart Lung Transplant.* **11:**1200–1208.
128. **Thiel, S., T. Vorup-Jensen, C. M. Stover, W. Schwaeble, S. B. Laursen, K. Poulsen, A. C. Willis, P. Eggelton, S. Hansen, U. Holmskov, K. B. M. Reid, and J. C. Jensenius.** 1997. A second serine protease associated with mannan-binding lectin that activates complement. *Nature* **386:**606–610.
129. **Thomas, T. C., S. A. Rollins, R. P. Rother, M. A. Giannoni, S. L. Hartman, E. A. Elliott, S. H. Nye, L. A. Matis, S. P. Squinto, and M. J. Evans.** 1996. Inhibition of complement activity by humanized anti-C5 antibody and single-chain Fv. *Mol. Immunol.* **33:**1389–1401.
130. **Ulanova, M., M. Hahn-Zoric, Y. L. Lau, A. Lucas, and L. A. Hanson.** 1996. Expression of *Haemophilus influenzae* type b idiotype 1 on naturally acquired antibodies. *Clin. Exp. Immunol.* **105:**422–428.
131. **van Emmerik, L. C., E. J. Kuijper, C. A. P. Fijen, J. Dankert, and S. Thiel.** 1994. Binding of mannan-binding protein to various bacterial pathogens of meningitis. *Clin. Exp. Immunol.* **97:**411–416.
132. **Vogel, C. W., and H. J. Müller-Eberhard.** 1982. The cobra venom factor-dependent C3 convertase of human complement. *J. Biol. Chem.* **257:**8292–8299.
133. **Volanakis, J. E., and M. M. Frank (ed.).** 1998. *The Human Complement System in Health and Disease*. Marcel Dekker, Inc., New York, N.Y.
134. **Wagner, E., and M. M. Frank.** 1998. Development of clinically useful agents to control complement-mediated tissue damage, p. 527–546. *In* J. E. Volanakis and M. M. Frank (ed.), *The Human Complement System in Health and Disease*. Marcel Dekker, Inc., New York, N.Y.

135. **Wagner, E., J. L. Platt, and M. M. Frank.** 1998. High dose intravenous immunoglobulin does not affect complement-bacteria interactions. *J. Immunol.* **160:**1936–1943.
136. **Wang, Y., Q. L. Hu, J. A. Madri, S. A. Rollins, A. Chodera, and L. A. Matis.** 1995. Amelioration of lupus-like autoimmune disease in NZB/WF1 mice after treatment with a blocking monoclonal antibody specific for complement component C5. *Proc. Natl. Acad. Sci. USA* **93:**8563–8568.
137. **Wang, Y., S. A. Rollins, J. A. Madri, and L. A. Matis.** 1995. Anti-C5 monoclonal antibody therapy prevents collagen-induced arthritis and ameliorates established disease. *Proc. Natl. Acad. Sci. USA* **92:**8955–8959.
138. **Waytes, A. T., F. S. Rosen, and M. M. Frank.** 1996. Treatment of angioedema with a vapor-heated C1 inhibitor concentrate. *N. Engl. J. Med.* **334:**1630–1634.
139. **Webster, A. D. B., G. P. Spickett, B. J. Thompson, and J. Farrant.** 1988. Viruses and antibody deficiency syndromes. *Immunol. Invest.* **17:**93–105.
140. **Weisman, H. F., T. Bartow, M. K. Leppo, H. C. Marsh, Jr., G. R. Carson, M. F. Concino, M. P. Boyle, K. H. Roux, M. L. Weisfeldt, and D. T. Fearon.** 1990. Soluble human complement receptor type 1: in vivo inhibitor of complement suppressing post-ischemic myocardial inflammation and necrosis. *Science* **249:**146–151.
141. **Wu, M. J., K. H. Shu, C. H. Cheng, and J. D. Lian.** 1997. Complications of membrane-filtration plasma exchange. *Chung Hua I Shueh Chih (Taipei)* **60:**147–154.
142. **Zhang, W., and P. J. Lachman.** 1994. Glycosylation of IgA is required for optimal activation of the alternative complement pathway by immune complexes. *Immunology* **81:**137–141.

Xenotransplantation
Edited by Jeffrey L. Platt

Chapter 8

Complement Regulation and the Host Response to Infection

B. Paul Morgan

The complement (C) system comprises some 15 soluble plasma proteins that interact with one another in three distinct enzymatic activation cascades (the classical, alternative, and lectin pathways) and in the nonenzymatic membrane attack pathway (Fig. 1). C is an important component of the host innate immune system. Activation of C on bacteria or other pathogens causes elimination of the pathogen either directly by causing lysis or indirectly by marking the pathogen for removal by phagocytes. C activation products also play a part in recruiting phagocytes to the site of disease. The importance of C in defense against infection is vividly illustrated in individuals lacking a functional C system (69). Most dramatically, deficiency of C3, a key component essential for function, causes a profound immunodeficiency characterized by numerous infections with pyogenic bacteria. Patients with deficiencies of the classical pathway commonly present with a syndrome that resembles closely the autoimmune disorder systemic lupus erythematosus (110). This is caused by a failure of the normal mechanisms of immune complex solubilization and transport, which depend heavily on the presence of a functional C system.

Activation of C generates numerous active products, which can, if produced at inappropriate sites or in an unregulated manner, cause damage to host cells. To protect host cells from these potentially damaging effects of C activation, numerous regulatory proteins exist both in the fluid phase and on cell membranes (Fig. 1). Nevertheless, C activation makes a substantial contribution to pathology in numerous diseases. The purpose of this chapter is to review briefly the main situations in vivo where C may cause disease, discuss recent strategies for regulating C activation in order to reduce C-mediated pathology, and address the potential problems related to therapies that inhibit the physiological effects of C activation.

CONTRIBUTION OF C TO PATHOLOGY

There is within the C system an enormous potential for self-harm, invoking the frequent description of C as a double-edged sword. In general, harm will result when C activation

B. Paul Morgan • Complement Biology Group, University of Wales College of Medicine, Heath Park, Cardiff, CF14 4XN, Wales, U.K.

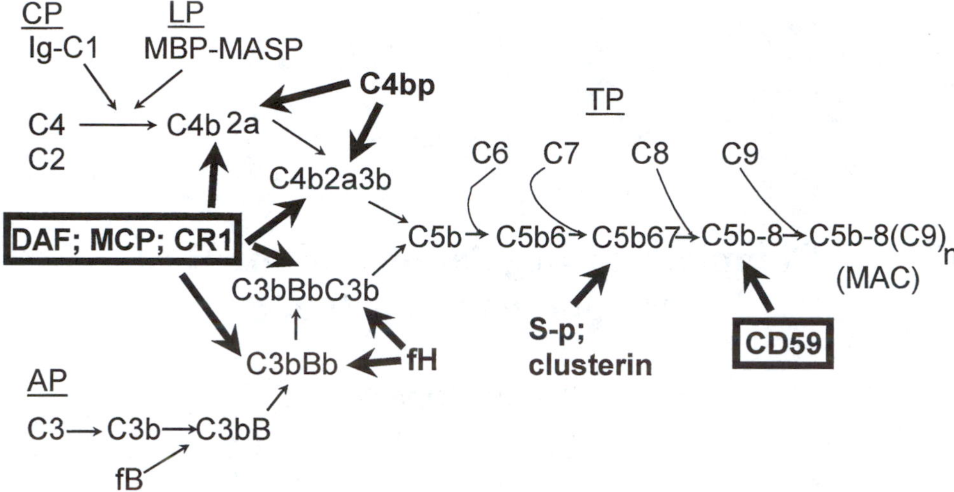

Figure 1. Complement and its control. The C system comprises three activation pathways—classical pathway (CP), alternative pathway (AP), and lectin pathway (LP) — and a common final terminal pathway (TP). The activation pathways and terminal pathway are tightly controlled by a number of fluid-phase and membrane-associated proteins acting either to inhibit the enzymes of the activation pathways (activated C1, C3 convertases, C5 convertases) or to restrict assembly of the MAC. Arrows indicate where in the system each of the regulators exerts its effect. Membrane-bound regulators are boxed, and fluid-phase inhibitors are in bold. Abbreviations as in footnotes to Table 1.

occurs in an uncontrolled manner and/or at an inappropriate site; the end result of this will be inflammation and tissue destruction. The C system contributes to tissue damage in a large number of autoimmune diseases. Autoantibodies and immune complexes deposit in the affected organs where they trigger activation of C and exacerbate inflammation. In many autoimmune diseases, from the organ specific (e.g., autoimmune thyroid disease) to the disseminated (e.g., systemic lupus erythematosus), C deposition can be detected in the affected tissues and products of C activation are found in the plasma (51, 94, 116). In all of these autoimmune diseases C is just one of several factors that contribute to tissue damage. Nevertheless, modulation of C activation may be of therapeutic benefit in these conditions. In systemic lupus erythematosus, autoantibodies are present that recognize DNA and other components of normal cells. Following any stimulus to cell death, these components will be released and immune complexes will form. Immune complexes deposit in capillary beds, particularly in skin and kidney, where they activate C to cause inflammation and further tissue destruction. A vicious cycle is triggered in which more cell killing drives the production of more immune complexes that in turn exacerbates C activation and tissue destruction.

"Iatrogenic" (treatment-precipitated) C activation is a common consequence of the many modern therapies that involve contact of blood with a foreign surface (63, 64). Such therapies include renal hemodialysis and cardiopulmonary bypass. Many of the materials used in the tubing and membrane components of the extracorporeal circuits are "bioincompatible" and will activate the clotting and C cascades in plasma. Exposure of blood to these materials in extracorporeal circuits is thus a frequent and potentially hazardous event (63). In hemodialysis, blood is in contact with a large surface area of dialysis membrane, which is usually made of cuprophane, a complex polysaccharide material that efficiently activates C via the alternative pathway. Release of active fragments, particularly C3a and C5a, causes activation of neutrophils and monocytes, which aggregate and become deposited in the lung. Release of toxic molecules from these cells causes the lung damage that is a common complication of long-term dialysis (46). Numerous modifications to the membrane surface have been investigated to reduce C activation. The most promising strategy involves coating the membrane with heparin, a simple procedure that renders the circuit much less C activating (12, 61, 64, 81).

Activation of C may also occur in transplanted organs. When a poorly matched organ is used for transplant, it is rapidly rejected due, in part, to C activation in the graft, the phenomenon of hyperacute rejection. C-mediated hyperacute rejection is an almost universal outcome of cross-species transplants and is thus a major barrier to the use of animal organs for human recipients in xenotransplantation, the subject of this volume.

INHIBITION OF C AS A THERAPEUTIC STRATEGY

Therapies that inhibit C activation may break the proinflammatory cycle and reduce inflammation in many and diverse diseases. Application of this attractive strategy has until recently been limited by the lack of specific and effective pharmacological inhibitors of C. Numerous agents have been proposed as C-inhibitory therapies based on their anti-C activities in vitro, but all have proved disappointing when tested in vivo. The naturally occurring C regulators (Table 1) are excellent inhibitors of C and have potential as therapeutic agents. Both soluble and membrane-associated C regulators have been shown to be potential therapeutics.

Soluble C Regulators

C1 inhibitor (C1inh) was the first of the naturally occurring C regulators to be used therapeutically as a replacement therapy in hereditary angioedema (HAE), a disease caused by an incomplete deficiency of this key C regulator (25). C1inh purified from plasma was a safe and effective therapy for acute attacks of HAE, rapidly inhibiting the activity of C1 and other proteolytic cascades and resolving edema. In experimental animals, C1inh was effective in therapy of rodent models of shock and acute pancreatitis (23, 75, 109), and in a feline model of myocardial infarction (6). High-dose therapy with C1inh has been shown to be of benefit in septic shock and the related vascular leak syndrome in humans (30) and in treatment of the toxic effects associated with administration of high doses of interleukin-2 (78). Large-scale trials of the efficacy of C1inh in shock syndromes and reperfusion injuries have yet to take place.

The fluid-phase inhibitors of the C3 convertases, factor H (fH) and C4b binding protein (C4bp), are present in plasma at high concentrations (fH, 450 mg/l; C4bp, 250 mg/l) and, together with the protease factor I (fI), are essential for restriction of C activation in the fluid phase. Despite their high concentration in plasma, fH and C4bp do not prevent activation of C on appropriate surfaces such as bacterial capsules. The fact that the fluid-phase C3 convertase inhibitors fail to inhibit C activation on surfaces despite their high concentration in plasma makes it unlikely that they would prove effective as therapeutics. To bring about

Table 1. Summary of human complement regulatory proteins[a]

Molecule	Structure	Concn (mg/liter)	Gene	Target
Plasma:				
C1inh	Single chain, 76 kDa	200	11	C1
fH	Single chain, 90 kDa	450	1 (RCA)	C3/C5 conv.
fI	2 chains: α, 50 kDa; β, 38 kDa	35	4	C3/C5 conv.
C4bp	6 or 7 α chains (70 kDa), 1 or 0 β chain (45 kDa)	250	1 (RCA) 1 (RCA)	CP C3 conv.
S-protein	Single chain, 83 kDa	500	17q	C5b-7
Clusterin	2 chains: α, 35 kDa; β, 38 kDa	50	8p	C5b-7
CPN (AI)	Dimeric heterodimer (85/50 kDa; total 290 kDa)	30	?	C3a, C4a, C5a
Membrane:				
MCP	Single chain, 60 kDa; TM	–	1 (RCA)	C3/C5 conv.
DAF	Single chain, 65 kDa; GPI	–	1 (RCA)	C3/C5 conv.
CR1	Single chain, 200 kDa; TM	–	1 (RCA)	C3/C5 conv.
HRF	Single chain, 65 kDa; GPI	–	?	C5b-8/C5b-9
CD59	Single chain, 20 kDa; GPI	–	11	C5b-8/C5b-9

[a]RCA, regulators of complement activation gene cluster; TM, transmembrane; GPI, glycosyl phosphatidylinositol; C1inh, C1 inhibitor; fH, factor H; fI, factor I; C4bp, C4b binding protein; CPN, carboxypeptidase N; AI, anaphylatoxin inactivator; MCP, membrane cofactor protein (CD46); DAF, decay-accelerating factor (CD55); CR1, C receptor 1; HRF, homologous restriction factor.

even a 50% increase in the plasma concentration of fH would require administration of several grams of protein! Nevertheless, modified forms of C4bp and/or fH with improved efficiencies of inhibition might yield agents of sufficient activity to be used as therapeutics.

The fluid-phase inhibitors of the terminal pathway, S-protein and clusterin, are multifunctional proteins present in plasma at high concentrations (S-protein, 500 mg/l; clusterin, 50 mg/l). Each binds C5b-7 complexes in a nonspecific manner, preventing association of the complex with membrane and formation of the lytic membrane attack complex. For reasons noted above, they are unlikely to make good targets for therapeutics.

Membrane C Regulators

The membrane regulators of C, decay-accelerating factor (DAF), membrane cofactor protein (MCP), C receptor 1 (CR1), and CD59, together effectively police the membranes of self cells to prevent damage by autologous C. Fearon in the late 1980s first advanced the concept that soluble forms of membrane C regulators might inhibit efficiently C activation from the fluid phase. A recombinant soluble form of CR1 (sCR1) was generated, comprising the 30 short consensus repeats but lacking the transmembrane and cytoplasmic portions of the molecule (Fig. 2) (65, 114, 115). Recombinant sCR1 expressed in mammalian cells was a potent inhibitor of activation of human C and also inhibited C from numerous other species, allowing testing of sCR1 in animal models of disease (43). In a rat model of myocardial infarction, a single dose of sCR1 markedly inhibited tissue damage (65). A beneficial effect of sCR1 has subsequently been demonstrated in numerous models of disease, many but not all of which involve ischemia-reperfusion injury (Table 2). In humans, clinical trials using sCR1 have begun in the adult respiratory distress syndrome, myocardial infarction,

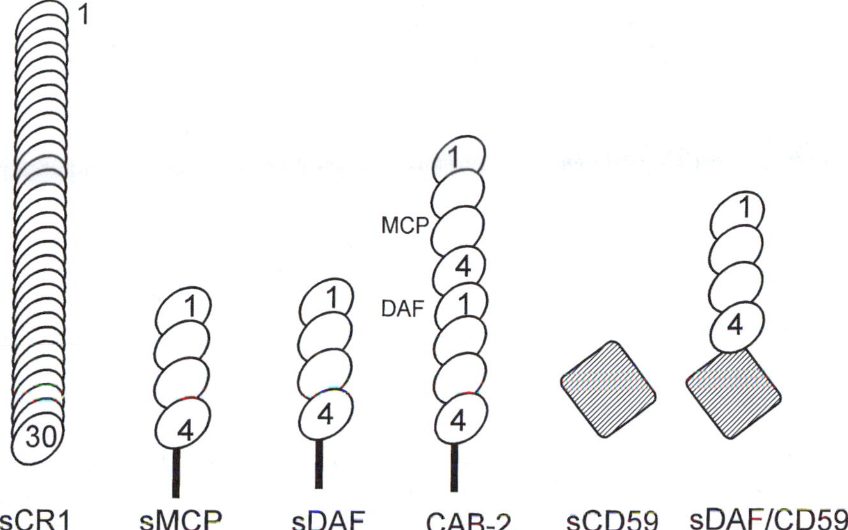

Figure 2. Recombinant soluble C regulators. Recombinant soluble forms of each of the major membrane C regulatory proteins have been generated. Recombinant soluble CR1 (sCR1) consists of the 30 short consensus repeats (SCRs, represented as overlapping ovals) of CR1, which represent almost all of the extracellular portion of this molecule (1 is N-terminal). Recombinant soluble MCP (sMCP) and DAF (sDAF) consist of the four SCRs that contain the C regulatory activities together with a portion of the rigid C-terminal STP region. CAB-2 is a chimeric molecule in which sMCP is attached through the C-terminus to the N-terminus of sDAF. CD59 is a globular molecule with no SCR structures. DAF/CD59 chimeras have been expressed on cells but not, to date, as the soluble molecules depicted here. (Modified from reference 69a.)

and lung transplantation. All of these disease targets are shock and/or ischemia-reperfusion injuries and all are acute. Future applications may extend to chronic autoimmune disorders such as multiple sclerosis and rheumatoid arthritis.

Recombinant soluble forms of DAF and MCP have also been engineered and expressed using a strategy similar to that described for sCR1 (15, 66). The recombinant molecules comprised the four short consensus repeats together with the serine-threonine-proline-rich (STP) region but without the membrane-anchoring regions (Fig. 2). Both sDAF and sMCP have been shown to inhibit C activation in vitro in human serum and in vivo in rodents (14, 15, 66). Unlike the other regulators, sCR1 combines both cofactor and decay-accelerating activities for the C3 convertases in a single molecule, which is likely to be advantageous. Indeed, in a comparison of the relative C inhibitory efficiencies of the three recombinant soluble convertase inhibitors, sCR1 was the most efficient on a molar basis, but a combination of sDAF and sMCP approached the efficacy of sCR1 (14). Further, a hybrid recombinant molecule in which DAF and MCP have been combined, termed CAB-2, was more effective as a C inhibitor in vitro and in vivo than either parent molecule or even a combination of the two parent molecules (38).

CD59 inhibits at the stage of assembly of the membrane attack complex (MAC) (18). Soluble forms of CD59 lacking the glycosyl phosphatidylinositol (GPI) anchor have been

Table 2. sCR1 in animal models of disease

Model disease	Effect of sCR1	Reference
Myocardial ischemia-reperfusion (rat)	Reduced infarct size	114, 115
Intestinal ischemia-reperfusion (rat)	Reduced local (gut) and remote (lung) inflammation and tissue destruction	39, 119
Skeletal muscle ischemia-reperfusion (mouse)	Improved muscle reperfusion and muscle viability, reduced lung injury	82
Liver ischemia-reperfusion (rat)	Improved liver function, reduced release of liver enzymes	11
Thermal injury (rat)	Reduced local (skin) and remote (lung) inflammation and tissue destruction	74
Xenograft rejection (guinea pig to rat; pig to primate)	Increased survival time of xenograft	89, 92
Allograft rejection (rat)	Reduced inflammation in renal allograft	88
Experimental demyelination (rat)	Reduced brain inflammation and myelin loss	84
Traumatic brain injury (rat)	Reduced neutrophil accumulation in brain	42
Experimental glomerulonephritis (rat)	Improved renal function, reduced glomerular damage and proteinuria	16
Hemodialysis (ex vivo)	Reduced neutrophil activation, reduced lung injury	13, 40
Acid instillation in lung (rat)	Decreased neutrophil accumulation in lung, decreased plasma TNF	77
Experimental myasthenia gravis (rat)	Reduced loss of acetylcholine receptors; improved muscle function	83
Experimental autoimmune neuritis (rat)	Improved nerve conduction, reduced incidence of paralysis	41

extracted from urine and generated by recombinant techniques (52, 62, 104). Soluble CD59 (sCD59) inhibits MAC formation and target lysis when tested in a serum-free reactive lysis system using purified C components, demonstrating that the soluble molecule can interact with and inhibit the forming MAC. However, sCD59 loses its inhibitory activity in the presence of serum, a consequence of its association with serum lipoproteins (104). This precludes the use of sCD59 as a therapeutic agent in vivo. However, it is possible that sCD59 can be modified to retain inhibitory activity in the presence of serum. Identification of the active site in CD59 may permit the creation of smaller, more active fragments or active site peptides with reduced binding to lipoproteins but retaining MAC inhibitory activity. It may also be possible to target sCD59 to specific tissue sites by generating chimeras of CD59 and antibody fragments. Perhaps simplest of all, CD59, either GPI-anchored or soluble, could be delivered directly to tissue sites such as the joint in arthritis or the brain in demyelination, thus avoiding the inhibitory influence of serum.

Numerous approaches are being investigated to optimize the soluble C regulators for therapy. Molecules are being developed that contain only the active sites by deleting the portions of the molecule redundant for activity in the plasma. A recent report described the generation of a truncated form of sCR1 lacking LHR-A within which resides the C4b binding site to generate a specific inhibitor of the alternative pathway (29, 99). Another approach involves the selective targeting of C regulators to areas of C activation. A form of sCR1 expressing multiple copies of the sialyl-Lewis-X carbohydrate epitope was generated to produce an agent that binds P-selectin expressed on activated endothelium at inflammatory sites (1, 53). Modifications that extend the half-life in vivo are also being explored. Fusion of the albumin-binding domains from protein G to the carboxy-terminus of sCR1 caused a doubling of the half-life in vivo in the rat without adversely affecting the activity of the protein (55). Other strategies for modifying sCR1 and other soluble recombinant C regulators to enhance activity and/or half-life in vivo will undoubtedly follow.

C-Inhibiting Antibodies

It has been realized for several years that some monoclonal antibodies (MAb) against key C components can effectively remove that component from serum and efficiently inhibit C. The therapeutic possibilities of this observation have not escaped notice. Most work has been done on antibody against C5. A MAb was identified that had the unique property of binding C5 in a manner that prevented its cleavage by the C5-convertases of the activation pathways, thus blocking generation of C5a and MAC (49, 95, 106, 111, 112). This MAb caused complete inhibition of serum C when added at a concentration sufficient to bind all the C5. The MAb was specific for human C5 so could not be tested in vivo in animals; however, blocking antibodies against rodent C5 have subsequently been produced and have proven effective in therapy of experimental diseases involving C activation (112). A humanized single-chain Fv (scFv) version of the anti-human C5 antibody has been developed that retains C5-binding activity, has a long half-life, and is well tolerated in vivo. This agent is in the early stages of testing in humans.

Blocking antibodies against other C components might also be of use in therapy. A MAb against C8 has been shown to be an excellent blocker of the terminal pathway in vitro but has yet to be tested in vivo. For blocking antibodies against C components to be effective, they must be administered in quantities sufficient to bind all of the target component. Antibodies that bind only activated C components or activation complexes could be effective at much lower concentrations because the target antigen is much less abundant and generated only during C activation. Such neoantigenic antibodies are already widely used for assays of C activation but have yet to be exploited in therapy.

Another possible target for anticomplement antibodies is the interaction of C5a with its receptor. MAbs targeting C5a or the C5a receptor have been developed as potential therapeutics (2, 71, 73). Comparison of the therapeutic effects of anti-C5 (blocking C5a and MAC) and anti-C5a or anti-C5a receptor (blocking C5a alone) in experimental disease will clarify the relative roles of these two effectors in pathology.

A potential problem with the use of antibodies against C components is that these large molecules will penetrate tissues poorly and may not be effective inhibitors of locally generated C, a major drive to pathology. The development of small antibody-derived agents such as the anti-C5 scFv described above might circumvent this problem.

Small Molecule Inhibitors of C

Improved understanding of the function and structure of the C components, regulators and receptors, has guided the design of small-molecule drugs capable of effectively inhibiting at various points in the C system. Small molecules offer substantial advantages over the large recombinant proteins and antibodies described above in that they will be substantially less expensive to produce, might be active when given orally, and may penetrate more readily into tissues. One attractive target for drug design is the interaction of the small chemotactic fragments C3a and C5a with their respective receptors. The receptors for C3a (C3aR) and C5a (C5aR) are members of the 7-transmembrane-spanning receptor family that includes receptors for many chemokines. Numerous strategies have been applied to blocking receptors of this family, many of which might be applicable to the C3aR and C5aR (4). Small peptides capable of efficiently antagonizing the binding of C5a with target have been generated and shown to be effective inhibitors of C5a-induced effects in vitro and in animal models (44, 47). Peptides are not ideal as therapeutic agents; they cannot be given orally because they are destroyed by enzymes in the gut and they have very short half-lives in vivo. Highly cationic nonpeptide agents based on 4,6-diaminoquinoline have also been shown to function as antagonists, although they are untested in vivo (50). Several other nonpeptide antagonists of the C5aR have recently been reported (3, 20, 121).

Other C components and receptors are also potential targets for small-molecule inhibitors. Of particular note is the recent description of a 13-residue cyclic peptide inhibitor of C3, termed compstatin (72, 76). The peptide binds C3 and prevents its cleavage by C3 convertases, thereby inhibiting C activation, and has proven effective in an ex vivo model of cardiopulmonary bypass. There is now enormous interest from the pharmaceutical sector in the development of better small-molecule inhibitors of C, and many such agents will no doubt emerge in the next few years.

POTENTIAL NEGATIVE CONSEQUENCES OF THERAPEUTIC INHIBITION OF C

The primary biological roles of C are to protect against infection and to aid the clearance of immune complexes. Individuals deficient in C thus have problems related to infection and immune complex disease, although the clinical picture is dependent on the precise location in the system of the deficiency. Those deficient in components of the classical pathway (C1, C4, C2) cannot process immune complexes and have a very high incidence of immune complex disease. Individuals deficient in C3 have a profound immunodeficiency and suffer severe, recurrent bacterial infections. In contrast, individuals deficient in components of the terminal pathway have as their sole deficit an increased susceptibility to meningococcal disease (70).

Administration of agents that inhibit C will render the individual C-deficient and may markedly increase susceptibility to infections. Immune complex disease may also be a problem if C inhibition is maintained for long periods. The agents inhibiting at the C3 convertase stage (sCR1, sDAF, sMCP) will not influence the deposition of C1, C4, and C2 on targets and are thus unlikely to interfere with immune complex handling. They will, however, inhibit the amplification loop essential for effective opsonization of bacteria, prevent the generation of chemotactic peptides, and block the membrane attack pathway, three events key to the efficient destruction of bacteria. Individuals given these agents or other agents acting at this stage of the C pathway, often already at high risk of infection because of the underlying pathology, are compromised still further in their ability to resist bacterial infection. Appropriate prophylaxis with antibiotics is thus an essential adjunct to therapy with sCR1 or related agents.

Therapy with agents inhibiting later in the C pathway offers some theoretical advantages. Many of the pathological effects of C are mediated by products of the terminal pathway (C5a and MAC), whereas the bulk of the physiological effects are mediated by products of the activation pathways (67, 68). Therefore, inhibitors acting in the terminal pathway are less likely to predispose to bacterial infections and immune complex disease, particularly when used for long-term therapy. Comparison of agents blocking both C5a and MAC (anti-C5 antibody), C5a alone (anti-C5a or anti-C5aR antibody), and MAC alone (CD59, anti-C8 antibody) in therapy of experimental disease models will provide valuable information on the relative importance of MAC and C5a in driving pathology.

INHIBITION OF C IN THE CONTEXT OF XENOTRANSPLANTATION

Transplants between distantly related or discordant species (e.g., pig–man; mouse–guinea pig) result in the rapid destruction of the donor organ as natural antibody and C from the recipient serum attack the endothelium (8, 35, 36). With the realization that hyperacute rejection was mediated by C attack (100) came the suggestion that the human C regulators might be utilized to overcome this hurdle (102, 118). The simplest approach to protecting the xenograft would be to utilize the fluid-phase C regulators described above. There is clear evidence that systemic inhibition of C, either using sCR1 or the C-depleting agent cobra venom factor, can markedly prolong the survival of a discordant xenograft (9, 89–92, 96). Indeed, a number of other agents that cause systemic inhibition of C, including the small-molecule C inhibitors FK506 (37) and K76-COOH (105), the monoclonal anti-C5 antibody described above (49), and intravenous immunoglobulin (54), significantly extend the lifetime of the xenotransplanted organ. In many cases, survival was extended beyond the period of C inhibition, suggesting that the vigorous attack characteristic of hyperacute rejection does not occur if the organ has been present in the C-inhibited host for several days, even when host C levels return to normal. This phenomenon, known as accommodation, remains somewhat mysterious but probably relates to changes in the endothelium of the organ that render it unreactive with natural antibody and much less C activating (26, 85). These data indicate that relatively short-term inhibition of C using sCR1 or other inhibitors might be sufficient to circumvent hyperacute rejection in pig–human transplants.

To better protect the grafted organ or cells from C, a dramatically different approach has received much attention and is described in more detail elsewhere in this volume. The basic concept is to generate by transgenesis pigs (or other donor species) expressing human C regulators on endothelia and other exposed sites. The validity of this approach was first demonstrated by transfection of cultured cells with human MCP (79, 80) and later confirmed by creating transgenic mice abundantly expressing human DAF, CD59, or MCP on endothelium and at other sites (22, 28, 48, 60). Hearts harvested from each of these transgenic strains could be perfused ex vivo with human blood or serum for prolonged periods whereas nontransgenic hearts were rapidly destroyed by C activation. Encouraged by these results, several groups have gone on to generate by transgenesis pigs expressing human C regulators on endothelium and at other sites (7, 17, 21). Organs from pigs transgenic for human DAF were resistant to C damage when perfused with human blood ex vivo and when transplanted into primates (10, 17, 27, 87). Others have generated pigs expressing human MCP and/or CD59 and have shown similar protection against human C in ex vivo perfused hearts (21, 58, 59). Even when engineered organs expressing human C regulators are used, there is certainly a case for the concomitant administration of systemic inhibitors of C to reduce further the risk of damage to the endothelium.

A second molecular approach has involved the engineering of pigs such that the endothelium is no longer a target for natural antibody. The major target on pig endothelium for human IgM natural antibody is the carbohydrate epitope Galα1-3Gal, present in pigs and other non-primate mammals but absent in man and other primates (107, 108). A clever tactic has been adopted to eliminate this epitope. The enzyme fucosyl transferase, hyperexpressed in transgenic pigs, competes with the natural glycosylation system to replace the Galα1-3Gal epitope with a fucosylated sugar not recognized by natural antibody (97, 98). The success of this strategy is dependent on the assumption that classical pathway activation triggered by natural antibody is the primary route for C activation. However, there is considerable evidence that the porcine endothelium also triggers activation of the alternative pathway, even in the absence of natural antibody (86, 93, 117). Nevertheless, a combination of these two complementary approaches—hyperexpressing human CRP and eliminating binding of natural antibody—holds enormous promise for the future.

POTENTIAL NEGATIVE CONSEQUENCES OF EXPRESSION OF HUMAN C REGULATORS ON XENOGRAFTS

The human C regulators have properties that might be undesirable for the grafted organ. C regulators are utilized by several viruses and other microorganisms as a receptor. Of particular importance in this context is the demonstration that the measles virus utilizes human MCP as receptor (56, 57). A xenograft hyperexpressing human MCP might thus be rendered highly susceptible to infection with measles virus with consequences for the graft that are not predictable from current knowledge. DAF is utilized as receptor by numerous viruses, including members of the echovirus and enterovirus family, and by pathogenic strains of *Escherichia coli* (5, 45, 113). Again, consequences for infection of hyperexpression of DAF on the xenograft remain unknown. Several enveloped viruses, notably cytomegalovirus and the human immunodeficiency virus type 1, are protected from C attack by C regulators "pirated" from host cells during budding (24, 101, 103). Budding from cells hyperexpressing C regulators could conceivably yield viruses with enhanced resistance to host C, which might render them more pathogenic. CD59 has been implicated in binding CD2 (19, 31), and it has recently been reported that DAF is the ligand for CD97, a surface receptor upregulated on activated lymphocytes (33, 34). Hyperexpression of CD59 and DAF might thus make the graft attractive for activated lymphocytes that will express both CD2 and CD97. The consequences of this for graft survival are uncertain.

A current controversy in xenotransplantation concerns the potential for endogenous retroviruses in the pig cells to cause disease in the recipient and in the population at large (described elsewhere in this volume). A further cause for concern is that enveloped viruses budding from pig cells hyperexpressing human C regulators will take with them in the envelope a high concentration of the regulators that might render the virus particles resistant to C killing and increase virulence. Tumors arising from the grafted tissue might similarly be protected against C attack. C is activated in many human tumors, and C regulator expression is frequently elevated in tumor tissue (32, 120). Tumors arising from pig cells hyperexpressing C regulators might therefore be extremely resistant to C, increasing malignancy.

CONCLUSION

The novel anti-C therapies described here are still far from ideal as therapeutic agents, but ongoing developments will produce better anti-C agents for use in therapy of disease and in the protection of bioincompatible surfaces, including transplanted cells and organs. The strategies are not without risk, and the effects of inhibiting C must always be considered when embarking on a course of C inhibition. With systemic agents the risk relates to infection and immune complex disease and is manageable with appropriate precautions. The risks of expression of human C regulators in transplanted tissue are rather more complex and require further thought and experimentation.

REFERENCES

1. **Akahori, T., Y. Yuzawa, K. Nishikawa, T. Tamatani, R. Kannagi, M. Miyasaka, H. Okada, N. Hotta, and S. Matsuo.** 1997. Role of a sialyl Lewis(x)-like epitope selectively expressed on vascular endothelial cells in local skin inflammation of the rat. *J. Immunol.* **158:**5384–5392.
2. **Amsterdam, E. A., G. L. Stahl, H. L. Pan, S. V. Rendig, M. P. Fletcher, and J. C. Longhurst.** 1995. Limitation of reperfusion injury by a monoclonal antibody to C5a during myocardial infarction in pigs. *Am. J. Physiol.* **268:**H448–H457.
3. **Astles, P. C., T. J. Brown, P. Cox, F. Halley, P. M. Lockey, C. McCarthy, I. M. McLay, T. N. Majid, A. D. Morley, B. Porter, A. J. Ratcliffe, and R. J. A. Walsh.** 1997. New nonpeptidic C5a receptor antagonists. *Bioorg. Med. Chem. Lett.* **7:**907–912.
4. **Baggiolini, M., and B. Moser.** 1997. Blocking chemokine receptors. *J. Exp. Med.* **186:**1189–1191.
5. **Bergelson, J. M., M. Chan, K. R. Solomon, N. F. St. John, H. Lin, and R. W. Finberg.** 1994. Decay-accelerating factor (CD55), a glycosylphosphatidylinositol-anchored complement regulatory protein, is a receptor for several echoviruses. *Proc. Natl. Acad. Sci. USA* **91:**6245–6249.
6. **Buerke, M., T. Murohara, and A. M. Lefer.** 1995. Cardioprotective effects of a C1 esterase inhibitor in myocardial ischemia and reperfusion [see comments]. *Circulation* **91:**393–402.
7. **Byrne, G., K. McCurry, M. Martin, J. Platt, and J. Logan. 1996.** Development and analysis of transgenic pigs expressing the human complement regulatory protein CD59 and DAF. *Transplant. Proc.* **28:**759.
8. **Calne, R. Y.** 1970. Organ transplantation between widely disparate species. *Transplant. Proc.* **2:**550–553.
9. **Candinas, D., B. A. Lesnikoski, S. C. Robson, S. M. Scesney, I. Otsu, T. Myiatake, H. C. Marsh, Jr., U. S. Ryan, W. W. Hancock, and F. H. Bach.** 1996. Soluble complement receptor type 1 and cobra venom factor in discordant xenotransplantation. *Transplant. Proc.* **28:**581.
10. **Carrington, C. A., A. C. Richards, E. Cozzi, G. Langford, N. Yannoutsos, and D. J. White.** 1995. Expression of human DAF and MCP on pig endothelial cells protects from human complement. *Transplant. Proc.* **27:**321–323.
11. **Chavez-Cartaya, R., E. Cozzi, G. Pino-DeSola, N. V. Jamieson, and D. J. White.** 1995. Regulation of complement activation in rat liver ischemia and reperfusion: expression of endothelial CD59 (RIP). *Transplant. Proc.* **27:**2852–2854.
12. **Cheung, A. K.** 1994. Complement activation as index of haemodialysis membrane biocompatibility: the choice of methods and assays. *Nephrol. Dialysis Transplant.* **9:**96–103.
13. **Cheung, A. K., C. J. Parker, and M. Hohnholt.** 1994. Soluble complement receptor type 1 inhibits complement activation induced by hemodialysis membranes in vitro. *Kidney Int.* **46:**1680–1687.
14. **Christiansen, D., J. Milland, B. R. Thorley, I. F. McKenzie, and B. E. Loveland.** 1996. A functional analysis of recombinant soluble CD46 in vivo and a comparison with recombinant soluble forms of CD55 and CD35 in vitro. *Eur. J. Immunol.* **26:**578–585.
15. **Christiansen, D., J. Milland, B. R. Thorley, I. F. McKenzie, P. L. Mottram, L. J. Purcell, and B. E. Loveland.** 1996. Engineering of recombinant soluble CD46: an inhibitor of complement activation. *Immunology* **87:**348–354.
16. **Couser, W. G., R. J. Johnson, B. A. Young, C. G. Yeh, C. A. Toth, and A. R. Rudolph.** 1995. The effects of soluble recombinant complement receptor 1 on complement-mediated experimental glomerulonephritis. *J. Am. Soc. Nephrol.* **5:**1888–1894.
17. **Cozzi, E., G. A. Langford, A. Richards, K. Elsome, R. Lancaster, P. Chen, N. Yannoutsos, and D. J. White.** 1994. Expression of human decay accelerating factor in transgenic pigs. *Transplant. Proc.* **26:**1402–1403.
18. **Davies, A.** 1996. Policing the membrane: cell surface proteins which regulate complement. *Res. Immunol.* **147:**82–87.
19. **Deckert, M., J. Kubar, D. Zoccola, G. Bernard-Pomier, P. Angelisova, V. Horejsi, and A. Bernard.** 1992. CD59 molecule: a second ligand for CD2 in T cell adhesion. *Eur. J. Immunol.* **22:**2943–2947.

20. **De Laszlo, S. E., E. E. Allen, B. Li, D. Ondeyka, R. Rivero, L. Malkowitz, C. Molineaux, S. J. Siciliano, M. S. Springer, W. J. Greenlee, and N. Mantlo.** 1997. A nonpeptidic agonist ligand of the human C5a receptor: synthesis, binding affinity optimization and functional characterization. *Bioorg. Med. Chem. Lett.* **7:**213–218.

21. **Diamond, L. E., K. R. McCurry, M. J. Martin, S. B. McClellan, E. R. Oldham, J. L. Platt, and J. S. Logan.** 1996. Characterization of transgenic pigs expressing functionally active human CD59 on cardiac endothelium. *Transplantation* **61:**1241–1249.

22. **Diamond, L. E., K. R. McCurry, E. R. Oldham, M. Tone, H. Waldmann, J. L. Platt, and J. S. Logan.** 1995. Human CD59 expressed in transgenic mouse hearts inhibits the activation of complement. *Transplant. Immunol.* **3:**305–312.

23. **Dickneite, G.** 1993. Influence of C1-inhibitor on inflammation, edema and shock. *Behring Inst. Mitteilung.* **93:**299–305.

24. **Dierich, M. P., H. Stoiber, and A. Clivio.** 1996. A "complement-ary" AIDS vaccine. *Nature Med.* **2:**153–155.

25. **Donaldson, V. H., and R. R. Evans.** 1963. A biochemical abnormality in hereditary angioneurotic edema. Absence of serum inhibitor of C1′-esterase. *Am. J. Med.* **35:**37–44.

26. **Dorling, A., C. Stocker, T. Tsao, D. O. Haskard, and R. I. Lechler.** 1996. In vitro accommodation of immortalized porcine endothelial cells: resistance to complement mediated lysis and down-regulation of VCAM expression induced by low concentrations of polyclonal human IgG antipig antibodies. *Transplantation* **62:**1127–1136.

27. **Dunning, J., P. C. Braidley, J. Wallwork, and D. J. White.** 1994. Analysis of hyperacute rejection of pig hearts by human blood using an ex vivo perfusion model. *Transplant. Proc.* **26:**1016–1017.

28. **Fodor, W. L., B. L. Williams, L. A. Matis, J. A. Madri, S. A. Rollins, J. W. Knight, W. Velander, and S. P. Squinto.** 1994. Expression of a functional human complement inhibitor in a transgenic pig as a model for the prevention of xenogeneic hyperacute organ rejection. *Proc. Natl. Acad. Sci. USA* **91:**11153–11157.

29. **Gralinski, M. R., B. C. Wiater, A. N. Assenmacher, and B. R. Lucchesi.** 1996. Selective inhibition of the alternative complement pathway by sCR1[desLHR-A] protects the rabbit isolated heart from human complement-mediated damage. *Immunopharmacology* **34:**79–88.

30. **Hack, C. E., A. C. Ogilvie, B. Eisele, A. J. Eerenberg, J. Wagstaff, and L. G. Thijs.** 1993. C1-inhibitor substitution therapy in septic shock and in the vascular leak syndrome induced by high doses of interleukin-2. *Intens. Care Med.* **19:**S19–S28.

31. **Hahn, W. C., E. Menu, A. L. Bothwell, P. J. Sims, and B. E. Bierer.** 1992. Overlapping but nonidentical binding sites on CD2 for CD58 and a second ligand CD59. *Science* **256:**1805–1807.

32. **Hakulinen, J., and S. Meri.** 1994. Expression and function of the complement membrane attack complex inhibitor protectin (CD59) on human breast cancer cells. *Lab. Invest.* **71:**820–827.

33. **Hamann, J., W. Eichler, D. Hamann, H. M. J. Kerstens, P. J. Poddighe, J. M. N. Hoovers, E. Hartmann, M. Strauss, and R. A. W. van Lier.** 1995. Expression cloning and chromosomal mapping of the leucocyte activation antigen CD97, a new seven-span transmembrane molecule of the secretin receptor superfamily with an unusual extracellular domain. *J. Immunol.* **155:**1942–1950.

34. **Hamann, J., B. Vogel, G. M. van Schijndel, and R. A. van Lier.** 1996. The seven-span transmembrane receptor CD97 has a cellular ligand (CD55, DAF). *J. Exp. Med.* **184:**1185–1189.

35. **Hammer, C.** 1994. Fundamental problems of xenotransplantation. *Pathol. Biol.* **42:**203–207.

36. **Hammer, C., M. Suckfull, and D. Saumweber.** 1992. Evolutionary and immunological aspects of xenotransplantation. *Transplant. Proc.* **24:**2397–2400.

37. **Hayashi, S., M. Ito, M. Yasutomi, Y. Namii, I. Yokoyama, K. Uchida, and H. Takagi.** 1995. Evidence that donor pretreatment with FK506 has a synergistic effect on graft prolongation in hamster-to-rat heart xenotransplantation. *J. Heart Lung Transplant.* **14:**579–584.

38. **Higgins, P. J., J. L. Ko, R. Lobell, C. Sardonini, M. K. Alessi, and C. G. Yeh.** 1997. A soluble chimeric complement inhibitory protein that possesses both decay-accelerating and factor I cofactor activities. *J. Immunol.* **158:**2872–2881.

39. **Hill, J., T. F. Lindsay, F. Ortiz, C. G. Yeh, H. B. Hechtman, and F. D. Moore, Jr.** 1992. Soluble complement receptor type 1 ameliorates the local and remote organ injury after intestinal ischemia-reperfusion in the rat. *J. Immunol.* **149:**1723–1728.

40. **Himmelfarb, J., E. McMonagle, D. Holbrook, and C. Toth.** 1995. Soluble complement receptor 1 inhibits both complement and granulocyte activation during ex vivo hemodialysis. *J. Lab. Clin. Med.* **126:**392–400.

41. **Jung, S., K. V. Toyka, and H. P. Hartung.** 1995. Soluble complement receptor type 1 inhibits experimental autoimmune neuritis in Lewis rats. *Neurosci. Lett.* **200:**167–170.
42. **Kaczorowski, S. L., J. K. Schiding, C. A. Toth, and P. M. Kochanek.** 1995. Effect of soluble complement receptor-1 on neutrophil accumulation after traumatic brain injury in rats. *J. Cereb. Blood Flow Metab.* **15:**860–864.
43. **Kalli, K. R., P. Hsu, and D. T. Fearon.** 1994. Therapeutic uses of recombinant complement protein inhibitors. *Springer Semin. Immunopathol.* **15:**417–431.
44. **Kaneko, Y., N. Okada, L. Baranyi, T. Azuma, and H. Okada.** 1995. Antagonistic peptides against human anaphylatoxin c5a. *Immunology* **86:**149–154.
45. **Karnauchow, T. M., D. L. Tolson, B. A. Harrison, E. Altman, D. M. Lublin, and K. Dimock.** 1996. The HeLa cell receptor for enterovirus 70 is decay-accelerating factor (CD55). *J. Virol.* **70:**5143–5152.
46. **Kirklin, J. K., D. E. Chenoweth, D. C. Naftel, E. H. Blackstone, J. W. Kirklin, D. D. Bitran, J. G. Curd, J. G. Reves, and P. N. Samuelson.** 1986. Effects of protamine administration after cardiopulmonary bypass on complement, blood elements, and the hemodynamic state. *Ann. Thorac. Surg.* **41:**193–199.
47. **Konteatis, Z. D., S. J. Siciliano, G. Van Riper, C. J. Molineaux, S. Pandya, P. Fischer, H. Rosen, R. A. Mumford, and M. S. Springer.** 1994. Development of C5a receptor antagonists: differential loss of functional responses. *J. Immunol.* **153:**4200–4205.
48. **Kroshus, T. J., R. M. Bolman III, A. P. Dalmasso, S. A. Rollins, E. R. Guilmette, B. L. Williams, S. P. Squinto, and W. L. Fodor.** 1996. Expression of human CD59 in transgenic pig organs enhances organ survival in an ex vivo xenogeneic perfusion model. *Transplantation* **61:**1513–1521.
49. **Kroshus, T. J., S. A. Rollins, A. P. Dalmasso, E. A. Elliott, L. A. Matis, S. P. Squinto, and R. M. Bolman 3rd.** 1995. Complement inhibition with an anti-C5 monoclonal antibody prevents acute cardiac tissue injury in an ex vivo model of pig-to-human xenotransplantation. *Transplantation* **60:**1194–1202.
50. **Lanza, T. J., P. L. Durette, T. Rollins, S. Siciliano, D. N. Cianciarulo, S. V. Kobayashi, C. G. Caldwell, M. S. Springer, and W. K. Hagmann.** 1992. Substituted 4,6-diaminoquinolines as inhibitors of C5a receptor binding. *J. Med. Chem.* **35:**252–258.
51. **Laurell, A.-B.** 1986. Complement determinations in clinical diagnosis, p. 272–287. *In* K. Rother and G.O. Till (ed.), *The Complement System*. Springer, Berlin, Germany.
52. **Lehto, T., E. Honkanen, A. M. Teppo, and S. Meri.** 1995. Urinary excretion of protectin (CD59), complement SC5b-9 and cytokines in membranous glomerulonephritis. *Kidney Int.* **47:**1403–1411.
53. **Lowe, J. B., and P. A. Ward.** 1997. Therapeutic inhibition of carbohydrate-protein interactions in vivo. *J. Clin. Invest.* **99:**822–826.
54. **Magee, J. C., B. H. Collins, R. C. Harland, B. J. Lindman, R. R. Bollinger, M. M. Frank, and J. L. Platt.** 1995. Immunoglobulin prevents complement-mediated hyperacute rejection in swine-to-primate xenotransplantation. *J. Clin. Invest.* **96:**2404–2412.
55. **Makrides, S. C., P. A. Nygren, B. Andrews, P. J. Ford, K. S. Evans, E. G. Hayman, H. Adari, M. Uhlen, and C. A. Toth.** 1996. Extended in vivo half-life of human soluble complement receptor type 1 fused to a serum albumin-binding receptor. *J. Pharmacol. Exp. Therap.* **277:**534–542.
56. **Manchester, M., J. E. Gairin, J. B. Patterson, J. Alvarez, M. K. Liszewski, D. S. Eto, J. P. Atkinson, and M. B. Oldstone.** 1997. Measles virus recognizes its receptor, CD46, via two distinct binding domains within SCR1-2. *Virology* **233:**174–184.
57. **Manchester, M., M. K. Liszewski, J. P. Atkinson, and M. B. Oldstone.** 1994. Multiple isoforms of CD46 (membrane cofactor protein) serve as receptors for measles virus. *Proc. Natl. Acad. Sci. USA* **91:**2161–2165.
58. **McCurry, K. R., L. E. Diamond, D. L. Kooyman, G. W. Byrne, M. J. Martin, J. S. Logan, and J. L. Platt.** 1996. Human complement regulatory proteins expressed in transgenic swine protect swine xenografts from humoral injury. *Transplant. Proc.* **28:**758.
59. **McCurry, K. R., D. L. Kooyman, C. G. Alvarado, A. H. Cotterell, M. J. Martin, J. S. Logan, and J. L. Platt.** 1995. Human complement regulatory proteins protect swine-to-primate cardiac xenografts from humoral injury [see comments]. *Nature Med.* **1:**423–427.
60. **McCurry, K. R., D. L. Kooyman, L. E. Diamond, G. W. Byrne, J. S. Logan, and J. L. Platt.** 1995. Transgenic expression of human complement regulatory proteins in mice results in diminished complement deposition during organ xenoperfusion. *Transplantation* **59:**1177–1182.
61. **Mellbye, O. J., S. S. Froland, P. Lilleaasen, J. L. Svennevig, and T. E. Mollnes.** 1988. Complement activation during cardiopulmonary bypass: comparison between the use of large volumes of plasma and dextran 70. *Eur. Surg. Res.* **20:**101–109.

62. **Meri, S., T. Lehto, C. W. Sutton, J. Tyynela, and M. Baumann.** 1996. Structural composition and functional characterization of soluble CD59: heterogeneity of the oligosaccharide and glycophosphoinositol (GPI) anchor revealed by laser-desorption mass spectrometric analysis. *Biochem. J.* **316:**923–935.
63. **Mollnes, T. E.** 1997. Biocompatibility: complement as mediator of tissue damage and as indicator of incompatibility. *Exp. Clin. Immunogenet.* **14:**24–29.
64. **Mollnes, T. E., V. Videm, J. Riesenfeld, P. Garred, J. L. Svennevig, E. Fosse, K. Hogasen, and M. Harboe.** 1991. Complement activation and bioincompatibility. *Clin. Exp. Immunol.* **86**(Suppl. 1):21–26.
65. **Moore, F. D., Jr.** 1994. Therapeutic regulation of the complement system in acute injury states. *Adv. Immunol.* **56:**267–299.
66. **Moran, P., H. Beasley, A. Gorrell, E. Martin, P. Gribling, H. Fuchs, N. Gillett, L. E. Burton, and I. W. Caras.** 1992. Human recombinant soluble decay accelerating factor inhibits complement activation in vitro and in vivo. *J. Immunol.* **149:**1736–1743.
67. **Morgan, B. P.** 1989. Complement membrane attack on nucleated cells: resistance, recovery and non-lethal effects. *Biochem. J.* **264:**1–14.
68. **Morgan, B. P.** 1989. Mechanisms of tissue damage by the membrane attack complex of complement. *Complement Inflammat.* **6:**104–111.
69. **Morgan, B. P.** 1994. Clinical complementology: recent progress and future trends. *Eur. J. Clin. Invest.* **24:**219–228.
69a. **Morgan, B. P., and C. L. Harris.** 1999. *Complement Regulatory Proteins*. Academic Press, London, United Kingdom.
70. **Morgan, B. P., and M. J. Walport.** 1991. Complement deficiency and disease. *Immunol. Today* **12:**301–306.
71. **Morgan, E. L., J. A. Ember, S. D. Sanderson, W. Scholz, R. Buchner, R. D. Ye, and T. E. Hugli.** 1993. Anti-C5a receptor antibodies. Characterization of neutralizing antibodies specific for a peptide, C5aR-(9-29), derived from the predicted amino-terminal sequence of the human C5a receptor. *J. Immunol.* **151:**377–388.
72. **Morikis, D., N. Assa-Munt, A. Sahu, and J. D. Lambris.** 1998. Solution structure of compstatin, a potent complement inhibitor. *Protein Sci.* **7:**619–627.
73. **Mulligan, M. S., E. Schmid, B. Beck-Schimmer, G. O. Till, H. P. Friedl, R. B. Brauer, T. E. Hugli, M. Miyasaka, R. L. Warner, K. J. Johnson, and P. A. Ward.** 1996. Requirement and role of C5a in acute lung inflammatory injury in rats. *J. Clin. Investig.* **98:**503–512.
74. **Mulligan, M. S., C. G. Yeh, A. R. Rudolph, and P. A. Ward.** 1992. Protective effects of soluble CR1 in complement- and neutrophil-mediated tissue injury. *J. Immunol.* **148:**1479–1485.
75. **Niederau, C., R. Brinsa, M. Niederau, R. Luthen, G. Strohmeyer, and L. D. Ferrell.** 1995. Effects of C1-esterase inhibitor in three models of acute pancreatitis. *Int. J. Pancreatol.* **17:**189–196.
76. **Nilsson, B., R. Larsson, J. Hong, G. Elgue, K. N. Ekdahl, A. Sahu, and J. D. Lambris.** 1998. Compstatin inhibits complement and cellular activation in whole blood in two models of extracorporeal circulation. *Blood* **92:**1661–1667.
77. **Nishizawa, H., H. Yamada, H. Miyazaki, M. Ohara, K. Kaneko, T. Yamakawa, J. Wiener-Kronish, and I. Kudoh.** 1996. Soluble complement receptor type 1 inhibited the systemic organ injury caused by acid instillation into a lung. *Anesthesiology* **85:**1120–1128.
78. **Ogilvie, A. C., J. W. Baars, A. J. Eerenberg, C. E. Hack, H. M. Pinedo, L. G. Thijs, and J. Wagstaff.** 1994. A pilot study to evaluate the effects of C1 esterase inhibitor on the toxicity of high-dose interleukin 2. *Br. J. Cancer* **69:**596–598.
79. **Oglesby, T. J., C. J. Allen, M. K. Liszewski, D. J. White, and J. P. Atkinson.** 1992. Membrane cofactor protein (CD46) protects cells from complement-mediated attack by an intrinsic mechanism. *J. Exp. Med.* **175:**1547–1551.
80. **Oglesby, T. J., D. White, I. Tedja, K. Liszewski, L. Wright, J. Van den Bogarde, and J. P. Atkinson.** 1991. Protection of mammalian cells from complement-mediated lysis by transfection of human membrane cofactor protein and decay-accelerating factor. *Transact. Assoc. Am. Physic.* **104:**164–172.
81. **Ovrum, E., T. E. Mollnes, E. Fosse, E. A. Holen, G. Tangen, M. A. Ringdal, and V. Videm.** 1995. High and low heparin dose with heparin-coated cardiopulmonary bypass: activation of complement and granulocytes. *Ann. Thorac. Surg.* **60:**1755–1761.
82. **Pemberton, M., G. Anderson, V. Vetvicka, D. E. Justus, and G. D. Ross.** 1993. Microvascular effects

of complement blockade with soluble recombinant CR1 on ischemia/reperfusion injury of skeletal muscle. *J. Immunol.* **150:**5104–5113.

83. **Piddlesden, S. J., S. Jiang, J. L. Levin, A. Vincent, and B. P. Morgan.** 1996. Soluble complement receptor 1 (sCR1) protects against experimental autoimmune myasthenia gravis. *J. Neuroimmunol.* **71:**173–177.
84. **Piddlesden, S. J., M. K. Storch, M. Hibbs, A. M. Freeman, H. Lassmann, and B. P. Morgan.** 1994. Soluble recombinant complement receptor 1 inhibits inflammation and demyelination in antibody-mediated demyelinating experimental allergic encephalomyelitis. *J. Immunol.* **152:**5477–5484.
85. **Platt, J. L.** 1994. A perspective on xenograft rejection and accommodation. *Immunol. Rev.* **141:**127–149.
86. **Platt, J. L.** 1996. The immunological barriers to xenotransplantation. *Crit. Rev. Immunol.* **16:**331–358.
87. **Pohlein, C., A. Pascher, M. Storck, V. K. Young, W. Konig, D. Abendroth, M. Wick, J. Thiery, D. J. White, and C. Hammer.** 1996. Transgenic human DAF-expressing porcine livers: their function during hemoperfusion with human blood. *Transplant. Proc.* **28:**770–771.
88. **Pratt, J. R., M. J. Hibbs, A. J. Laver, R. A. Smith, and S. H. Sacks.** 1996. Effects of complement inhibition with soluble complement receptor-1 on vascular injury and inflammation during renal allograft rejection in the rat. *Am. J. Pathol.* **149:**2055–2066.
89. **Pruitt, S. K., and R. R. Bollinger.** 1991. The effect of soluble complement receptor type 1 on hyperacute allograft rejection. *J. Surg. Res.* **50:**350–355.
90. **Pruitt, S., R. R. Bollinger, B. H. Collins, H. C. Marsh, J. L. Levin, A. R. Rudolph, W. M. Baldwin 3rd, and F. Sanfilippo.** 1996. Continuous complement (C) inhibition using soluble C receptor type 1 (sCR1): effect on hyperacute rejection (HAR) of pig-to-primate cardiac xenografts. *Transplant. Proc.* **28:**756.
91. **Pruitt, S. K., R. R. Bollinger, B. H. Collins, H. C. Marsh, Jr., J. L. Levin, A. R. Rudolph, W. M. Baldwin 3rd, and F. Sanfilippo.** 1997. Effect of continuous complement inhibition using soluble complement receptor type 1 on survival of pig-to-primate cardiac xenografts. *Transplantation* **63:**900–902.
92. **Pruitt, S. K., A. D. Kirk, R. R. Bollinger, H. C. Marsh, Jr., B. H. Collins, J. L. Levin, J. R. Mault, J. S. Heinle, S. Ibrahim, A. R. Rudolph, W. M. Baldwin, 3rd, and F. Sanfilippo.** 1994. The effect of soluble complement receptor type 1 on hyperacute rejection of porcine xenografts. *Transplantation* **57:**363–370.
93. **Rajasinghe, H. A., V. M. Reddy, W. W. Hancock, M. H. Sayegh, and F. L. Hanley.** 1996. Key role of the alternate complement pathway in hyperacute rejection of rat hearts transplanted into fetal sheep. *Transplantation* **62:**407–411.
94. **Rauterberg, E. W.** 1986. Demonstration of complement deposits in tissues, p. 287–326. *In* K. Rother and G. O. Till (ed.), *The Complement System*. Springer, Berlin, Germany.
95. **Rollins, S. A., L. A. Matis, J. P. Springhorn, E. Setter, and D. W. Wolff.** 1995. Monoclonal antibodies directed against human C5 and C8 block complement-mediated damage of xenogeneic cells and organs. *Transplantation* **60:**1284–1292.
96. **Ryan, U. S.** 1995. Complement inhibitory therapeutics and xenotransplantation. *Nature Med.* **1:**967–968.
97. **Sandrin, M. S., W. L. Fodor, E. Mouhtouris, N. Osman, S. Cohney, S. A. Rollins, E. R. Guilmette, E. Setter, S. P. Squinto, and I. F. McKenzie.** 1995. Enzymatic remodelling of the carbohydrate surface of a xenogenic cell substantially reduces human antibody binding and complement-mediated cytolysis [see comments]. *Nature Med.* **1:**1261–1267.
98. **Sandrin, M. S., and I. F. McKenzie.** 1994. Gal alpha (1,3)Gal, the major xenoantigen(s) recognised in pigs by human natural antibodies. *Immunol. Rev.* **141:**169–190.
99. **Scesney, S. M., S. C. Makrides, M. L. Gosselin, P. J. Ford, B. M. Andrews, E. G. Hayman, and H. C. Marsh, Jr.** 1996. A soluble deletion mutant of the human complement receptor type 1, which lacks the C4b binding site, is a selective inhibitor of the alternative complement pathway. *Eur. J. Immunol.* **26:**1729–1735.
100. **Schilling, A., W. Land, E. Pratschke, K. Pielsticker, and W. Brendel.** 1976. Dominant role of complement in the hyperacute xenograft rejection reaction. *Surg. Gynecol. Obstetr.* **142:**29–32.
101. **Spiller, O. B., S. M. Hanna, D. V. Devine, and F. Tufaro.** 1997. Neutralization of cytomegalovirus virions: the role of complement. *J. Infect. Dis.* **176:**339–347.
102. **Stevens, R. B., and J. L. Platt.** 1992. The pathogenesis of hyperacute xenograft rejection. *Am. J. Kidney Dis.* **20:**414–421.
103. **Stoiber, H., A. Clivio, and M. P. Dierich.** 1997. Role of complement in HIV infection. *Annu. Rev. Immunol.* **15:**649–674.
104. **Sugita, Y., K. Ito, K. Shiozuka, H. Suzuki, H. Gushima, M. Tomita, and Y. Masuho.** 1994. Recombinant soluble CD59 inhibits reactive haemolysis with complement. *Immunology* **82:**34–41.

105. **Tanaka, M., N. Murase, Q. Ye, W. Miyazaki, M. Nomoto, H. Miyazawa, R. Manez, Y. Toyama, A. J. Demetris, S. Todo, and T. E. Starzl.** 1996. Effect of anticomplement agent K76 COOH on hamster-to-rat and guinea pig-to-rat heart xenotransplantation. *Transplantation* **62:**681–688.

106. **Thomas, T. C., S. A. Rollins, R. P. Rother, M. A. Giannoni, S. L. Hartman, E. A. Elliott, S. H. Nye, L. A. Matis, S. P. Squinto, and M. J. Evans.** 1996. Inhibition of complement activity by humanized anti-C5 antibody and single-chain Fv. *Molec. Immunol.* **33:**1389–1401.

107. **Vaughan, H. A., B. E. Loveland, and M. S. Sandrin.** 1994. Gal alpha(1,3)Gal is the major xenoepitope expressed on pig endothelial cells recognized by naturally occurring cytotoxic human antibodies. *Transplantation* **58:**879–882.

108. **Vaughan, H. A., I. F. McKenzie, and M. S. Sandrin.** 1995. Biochemical studies of pig xenoantigens detected by naturally occurring human antibodies and the galactose alpha(1-3)galactose reactive lectin. *Transplantation* **59:**102–109.

109. **Vesentini, S., L. Benetti, C. Bassi, A. Bonora, A. Campedelli, G. Zamboni, P. Castelli, and P. Pederzoli.** 1993. Effects of choline-esterase inhibitor in experimental acute pancreatitis in rats. Preliminary results. *Int. J. Pancreatol.* **13:**217–220.

110. **Walport, M. J., and P. J. Lachmann.** 1990. Complement deficiencies and abnormalities of the complement system in systemic lupus erythematosus and related disorders. *Curr. Opin. Rheumatol.* **2:**661–663.

111. **Wang, Y., Q. Hu, J. A. Madri, S. A. Rollins, A. Chodera, and L. A. Matis.** 1996. Amelioration of lupus-like autoimmune disease in NZB/WF1 mice after treatment with a blocking monoclonal antibody specific for complement component C5. *Proc. Nat. Acad. Sci. USA* **93:**8563–8568.

112. **Wang, Y., S. A. Rollins, J. A. Madri, and L. A. Matis.** 1995. Anti-C5 monoclonal antibody therapy prevents collagen-induced arthritis and ameliorates established disease. *Proc. Nat. Acad. Sci. USA* **92:**8955–8959.

113. **Ward, T., P. A. Pipkin, N. A. Clarkson, D. M. Stone, P. D. Minor, and J. W. Almond.** 1994. Decay-accelerating factor CD55 is identified as the receptor for echovirus 7 using CELICS, a rapid immuno-focal cloning method. *EMBO J.* **13:**5070–5074.

114. **Weisman, H. F., T. Bartow, M. K. Leppo, M. P. Boyle, H. C. Marsh, Jr., G. R. Carson, K. H. Roux, M. L. Weisfeldt, and D. T. Fearon.** 1990. Recombinant soluble CR1 suppressed complement activation, inflammation, and necrosis associated with reperfusion of ischemic myocardium. *Transact. Assoc. Am. Physic.* **103:**64–72.

115. **Weisman, H. F., T. Bartow, M. K. Leppo, H. C. Marsh, Jr., G. R. Carson, M. F. Concino, M. P. Boyle, K. H. Roux, M. L. Weisfeldt, and D. T. Fearon.** 1990. Soluble human complement receptor type 1: in vivo inhibitor of complement suppressing post-ischemic myocardial inflammation and necrosis. *Science* **249:**146–151.

116. **Whaley, K.** 1989. Measurement of complement activation in clinical practice. *Complement Inflammat.* **6:**96–103.

117. **White, D.** 1996. Alteration of complement activity: a strategy for xenotransplantation. *Trends Biotechnol.* **14:**3–5.

118. **White, D. J.** 1992. Transplantation of organs between species. *Int. Arch. Allergy Immunol.* **98:**1–5.

119. **Xiao, F., M. J. Eppihimer, B. H. Willis, and D. L. Carden.** 1997. Complement-mediated lung injury and neutrophil retention after intestinal ischemia- reperfusion. *J. Appl. Physiol.* **82:**1459–1465.

120. **Yamakawa, M., K. Yamada, T. Tsuge, H. Ohrui, T. Ogata, M. Dobashi, and Y. Imai.** 1994. Protection of thyroid cancer cells by complement-regulatory factors. *Cancer* **73:**2808–2817.

121. **Zhang, X., W. Boyar, N. Galakatos, and N. C. Gonnella.** 1997. Solution structure of a unique C5a semi-synthetic antagonist: implications in receptor binding. *Protein Sci.* **6:**65–72.

Xenotransplantation
Edited by Jeffrey L. Platt

Chapter 9

Recognition of Foreign Antigen and Foreign Major Histocompatibility Complex

Adriana Colovai, Rodica Ciubotariu, Raffaello Cortesini, and Nicole Suciu-Foca

Over the last 50 years, advances in controlling immunological rejection of organ allografts have rendered transplantation of tissues and organs from allogeneic human donors the preferred treatment for chronic failure of the kidney, heart, liver, and lung. However, the severe shortage of donor organs and tissues limits dramatically the number of patients who may receive a graft. An obvious solution to this problem would be the use of animal donors, such as the pig (2, 29, 30, 75, 86, 97). The pig offers the advantage of having favorable breeding characteristics, showing anatomical and physiological similarities with humans, and posing fewer ethical problems than do primates. Xenotransplantation using pigs as donors could provide an unlimited supply of good quality organs.

However, due to major obstacles that must be overcome to achieve xenograft tolerance, clinical application of xenotransplantation still belongs to the future.

Xenografts from discordant species, such as pig, are susceptible to hyperacute rejection, which is initiated by the binding of naturally occurring antibodies to carbohydrate determinants (i.e., α-Gal) on the surface of xenogeneic cells (76, 87). The generation of transgenic pigs expressing human complement-regulatory molecules on vascular endothelium may solve this critical problem (30). The next immunological barrier is acute vascular rejection, which involves multiple pathways, such as antibody binding and endothelial cell activation (3, 97). However, the exact mechanisms underlying this process are not fully understood. Attempts to prevent acute vascular rejection by blocking B-cell responses or, more recently, by blocking endothelial cell activation, have been only moderately effective (36, 103).

However, even in the absence of hyperacute and acute vascular rejection, cell-mediated immune responses against xenogeneic antigens are strong enough to cause graft destruction (46, 62). The role of T cells appears to be critical for rejection since in the absence of

Adriana Colovai, Rodica Ciubotariu, and Nicole Suciu-Foca • Department of Pathology, College of Physicians and Surgeons of Columbia University, 630 West 168th Street, New York, NY 10032. ***Raffaello Cortesini*** • Department of Surgery, Servizio Trapianti d'Organo, Instituto di II Clinica Chirurgica, Università Degli Studi di Roma "La Sapienza," Rome, Italy.

functional T cells (i.e., in nude mice), xenogeneic tissues can be successfully transplanted, while in normal animals they are invariably rejected (98).

Human anti-pig cellular responses measured in vitro are as strong or stronger than allogeneic immune responses (104). Thus, it is likely that conventional immunosuppressive drugs, used efficiently to prevent the rejection of allografts, will be insufficient to control the cellular immune response against pig xenografts. Furthermore, since nonspecific immunosuppressive drugs impair the host immune response against pathogens, the use of excessively high doses would make infectious complications unavoidable. This problem is of particular concern in view of the recent finding that pigs, the current donor of choice, harbor endogenous retroviruses that can infect human cells (70). Immunosuppression may facilitate the transfer of viruses from animal to human recipients, thus creating the risk of viral epidemics.

These considerations imply that successful xenotransplantation will require the development of strategies that permit specific suppression of the immune response to the graft, keeping intact the ability of the host to react against infectious agents. It is, therefore, important to understand the mechanisms that result in activation and suppression of T-cell responses against xenograft antigens and viruses. We will focus our discussion on human anti-pig T-cell responses as this system is particularly relevant to clinical transplantation.

T-CELL RESPONSES MEDIATED VIA THE DIRECT RECOGNITION PATHWAY

T-cell recognition of foreign major histocompatibility complex (MHC) antigens has represented a challenging enigma for cellular immunologists over more than three decades. The response to MHC allo- and xenoantigens differs in two important ways from the classical reactivity that T cells display against nominal antigens. First, T-cell reactivity to nominal antigens can be detected only if the individual had been primed in vivo with the respective antigen, or after in vitro immunization by multiple antigenic stimulations. In contrast, T cells from nonimmunized individuals respond vigorously in primary MLC against stimulating cells from an allogeneic or xenogeneic (swine) donor (34, 70, 104). This is due to the remarkably higher frequency of precursor T cells (>100-fold) that recognize foreign MHC-bearing cells.

The second major difference between T-cell responses to allogeneic or xenogeneic cells and reactivity to nominal antigens resides in the lack of self-MHC restriction and processing requirements for recognition of foreign cell surface MHC antigens. This situation is unique since in all other cases antigen-specific T lymphocytes recognize native protein antigens only after the antigen has been proteolysed and the resulting peptides have been presented by an MHC class II molecule expressed by self antigen-presenting cells (APCs) (39). APCs from individuals carrying MHC class II molecules that are different from those expressed by the T-cell donor cannot present efficiently the antigen to self-restricted T-cell clones. Direct recognition of foreign MHC antigens, therefore, violates the rule of self-MHC restriction, since the T-cell response is elicited in this case by allogeneic or xenogeneic MHC/peptide complexes.

The participation of such a high number of T cells (1 to 10% of the total population of unprimed T cells) in the direct recognition of alloantigens has been explained by two alternative yet not mutually exclusive hypotheses. The first proposes that multiple T-cell clones, each responsive to the same allogeneic MHC molecule complexed to a different self peptide, become activated by "multiple binary complexes" (64). This would explain the high heterogeneity of T cells responding to allogeneic cells. There is evidence that molecular mimicry plays an important role in driving the proliferation of this large population of T cells since there are numerous examples of T-cell clones that utilize the same T-cell receptor ($\alpha\beta$TCR) to recognize both a nominal antigen and an allogeneic MHC protein (59, 83). This indicates that T cells are activated by MHC/peptide complexes expressed on the surface of allogeneic (or xenogeneic) APCs, which mimic MHC/peptide complexes derived from the processing of nominal antigens by the self APCs.

The second hypothesis attributes the magnitude of the T-cell response to the high density of allogeneic MHC molecules on the surface of a foreign APC (16). Elucidation of the three-dimensional structure of class I (11) and class II MHC (17) molecules, together with major advances in our understanding of antigen processing and presentation, had clarified considerably the molecular basis of direct T-cell recognition. The emerging picture is that both the allogeneic MHC molecule itself and the bound peptides may each independently contribute to reactivity and, furthermore, that peptide binding to MHC may induce conformational changes in the MHC molecule itself that affect recognition (11, 17, 82, 102).

The most potent stimulators of the direct recognition pathways and acute rejection are bone marrow–derived dendritic cells, which express abundantly MHC class I and class II antigens as well as the costimulatory molecules required for T-cell activation (49, 94). Thus, while the first signal for T-cell activation comes from the engagement of the TCR with the MHC-peptide complex on the APC, the second signal is provided by the engagement of costimulatory molecules, such as CD80 and CD86, on the surface of the APC, with CD28 and CTLA4 (CD152) on the surface of T cells. Activated T cells express CD154 (CD40L), which interacts with CD40 expressed by APCs, inducing prolonged survival of dendritic cells and upregulated expression of CD58, CD80, and CD86 (19, 20, 72). Ligation of CD40 on the surface of APC, with CD154 expressed by activated T cells, augments the ability of APC to induce T-cell proliferation and IFN-γ production. Moreover, ligation of CD40 with CD154 results in the production of cytokines, such as IL-8, macrophage inflammatory protein (MIP)-1α, tumor necrosis factor (TNF)-α, and IL-12 (20, 45, 72). These cytokines amplify the inflammatory response, recruiting immune cells at the site of inflammation (i.e., MIP-1α and IL-8), and upregulating costimulatory activity on naive APC (i.e., TNF). Hence, activation of APCs via the CD40–CD154 interaction may be an important step in the induction of inflammation and anti-donor reactivity.

Comparison of the strength of direct recognition in the allogeneic (human–anti-human) and xenogeneic (human–anti-pig) MLC reactions showed that the human–anti-pig reactivity is similar to or greater than the human–anti-human response, implying that many molecular interactions involved in T-cell activation are functional in this species combination (15, 26, 88, 104). Indeed, several studies have shown that the following interactions are, at least partially, operating: CD4/class II, CD8/class I, CD2/LFA3, CD28/B7, CD40L/CD40, LFA-1/ICAM, VLA-4/VCAM, and Fas/FasL (10, 26, 61, 68). Human CD4$^+$ T cells were shown to specifically recognize polymorphic variants of DRβ chains on pig APCs, demonstrating that the TCR repertoire, accessory molecule interactions, and cytokine production required for direct recognition are functional (104). Similarly, human CD8$^+$ T cells were shown to be able to lyse pig targets in an MHC class I–specific fashion, a finding consistent with the notion that the molecular interactions between human T-cell receptor and coreceptor (CD8) and pig MHC class I antigens are, at least in part, functional in this xenogeneic combination (22, 88, 92, 105).

However, several interactions that are critical for immunoregulatory mechanisms, such as recognition of SLA class I molecules by human natural killer (NK) inhibitory receptors, or interaction of certain human cytokines such as IFN-γ with their receptors on pig cells, appear to be deficient in this xenogeneic system (5, 91). The incompatibility between human NK inhibitory receptors and their corresponding ligands on pig target cells may be responsible for the strength of the NK response against pig xenografts (41, 43, 58).

Human T cells show significantly stronger reactivity to pig than to human endothelial cells (15, 61). This is due to the fact that in addition to MHC class II molecules, pig endothelial cells also express B7 molecules (which are not present on human endothelial cells), costimulating efficiently xenoreactive T cells (61). Additional costimulatory signals are provided by the interaction of CD2 and LFA1 on human T cells with their porcine ligands (10, 26, 61, 68). Hence, it is likely that endothelial cells from pig xenografts will elicit a vigorous T-cell response in human recipients via the direct xenorecognition pathway.

Direct recognition of xenogeneic MHC antigens is, therefore, likely to initiate and perpetuate rejection since it can be triggered not only by "passenger" dendritic cells from the donor, but also by graft endothelial cells. This situation is different from that encountered in allotransplantation, where T cells recognizing donor MHC alloantigen on nonprofessional APCs (such as endothelial and epithelial cells), which are defective in the expression of costimulatory molecules, become anergized, failing to proliferate and produce IL-2 (49, 91).

Several studies have examined the human anti-porcine T-cell repertoire (43; Pennesi, G., in preparation), using in vitro assays to measure T-cell function and TCR spectratyping to identify the Vβ families involved. Human CD4$^+$ Th cell lines, which specifically recognize pig APCs, showed a skewed distribution of TCR Vβ gene expression. Interestingly, the TCR repertoire of xenoreactive Th cells was more restricted than the repertoire of allospecific Th cells (derived from the same human responder), indicating that a more stringent selection of T cells had taken place during expansion of xenoreactive CD4$^+$ T cells (Pennesi, G., in preparation). This finding can be explained by the limited number of human TCR molecules able to bind with favorable affinity to MHC from discordant species. It is possible that the self-MHC–driven selection of T cells in the thymus leads to a T-cell repertoire that mainly recognizes closely related MHC structures.

Alternatively, molecular incompatibility between certain cell membrane receptors and ligands expressed by human and pig cells may restrict the number of high-affinity T-cell clones able to proliferate in response to pig APCs. In any event, the limited TCR repertoire expressed by xenospecific T cells raises the possibility of a targeted immunosuppressive strategy, aimed at deleting distinct TCR families.

Similar to human xenoreactive Th lines, human T-suppressor (Ts) cells, which specifically recognize MHC class I molecules on the surface of xenogeneic cells, show a fairly restricted repertoire of TCR-Vβ families (26; Pennesi, G., in preparation). Xenospecific Ts cells derive from a subset of the CD8 population, which does not express the CD28 molecule. These CD8$^+$CD28$^-$ cells can be immunized in vitro against human or pig APCs by multiple stimulations performed in strictly controlled culture conditions (26, 57). The characteristics of xenospecific Ts cells are summarized in Table 1. Human Ts cells recognize

Table 1. Characteristics of human anti-pig suppressor cells (37)[a]

Phenotype	$CD3^+$, $CD8^+$, $CD45RO^+$, $CD28^-$
Specificity	Pig MHC class I antigens
TCR usage	Oligoclonal
Function	Inhibit IL-2 production and proliferation of human xenoreactive T-helper cells
Mechanism of action	Prevent upregulation of costimulatory molecules on xenogeneic APC by cell-to-cell interaction

[a]TCR, T-cell receptor; APC, antigen-presenting cell.

MHC class I antigens on allogeneic and xenogeneic APCs and block the response of T-helper cells to MHC class II antigens coexpressed by the APCs used for priming. This inhibitory effect is not mediated by lymphokines, but instead requires cell- to-cell interaction between $CD8^+CD28^-$ T-suppressor cells and allogeneic or xenogeneic APCs expressing antigens against which the T cells were primed. MHC class I–specific Ts cells were shown to inhibit Th activation by suppressing the CD40/40L and CD28/B7 costimulatory pathways and, thus, modulating the stimulatory function of the APCs (26, 57).

It has been recently demonstrated that, by recognizing antigen on APCs, T-helper cells deliver a series of signals that activate the APCs, which are then "licensed" to stimulate directly T-killer cells (9, 81, 90). One critical signal involves the CD40L expressed by antigen-stimulated T-helper cells and CD40, a surface receptor present on dendritic cells and other APCs. T-suppressor cells have the opposite effect, inhibiting the function of APC, and thereby interfering with the immune response to allo- or xenoantigens.

Several studies have shown that there is cross-talk between the MHC class I and class II pathways of peptide processing, supporting the notion that the same APCs present both helper- and suppressor-inducing peptides (12, 38, 69). It is possible that recognition by Ts cells of MHC class I–bound peptides helps control local inflammation caused by antigen-specific Th cells. Identification of suppressor-inducing peptides may be useful for the induction of unresponsiveness to allo- or xenoantigens.

The possibility of manipulating the activation of APCs will open new avenues for xenotransplantation. This possibility is supported by the finding that improved allo- and xenograft survival in rodents and preclinical model systems can be achieved by blockade of costimulation, using soluble ligands that bind to B7 molecules (i.e., CTLA4-Ig), making them unavailable for engagement by the CD28 molecule (52, 71, 99). More recently, attempts to block the CD40/CD40L costimulatory pathway by use of anti-CD40L antibodies yielded significantly improved results in the prevention of allogeneic graft rejection and reversal of ongoing rejection episodes (47).

Furthermore, simultaneous administration of CTLA4-Ig and anti-CD40L was shown to effectively abort clonal expansion of T cells in long-term survival of allogeneic grafts (44, 48). The efficiency of such immunosuppressive strategies, aimed at costimulation blockade by use of specific blocking agents or by "adoptive transfer" of suppressor cells, remains to be explored in the xenogeneic transplantation system. In vitro results obtained thus far indicate that xenospecific Ts cells are more efficient inhibitors of xenoreactive Th costimulation than specific antibodies to costimulatory molecules (26). The use of such regulatory T cells may, therefore, represent an attractive therapy for prevention and/or suppression of cellular rejection.

T-CELL RESPONSES MEDIATED VIA THE INDIRECT RECOGNITION PATHWAY

Over the past decade evidence has been accumulated that both allo- and xenorecognition occur not only via the direct but also via the indirect pathway, which defines T-cell responses against donor MHC molecules, which are processed by host APCs and presented as peptides bound to self-MHC class II molecules (14, 24, 31, 67, 74, 104).

Episodes of acute allograft rejection can be reversed by increased immunosuppression. However, if the host develops antibodies against the MHC antigens of the graft, rejection becomes irreversible (96). The production of alloantibodies is mediated by T-helper cells, which produce the lymphokines required for B-cell growth and maturation. Such T-helper cells recognize processed forms of allogeneic MHC molecules presented by host APCs, via the indirect route, which corresponds to the classical pathway of nominal antigen recognition. Most of our knowledge about the mechanism of indirect recognition derives from studies in the allogeneic system.

The stimulation of self-restricted IL-2 producing $CD4^+$ T cells by alloantigen has been documented both in human and animal systems (1, 7, 8, 27, 33, 50, 54, 55, 79). Peptides derived from the polymorphic regions of allogeneic MHC antigens were shown to induce T-cell alloreactivity when presented by self-MHC class II molecules. The T-cell response was specific for the native allogeneic MHC molecule and was mediated by $CD4^+$ T cells. Factors that determine the size of a T-cell response to a given MHC-bound peptide include the efficiency with which the peptide is generated from its parent protein, the affinity of binding to the MHC molecule, and the available TCR repertoire (56).

Experiments in mice and rats have demonstrated that host sensitization with allopeptides results in accelerated allograft rejection, delayed-type hypersensitivity (DTH) to the alloantigen, and production of specific alloantibodies (1, 8, 33, 50). The reverse was also shown to be true, e.g., immunization with allogeneic cells or tissues resulted in T-cell reactivity against MHC-derived allopeptides (7). Stimulation of antibody production by indirect presentation of allopeptides seems to be resistant to cyclosporin A administration, a finding consistent with the irreversible character of chronic rejection (89). T cells that recognize allopeptides presented by self-MHC provide help for alloreactive Cytotoxic Tlymphocytes (CTLs) and also stimulate macrophages, which are present in the same environment (1, 7, 27, 50, 54, 55, 56, 79, 89, 95). Furthermore, alloreactive $CD4^+$ T cells were shown to induce donor-specific cytotoxic T cells in CD8-depleted mice and, thus, to initiate graft rejection (50).

Hierarchies of antigen-specific T-helper cell responses have been observed following allotransplantation both in mice and humans (6, 27, 100). At the onset of a primary rejection episode, T cells from human recipients of organ allografts react against a sole immunodominant determinant of a donor HLA-DR molecule. The response spreads, however, to cryptic determinants of the same molecule or to other donor DR antigen during secondary acute rejection and/or chronic rejection.

Epitope spreading is a process whereby epitopes distinct from, and non-cross-reactive with, an inducing epitope become major targets of an ongoing immune response. This phenomenon accompanies chronic tissue destruction and has been extensively characterized in different experimental models of autoimmune diseases (51, 53). In human allotransplantation, persistent allopeptide reactivity and epitope spreading were shown to be crucial to the development of anti-HLA antibodies and chronic rejection (27).

Indirect recognition of xenogeneic antigens, however, is likely to induce more powerful immune responses than human allogeneic MHC antigens, because of the larger number of foreign antigenic peptides that result from the processing of xenogeneic proteins. Indeed, studies on indirect recognition of xenoantigens performed in mouse models of xenotransplantation have established that the recognition of processed forms of xenoantigens by self-restricted $CD4^+$ T cells is sufficient to cause unusually strong xenograft rejection (24, 31, 63, 67, 74).

The role of the indirect pathway of xenorecognition could be extensively studied in mice recipients of xenografts from discordant species, such as pig or monkey. In this model, xenograft rejection is primarily mediated by indirect recognition because of the molecular incompatibilities between critical receptors and ligands, which prevent direct activation of T cells by xenogeneic APCs (24, 31, 67, 74). Even under such conditions, the strength of xenograft rejection is markedly higher than that of allograft rejection, as indicated by the difficulty of prolonging xenograft survival by using standard immunosuppressive drugs. Furthermore, xenografts lacking MHC antigen expression are also rapidly rejected, providing evidence that the indirect pathway is not limited to T-cell recognition of xenogeneic MHC-derived peptides but includes the recognition of peptides derived from other proteins of xenogeneic origin (63).

In view of the significant contribution of the indirect recognition pathway, the effect of $CD4^+$ T-cell depletion has been tested in mice receiving xeno- or allografts (62, 74). Treatment with a depleting anti-CD4 monoclonal antibody resulted in better xeno- than allograft survival, consistent with the notion that xenograft rejection is more dependent on $CD4^+$ T-cell response than allograft rejection. The absence of $CD4^+$ T cells was accompanied by the lack of eosinophils in the xenograft site, suggesting that the heavy eosinophilic infiltrate, usually present in xenografts, is a CD4-dependent phenomenon (62).

Several studies have shown that macrophages are also present in high numbers in the xenograft infiltrate during rejection (46, 62). It is likely that macrophages play an important role in antigen processing and presentation, promoting indirect recognition of xenoantigens. In addition, macrophages also produce large amounts of IL-1 as well as other cytokines, such as TNF, which may contribute to the damage of graft cells. Thus, blocking macrophage function may be an important element in controlling xenograft rejection. Among several antimacrophage drugs that have been tested, dichloromethylene diphosphonate (Clodronate) significantly prolonged the survival of allogeneic islets in rats (13). However, strategies such as $CD4^+$ T-cell depletion or blocking the macrophage function represent nonspecific immunosuppressive therapies, which may severely impair the immune response to pathogens in a xenotransplant host.

An attractive strategy to inhibit in a specific fashion the indirect recognition of allo- and xenogeneic antigens consists of the generation of regulatory cells able to suppress the self-restricted T-cell response of the host against graft-derived antigens. In vitro generation and propagation of T-suppressor cells, which inhibit indirect recognition of an allogeneic HLA-derived peptide, have been recently reported (42). The structure of this peptide corresponded to the dominant epitope of the HLA-DR4 molecule presented in the context of DR11 protein and recognized by self MHC-restricted Th cells. Similar to allo- and xenospecific suppressor cells that inhibit the direct pathway of recognition (26, 57), allopeptide-specific Ts cells expressed the $CD8^+CD28^-$ phenotype and showed the following characteristics: (i) antigen specificity and restriction by self MHC class I molecules; (ii) limited TCR V beta gene usage; (iii) ability to inhibit antigen-specific, MHC class II–restricted Th proliferative responses; and (iv) capacity to downregulate and/or inhibit the upregulation by Th of CD40, CD80, and CD86 molecules on APCs.

In the xenogeneic system, however, the identification of dominant determinants derived from the processing of pig proteins and presented by host APC appears to be an overwhelming task, given the huge numbers of peptide candidates. Thus, the generation of Ts cells able to inhibit the response of human T cells against particular xenogeneic peptides has no practical relevance for inhibition of xenograft rejection. Nevertheless, strategies for generating Ts cells can be envisioned. For example, Ts cells that inhibit the response of human T cells to a whole spectrum of xenogeneic peptides could be generated in vitro under conditions that direct the human T-cell response toward recognition of foreign peptides in the context of self APC. This can be achieved by performing multiple stimulations of human T cells with APC-depleted pig cells in the presence of human APC and cytokines, which drive the expansion of Ts cells, such as IL-2, IL-7, and IL-10. Ts cells generated in this manner could be subsequently used for adoptive transfer to inhibit in vivo recognition of xenogeneic peptides.

In vivo induction of regulatory cells may be the mechanism underlying the beneficial effect of bone marrow transplantation (BMT) on allograft and xenograft survival (37, 80). A current hypothesis is that BMT provides selected donor cell subsets that may induce immunoregulatory networks (37). The nature of such cells is not yet known, although it is likely that donor dendritic cells may play a role in inducing the state of specific immune hyporesponsiveness (37, 80).

Attempts to induce mixed hematopoietic chimerism as a means of specifically eliminating the immune response to xenotransplants in primates are currently in progress (37). The results reported so far indicate that specific suppression of the T-cell response to miniswine antigens could be achieved in chimeric primates, raising optimism for a successful strategy of inducing specific tolerance of xenografts.

RECOGNITION OF VIRAL ANTIGENS PRESENT IN XENOGENEIC CELLS

The risk of cross-species transfer of infectious agents by transplantation of xenogeneic organs into humans represents a serious reason for concern, which has considerably delayed the initiation of clinical trials for xenotransplantation (18, 23, 66). Although relatively little is known about the characteristics that confer the ability of a pathogen to cross species barriers and about the possible outcomes of the infection, it is likely that the host response to such agents will occur through one of the following mechanisms:

1. Peptides derived from viral proteins will be recognized by human CTL in the context of pig MHC class I molecules via the direct recognition pathway, potentially leading to the killing of xenogeneic cells. However, viral recognition through this pathway is likely to be obscured by the direct recognition of peptides derived from pig proteins, which are presented by SLA class I molecules. Thus, inhibition of this recognition pathway by conventional or other means of immunosuppression may result in inhibition of the CTL response to either pig or viral peptides on the surface of pig cells.

2. Similar to pig proteins, viral proteins shed from a pig transplant will be processed and presented by human APCs in the context of HLA class II, via the indirect pathway of allo- and xenorecognition. Such viral peptides may elicit reactivity of $CD4^+$ T cells, which may, in turn, contribute to the immune attack against the graft. This possibility is supported by the finding that viral infections, such as cytomegalovirus, increase the risk of allograft rejection (101). However, by inhibiting the indirect recognition of graft-derived antigens (i.e., using adoptive transfer of suppressor cells or using agents that inhibit the processing ability of APC), Th reactivity against peptides derived from either pig or viral proteins and presented by host APC will be suppressed. While this strategy may work at preventing Th-mediated events that cause graft rejection, such as CTL attack or production of anti-graft antibodies, it may also diminish the ability of the host to develop a potent immune response to viral antigens.
3. Viruses carried by cells of a xenograft may be transferred into human cells. This possibility raises the most serious concern, given the increased vulnerability of the immunosuppressed host to infectious agents and the general risk posed to society by the spread of such viral infections.

Many viruses are considered "species-specific," being unable to cross interspecies barriers (84). If true, then xenotransplantation would carry less risk of donor-transmitted infections than allotransplantation, where infections caused by cytomegalovirus, hepatitis B and C viruses, Epstein-Barr virus, human immunodeficiency virus, or other infectious agents, passaged from the donor tissue into the recipient, often cause complications in immunosuppressed patients (25, 70, 84). However, cross-species barriers for viral transmission are not absolute. Some viral agents, including retroviruses, have the ability to infect cells from other species (75). Although transplantation of pig organs into humans has been considered to carry less risk than transplantation of non-human primate organs, given the lower chance of virus transmission between discordant compared to concordant species, recent studies have demonstrated that retroviruses expressed by pig cells can infect human cells (70). This finding prompted the fear that a porcine retrovirus from a transplanted organ might infect human recipients, and that viral recombination may create a hybrid better adapted to survival, replication, and pathogenicity in the human host.

Frequent contact between pigs and humans has apparently never led to retrovirally induced disease. However, in the particular situation of a transplant—close proximity and long-term contact—this barrier could be overcome, especially under the conditions of immunosuppression. It has recently been shown that α-Gal antigens are responsible not only for the development of hyperacute rejection, but also for the sensitivity of mammalian C-type retroviruses to inactivation by human serum (84). This sensitivity is thought to protect humans from transmission of C-type oncoviruses from other mammals. There may be, therefore, an increased chance for a pig endogenous retrovirus to be transmitted from the xenograft to the recipient when the anti-α-Gal response is compromised by the removal of anti-α-Gal antibodies from the patient's plasma, or by the use of transgenic pigs expressing human complement-regulatory proteins (2, 29, 30, 75, 86, 97). It is known that such proteins (i.e., CD46, CD55, and CD59) are present in the HIV envelope and can protect HIV from complement-mediated lysis (85).

A strategy that can be presently envisioned to minimize the threat posed by the transmission of porcine viruses would be to ensure that donor pigs do not carry infectious agents that could be passaged into human cells. However, there is still the risk of cross-species transmission of yet unknown endogenous viruses, rendering the benefit of breeding "clean" pigs questionable. Hybridization studies have unraveled the existence in the pig genome of about 50 related proviruses, one or more of which is expressed in a variety of tissue types, including heart and kidney—the two organs most likely to be transplanted (18). Since the envelope gene of a virus is the principal determinant of retroviral tropism, one could predict, based on the structure of this gene, whether a porcine endogenous retrovirus is capable of infecting human cells (85).

Attempts to immunize before transplantation primate recipients against such potentially infectious porcine viruses may be a necessary step toward safe xenotransplantation. Protective immunity against porcine viruses could be achieved, for example, by the use of vaccines that induce neutralizing antibodies directed to specific portions of the viral envelope protein. Vaccine-induced antibody responses, however, were shown to be insufficient in protecting monkeys or humans from HIV infection (4, 76, 93). Recent attempts to produce antiviral vaccines have, therefore, focused on generating CTL responses (35). Extensive evidence indicates that CTLs play a central role in the control of intracellular infections (65, 106). CTLs are able to kill virus-infected cells upon recognition of viral peptides in the context of host class I molecules. The effector function of CTL also includes the release of cytokines (i.e., IL-8, γ-IFN) (32, 60) and chemokines (i.e., MIP-1a, MIP-1b, RANTES) with antiviral activity (85).

It is generally accepted that strong CTL responses in the primary phase of retroviral infection play an important role in reducing the very high initial viremia (97). Hence, CTL responses induced prior to infection by an attenuated or a recombinant version of the virus could terminate or contain the viral infection more effectively. It is possible that a similar strategy applied for immunizing xenotransplant recipients against graft-carried viruses may result in the development of self-restricted cytotoxic T cells that will kill only the infected cells of the host and not xenograft cells. It is safe to assume that, given the MHC disparity between discordant species, such as human and pig, self-MHC-restricted responses will not expand to xenogeneic cells. Even if present at low frequency, cytotoxic T cells induced by antiviral immunization may be sufficient for clearing the viral infection and, thus, preventing the passage of an animal virus into the human recipient.

In conclusion, xenografts, like allografts, elicit T-cell–mediated immune responses against foreign antigens present in the graft, via the direct and indirect recognition pathways. However, xenografts induce more potent T-cell responses than do allografts because of the larger number of foreign antigens present in xenogeneic compared to allogeneic cells. For example, recognition of processed forms of xenogeneic proteins via the indirect recognition pathway will include a much more diverse set of foreign peptides. Furthermore, xenogeneic cells may carry species-specific viruses, which are also likely to elicit T-cell recognition. A very serious risk posed by xenotransplantation consists of the transmission of retroviruses into the immunocompromised host. Therefore, intense research has been focused on the induction of donor-specific tolerance, while keeping intact the ability of the host immune system to react against infections. Such strategies include transplantation of donor bone marrow cells and use of monoclonal antibodies able to block T-cell costimulatory pathways. Recently, the generation and expansion of human xenospecific T-suppressor cells, which effectively prevent the recognition of pig cells by human T-helper cells, opened new avenues to specific immunotherapy. Adoptive transfer of such cells into xenograft recipients may provide a successful alternative to achieve xenograft-specific tolerance.

REFERENCES

1. **Auchincloss, H., Jr., R. Lee, S. Shea, J. S. Markowitz, M. J. Grusby, and L. H. Glimcher.** 1993. The role of "indirect" recognition in initiating rejection of skin grafts from major histocompatibility complex class II-deficient mice. *Proc. Natl. Acad. Sci. USA* **90:**3373–3377.
2. **Auchincloss, H., Jr., and D. H., Sachs.** 1998. Xenogeneic transplantation. *Annu. Rev. Immunol.* **16:**433–470.
3. **Bach, F. H., H. Winkler, C. Ferran, W. W. Hancock, and S. C. Robson.** 1996. Delayed xenograft rejection. *Immunol. Today* **8:**379–384.
4. **Barin, F., M. F. McLane, J. S. Allan, T. H. Lee, J. E. Groopman, and M. Essex.** 1995. Virus envelope protein of HTLV-III represents major target antigen for antibodies in AIDS patients. *Science* **228:**1094–1096.
5. **Batten, P., M. H. Yacoub, and M. L. Rose.** 1996. Effect of human cytokines (IFN-γ, TNF-α, IL-1β, IL-4) on porcine endothelial cells: induction of MHC and adhesion molecules and functional significance of these changes. *Immunology* **87:**127–133.
6. **Benichou, G., and E. V. Fedoseyeva.** 1996. The contribution of peptides to T cell allorecognition and allograft rejection. *Int. Rev. Immunol.* **13:**231–245.
7. **Benichou, G., P. A. Takizawa, P. T. Ho, C. C. Killion, C. A. Olson, M. McMillan, and E. E. Sercarz.** 1990. Immunogenicity and tolerogenicity of self-major histocompatibility complex peptides. *J. Exp. Med.* **172:**1341–1346.
8. **Benichou, G., P. A. Takizawa, A. C. Olson, M. McMillan, and E. E. Sercarz.** 1992. Donor major histocompatibility complex (MHC) peptides are presented by recipient MHC molecules during graft rejection. *J. Exp. Med.* **175:**305–308.
9. **Bennett, S. R. M., F. R. Carbone, F. Karamalis, R. A. Flavell, J. F. Miller, and W. R. Heath.** 1998. Help for cytotoxic-T-cell responses is mediated by CD40 signaling. *Nature* **393:**478–480.
10. **Birmele, B., G. Thibault, H. Nivet, Y. Gruel, P. Bardos, and Y. Lebranchu.** 1996. Human lymphocyte adhesion to xenogeneic porcine endothelial cells: modulation by human TNF-α and involvement of NLA-4 and LFA-1. *Transplant. Immunol.* **4:**265–270.
11. **Bjorkman, P. J., M. A. Saper, B. Samraoui, W. S. Bennett, J. L. Strominger, and D. C. Wiley.** 1987. Structure of the human class I histocompatibility antigen HLA-A2. *Nature* **329:**506–512.
12. **Bohm, W., R. Schirmbeck, A. Elbe, K. Melber, D. Diminky, G. Kraal, N. van Rooijen, Y. Barenholz, and J. Reimann.** 1995. Exogenous hepatitis B surface antigen particles processed by dendritic cells or macrophages prime murine MHC class I-restricted cytotoxic T lymphocytes in vivo. *J. Immunol.* **155:**3313–3321.
13. **Bottino, R., L. A. Fernandez, C. Ricordi, R. Lehmann, M. F. Tsan, R. Oliver, and L. Inverardi.** 1998. Transplantation of allogeneic islet of Langerhans in the rat liver: effects of macrophage depletion on graft survival and microenvironment activation. *Diabetes* **47:**316–323.
14. **Bradley, J. A.** 1996. Indirect T cell recognition in allograft rejection. *Int. Rev. Immunol.* **13:**245–255.
15. **Bravery, C. A., P. Batten, M. H. Yacoub, and M. L. Rose.** 1995. Direct recognition of SLA- and HLA-like class II antigens on porcine endothelium by human T cells results in T cell activation and release of interleukin-2. *Transplantation* **60:**1024–1033.
16. **Brevan, M. J.** 1984. High determinant density may explain the phenomenon of alloreactivity. *Immunol. Today* **5:**128–130.
17. **Brown, J. H., T. S. Jardetzky, J. C., Gorga, L. J. Stern, R. G. Urban, J. L. Strominger, and D. C. Wiley.** 1993. Three-dimensional structure of the human class II histocompatibility antigen HLA-DR1. *Nature* **364:**33–39.
18. **Butler, D.** 1998. Last chance to stop and think on risk of xenotransplants. *Nature* **391:**320–325.
19. **Caux, C., C. Massacrier, B. Vanbervliet, B. Dubois, C. Van Kooten, I. Durand, and J. Banchereau.** 1994. Activation of human dendritic cells through CD40 cross-linking. *J. Exp. Med.* **180:**1263–1272.
20. **Cella, M., D. Scheidegger, K. Palmer-Lehman, P. Lane, A. Lanzavecchia, and G. Alber.** 1996. Ligation of CD40 on dendritic cells triggers production of high levels of interleuken-12 and enhances T cell stimulatory capacity: T-T help via APC activation. *J. Exp. Med.* **184:**747–752.

21. **Cen, H., M. C. Breinig, R. W. Atchinson, M. Ho, and J. L. C. McKnight.** 1991. Epstein-Barr virus transmission via the donor organs in solid organ transplantation: polymerase chain reaction and restriction fragment length polymorphism analysis of IR2, IR3, and IR4. *J. Virol.* **65:**976–980.
22. **Chan, D. V., and H. Auchincloss, Jr.** 1996. Human anti-pig cell-mediated cytotoxicity in vitro involves non-T as well as T cell components. *Xenotransplantation* **3:**158–165.
23. **Chapman, L. E., T. M. Folles, D. R. Salomon, A. P. Patterson, T. E. Eggerman, and P. D. Noguchi.** 1995. Xenotransplantation and xenogeneic infections. *N. Engl. J. Med.* **333:**1498–1501.
24. **Chitillan, H. V., T. M. Lauler, K. Stenger, S. Shea, and H. Auchincloss, Jr.** 1998. The strength of cell-mediated xenograft rejection in the mouse is due to the $CD4^+$ indirect response. *Xenotransplantation* **5:**93–98.
25. **Chou, S.** 1986. Acquisition of donor strains of cytomegalovirus by renal-transplant recipients. *N. Engl. J. Med.* **314:**1418–1423.
26. **Ciubotariu, R., A. I. Colovai, G. Pennesi, Z. Lui, D. Smith, P. Berlocco, R. Cortesini, and N. Suciu-Foca.** 1998. Specific suppression of human $CD4^+$ T helper cell responses to pig MHC antigens by $CD8^+CD28^-$ regulatory T cells. *J. Immunol.* **161:**5193–5202.
27. **Ciubotariu, R., Z. Liu, A. I. Colovai, E. Ho, S. Ravalli, S. Itescu, M. A. Hardy, R. Cortesini, E. A. Rose, and N. Suciu-Foca.** 1998. Persistent allopeptide reactivity and epitope spreading in chronic rejection of organ allografts. *J. Clin. Invest.* **101:**398–405.
28. **Cocchi, F., A. L. DeVico, D. A. Garzino, S. K. Arya, R. C. Gallo, and P. Lasso.** 1995. Identification of RANTES, MIP-1 alpha, and MIP-1 beta as the major HIV-suppressive factors produced by $CD8^+$ T cells. *Science* **270:**1811–1815.
29. **Cooper, D. K. C., Y. Ye, L. L. Rolf, Jr., and N. Zuhdi.** 1991. The pig as potential organ donor for man, p. 481. *In* D. K. C. Cooper, E. Kemp, K. Reemsta, and D. J. G. White (ed.), *Xenotransplantation*. Springer-Verlag, Heidelberg, Germany.
30. **Cozzi, E., and D. J. G. White.** 1995. The generation of transgenic pigs as potential organ donors for humans. *Nature Med.* **1:**964–966.
31. **Dorling, A., R. Binns, and R. I. Lechler.** 1996. Cellular xenoresponses: observation of significant primary indirect human T cell anti-pig xenoresponses using co-stimulator-deficient or SLA class II-negative porcine stimulators. *Xenotransplantation* **3:**112–119.
32. **Emilie, D., M. D. Maillot, J. F. Nicolas, R. Fior, and P. Galanand.** 1992. Antagonistic effect of interferon-gamma on tat-induced transactivation of HIV long terminal repeat. *J. Biol. Chem.* **267:**20565–20570.
33. **Fangmann, J., R. Dalchau, and J. W. Fabre.** 1992. Rejection of skin allografts by indirect allorecognition of donor class I major histocompatibility complex peptides. *J. Exp. Med.* **175:**1521–1529.
34. **Fischer Lindahl, K., and D. B. Wilson.** 1977. Histocompatibility antigen-activated cytotoxic T lymphocytes II. Estimates of frequency and specificity of precursors. *J. Exp. Med.* **145:**508–522.
35. **Gallimore, A., M. Cranage, N. Cook, N. Almond, J. Bootman, E. Rud, P. Silvera, M. Dennis, T. Corcoran, J. Stott, et al.** 1995. Early suppression of SIV replication by $CD8^+$ nef-specific cytotoxic T cells in vaccinated macaques. *Nature Med.* **1:**1167–1173.
36. **Goodman, D. J., M. A. von Albertini, A. Shea, C. J. Wrighton, and F. H. Bach.** 1996. Adenoviral-mediated overexpression of $\kappa B\alpha$ in endothelial cells inhibits natural killer cell-mediated endothelial cell activation. *Transplantation* **62:**967–972.
37. **Greenstein, J. L., and D. H. Sachs.** 1997. The use of tolerance for transplantation across xenogeneic barriers. *Nature Biotechnol.* **15:**235–238.
38. **Harding, C. V., and R. Song.** 1994. Phagocytic processing of exogenous particulate antigens by macrophages for presentation by class I MHC molecules. *J. Immunol.* **153:**4925–4933.
39. **Heber-Katz, E., R. H. Schwartz, L. A. Matis, C. Hannum, T. Fairwell, E. Apella, and D. Hansburg.** 1982. Contribution of antigen-presenting cell major histocompatibility complex gene products to the specificity of antigen-induced T cell activation. *J. Exp. Med.* **155:**1086–1099.
40. **Ildstad, S. T., and D. H. Sachs.** 1984. Reconstitution with syngeneic plus allogeneic or xenogeneic bone marrow leads to specific acceptance of allografts or xenografts. *Nature* **307:**168–170.
41. **Inverardi, L., M. Samaja, R. Motterlini, F. Mangili, J. R. Bender, and R. Pardi.** 1992. Early recognition of a discordant xenogeneic organ by human circulating lymphocytes. *J. Immunol.* **149:**1416–1423.
42. **Jiang, S., S. Tugulea, G. Pennesi, Z. Liu, A. Mulder, S. Lederman, P. Harris, R. Cortesini, and N. Suciu-Foca.** 1998. Induction of MHC-class I restricted human suppressor T cells by peptide priming in vitro. *Hum. Immunol.* **59:**690–699.

43. **Kirk, A. D., R. A. Li, M. S. Kinch, K. A. Abernethy, C. Doyle, and R. R. Bollinger.** 1993. The human antiporcine cellular repertoire: in vitro studies of acquired and innate cellular responsiveness. *Transplantation* **55:**924–931.
44. **Kirk, A. K., D. M. Harland, N. N. Armstrong, T. A. Davis, Y. Dong, G. S. Gray, X. Hong, D. Thomas, J. H. Fechner, Jr., and S. J. Knechtle.** 1997. CTLA4-Ig and anti-CD40 ligand prevent renal allograft rejection in primates. *Proc. Natl. Acad. Sci. USA* **194:**8789–8794.
45. **Koch, F., U. Stanzl, P. Jennewein, K. Janke, C. Heufler, E. Kampgen, N. Romani, and G. Schuler.** 1996. High level IL-12 production by murine dendritic cells: upregulation via MHC class II and CD40 molecules and downregulation by IL-10. *J. Exp. Med.* **184:**741–746.
46. **Korsgren, O.** 1997. Acute cellular xenograft rejection. *Xenotransplantation* **4:**11–19.
47. **Larsen, C. P., D. Z. Alexander, D. Hollenbaugh, E. T. Elwood, S. C. Ritchie, A. Aruffo, R. Hendrix, and T. C. Pearson.** 1996. CD40-gp30 interactions play a critical role during allograft rejection. Suppression of allograft rejection by blockade of the CD40-gp39 pathway. *Transplantation* **61:**4–9.
48. **Larsen, C. P., E. T. Elmwood, D. Z. Alexander, S. C. Ritchie, R. Hendrix, D. Tucker, C. Burden, H. R. Cho, A. Aruffo, D. Hollenbaugh, P. S. Linsley, K. J. Winn, and T. C. Pearson.** 1996. Long-term acceptance of skin and cardiac allografts after blocking CD40 and CD28 pathways. *Nature* **381:**434–438.
49. **Lechler, R. I., and J. R. Batchelor.** 1982. Restoration of immunogenicity to passenger cell depleted kidney allografts by the addition of donor strain dendritic cells. *J. Exp. Med.* **155:**31–41.
50. **Lee, R. S., M. J. Grusby, L. H. Glimcher, H. J. Winn, and H. Auchincloss, Jr.** 1994. Indirect recognition by helper cells can induce donor-specific cytotoxic T lymphocytes in vivo. *J. Exp. Med.* **179:**865–872.
51. **Lehmann, P. V., T. Forsthuber, A. Miller, and E. E. Sercarz.** 1992. Spreading of T cell autoimmunity to cryptic determinants of autoantigen. *Nature* **358:**155–157.
52. **Levisetti, M. G., P. A. Padrid, G. L. Szat, N. Mittal, S. M. Meehan, C. L. Wardrip, G. S. Gray, D. S. Bruce, J. R. Thistlewaite, Jr., and J. A. Bluestone.** 1997. Immunosuppressive effects of human CTLA4-Ig in a non-human primate model of allogeneic pancreatic islet transplantation. *J. Immunol.* **159:**5187–5191.
53. **Lipham, W. J., T. M. Redmond, H. Takahashi, J. A. Berzofsky, B. Wiggert, G. J. Chader, and I. Gery.** 1991. Recognition of peptides that are immunopathogenic but cryptic. Mechanisms that allow lymphocytes sensitized against cryptic peptides to initiate pathogenic autoimmune process. *J. Immunol.* **146:**3757–3762.
54. **Liu, Z., A. I. Colovai, S. Tugulea, E. F. Reed, P. E. Fisher, D. Mancini, E. A. Rose, R. Cortesini, R. E. Michler, and N. Suciu-Foca.** 1996. Indirect recognition of donor HLA-DR peptides in organ allograft rejection. *J. Clin. Invest.* **98:**1150–1157.
55. **Liu, Z., P. E. Harris, A. I. Colovai, E. F. Reed, A. Maffei, and N. Suciu-Foca.** 1996. Indirect recognition of donor MHC-class II antigens in human transplantation. *Clin. Immunol. Immunopathol.* **78:**228–235.
56. **Liu, Z., Y. K. Sun, Y. P. Xi, B. Hong, P. E. Harris, E. Reed, and N. Suciu-Foca.** 1993. Limited usage of TCR Vβ genes by allopeptide specific T cells. *J. Immunol.* **150:**3180–3186.
57. **Liu, Z., S. Tugulea, R. Cortesini, and N. Suciu-Foca.** 1998. Specific suppression of T helper alloreactivity by allo-MHC-class I restricted $CD8^+$ $CD28^-$ T cells. *Int. Immunol.* **10:**101–109.
58. **Lo, D., L. C. Burkly, R. A. Flavell, R. D. Palmiter, and R. L. Brinster.** 1989. Tolerance in transgenic mice expressing class II major histocompatibility complex on pancreatic acinar cells. *J. Exp. Med.* **170:**87–104.
59. **Lombardi, G., S. Sidhu, J. R. Batchelor, and R. I. Lechler.** 1989. Allorecognition of DR1 by T cells from a DR4/DRw13 responder mimics self-restricted recognition of endogenous peptides. *Proc. Natl. Acad. Sci. USA* **86:**4190–4194.
60. **Mackewicz, C. E., L. C. Yang, J. D. Lifson, and J. A. Levy.** 1994. Non-cytotoxic CD8 T-cell anti-HIV responses in primary HIV-1 infection. *Lancet* **344:**1671–1674.
61. **Maher, S. E., K. Karmann, W. Min, C. C. W. Hughes, J. S. Pober, and A. L. M. Bothwell.** 1996. Porcine endothelial CD86 is a major costimulator of xenogeneic human T cells. *J. Immunol.* **157:**3838–3844.
62. **Mandel, T. E., J. Kovarik, M. Koulmanda, and H. M. Georgiou.** 1997. Cellular rejection of fetal pancreas grafts: differences between allo- and xenografts rejection. *Xenotransplantation* **4:**2–10.
63. **Markmann, J. F., L. Campos, A. Bhandoola, J. I. Kim, N. M. Desai, H. Bassiri, B. R. Claytor, and C. F. Barker.** 1994. Genetically engineered grafts to study xenoimmunity: a role for indirect antigen presentation in the destruction of major histocompatibility complex antigen deficient xenografts. *Surgery* **116:**242–248.
64. **Matzinger, P., and M. J. Brevan.** 1977. Why do so many lymphocytes respond to major histocompatibility complex antigens? *Cell Immunol.* **29:**1–5.

65. **McMichael, A. J., F. M. Gotch, G. R. Noble, and P. A. S. Beare.** 1983. Cytotoxic T-cell immunity to influenza. *N. Engl. J. Med.* **309:**13–17.
66. **Michaels, M. G.** 1997. Infectious concerns of cross-species transplantation: xenozoonoses. *World J. Surg.* **21:**968–974.
67. **Moses, R. D., R. N. I. Pierson, H. J. Winn, and H. J. Auchincloss.** 1990. Xenogeneic proliferation and lymphokine production are dependent on CD4$^+$ helper T cells and self-antigen-presenting cells in the mouse. *J. Exp. Med.* **172:**567–575.
68. **Murray, A. G., M. M. Khodadoust, J. S. Pober, and A. L. M. Bothwell.** 1994. Porcine aortic endothelial cells activate human T cells: direct presentation of MHC antigens and costimulation by ligands for human CD2 and CD28. *Immunity* **1:**57–63.
69. **Nuchtern, J. G., W. E. Biddison, and R. D. Klausner.** 1990. Class II molecules can use the endogenous pathway of antigen presentation. *Nature* **343:**74–76.
70. **Patience, C., Y. Takeuchi, and R. A. Weiss.** 1997. Infection of human cells by an endogenous retrovirus of pigs. *Nature Med.* **3:**282–286.
71. **Pearson, T. C., D. Z. Alexander, K. J. Winn, P. S. Linsley, R. P. Lowry, and C. P. Larsen.** 1994. Transplantation tolerance induced by CTLA4-Ig. *Transplantation* **57:**1701–1706.
72. **Peguet-Navarro, J., C. Dalbiez-Gauthier, F. M. Rattis, C. Van Kooten, J. Banchereau, and D. Schmitt.** 1995. Functional expression of CD40 antigen on human epidermal Langerhans cells. *J. Immunol.* **155:**4241–4247.
73. **Pereira, B. J. G., E. L. Milford, R. L. Kirkman, and A. S. Levey.** 1991. Transmission of hepatitis C virus by organ transplantation. *N. Engl. J. Med.* **325:**454–460.
74. **Pierson, R. N., H. J. Winn, P. S. Russell, and H. Auchincloss, Jr.** 1989. Xenogeneic skin graft rejection is especially dependent on CD4$^+$ T cells. *J. Exp. Med.* **170:**991–996.
75. **Platt, J. L.** 1998. New directions for organ transplantation. *Nature* **392:**11–17.
76. **Platt, J. L., B. J. Lindman, R. L. Geller, H. J. Noreen, J. L. Swanson, A. P. Dalmasso, and F. H. Bach.** 1991. The role of natural antibodies in the activation of xenogeneic endothelial cells. *Transplantation* **52:**1037–1043.
77. **Purcell, D. F., C. M. Broscius, E. F. Vanin, C. E. Buckler, A. W. Nienhuis, and M. A. Martin.** 1996. An array of murine leukemia virus-related elements is transmitted and expressed in a primate recipient of retroviral gene transfer. *J. Virol.* **70:**887–897.
78. **Putney, S. D., T. J. Matthews, W. G. Robey, D. L. Lynn, M. R. Guroff, W. T. Mueller, A. J. Langlois, J. Ghrayeb, S. R. Petteway, K. J. Weinhold, et al.** 1986. HTLV-HI/LAV-neutralizing antibodies to an *E. coli*-produced fragment of the virus envelope. *Science* **234:**1392–1395.
79. **Renna Molajoni, E., P. Cinti, A. Orlandini, J. Molajoni, S. Tugulea, E. Ho, Z. Liu, N. Suciu-Foca, and R. Cortesini.** 1997. Mechanism of liver allograft rejection: the indirect recognition pathway. *Hum. Immunol.* **53:**57–63.
80. **Ricordi, C., S. T. Ildstad, A. J. Demetris, A. Y. Abou El-Ezz, N. Murase, and T. E. Styarzl.** 1992. Donor dendritic cells repopulation in recipients after rat-to-mouse bone-marrow transplantation. *Lancet* **339:**1610–1611.
81. **Ridge, J. P., F. DiRosa, and P. Matzinger.** 1998. A conditioned dendritic cell can be a temporal bridge between a CD4$^+$ T-helper and a T-killer cell. *Nature* **393:**474–478.
82. **Roetzchke, O., K. Falk, S. Faath, and H. G. Rammensee.** 1991. On the nature of peptides involved in T cell alloreactivity. *J. Exp. Med.* **174:**1059–1071.
83. **Rosenberg, A. S., T. Mizuochi, S. O. Sharrow, and A. Singer.** 1987. Phenotype, specificity, and function of T cell subsets and T cell interactions involved in skin allograft rejection. *J. Exp. Med.* **165:**1296–1315.
84. **Rother, R. P., W. L. Fodor, J. P. Springhorn, C. W. Birks, E. Setter, M. S. Sandrin, S. P. Squinto, and S. A. Rollins.** 1995. A novel mechanism of retrovirus inactivation in human serum mediated by anti-alpha-galactosyl natural antibody. *J. Exp. Med.* **182:**1345–1355.
85. **Rowland-Jones, S., R. Tan, and A. McMichael.** 1997. Role of cellular immunity in protection against HIV infection. *Adv. Immunol.* **65:**277–346.
86. **Sachs, D. H.** 1994. The pig as potential xenograft donor. *Vet. Immunol. Immunopathol.* **43:**185–191.
87. **Sandrin, M. S., H. A. Vaughan, and I. F. C. McKenzie.** 1994. Identification of Gal (α1.3) Gal as the major epitope for pig-to-human vascularized xenografts. *Transplant. Res.* **8:**134–149.
88. **Satake, M., N. Kawagishi, and E. Moller.** 1996. Direct activation of human responder T cells by porcine

stimulator cells leads to T cell proliferation and cytotoxic T cell development. *Xenotransplantation* **3:**198–206.

89. **Sawyer, G., R. Dalchau, and J. Fabre.** 1993. Indirect T cell allorecognition: a cyclosporin A resistant pathway for T cell help for antibody production to donor MHC antigens. *Transplant. Immunol.* **1:**77–81.
90. **Schoenberger, S. P., R. E. M. Toes, E. I. H. van der Voort, R. Offringa, and C. J. M. Melief.** 1998. T-cell help for cytotoxic T lymphocytes is mediated by CD40-CD40L interactions. *Nature* **393:**480–483.
91. **Seebach, J. D., C. Comrack, S. Germana, C. LeGuern, D. H. Sachs, and H. DerSimonian.** 1997. HLA-Cw3 expression on porcine endothelial cells protects against xenogeneic cytotoxicity mediated by a subset of human NK cells. *J. Immunol.* **159:**3655–3661.
92. **Shishido, S., B. Naziruddin, T. Howard, and T. Mohanakumar.** 1997. Recognition of porcine major histocompatibility complex class I antigens by human $CD8^+$ cytolytic T cell clones. *Transplantation* **64:**340–346.
93. **Steimer, K. S., C. J. Scendella, P. V. Skiles, and N. L. Haigwood.** 1991. Neutralization of divergent HIV-1 isolates by conformation-dependent human antibodies to Gp120. *Science* **254:**105–108.
94. **Steinman, R. M.** 1991. The dendritic cell system and its role in immunogenicity. *Annu. Rev. Immunol.* **9:**271–296.
95. **Stock, P. G., N. L. Ascher, S. Chen, J. Field, F. H. Bach, and D. E. Sutherland.** 1991. Evidence for direct and indirect pathways in the generation of the alloimmune response against pancreatic islets. *Transplantation* **52:**704–709.
96. **Suciu-Foca, N., E. Reed, C. Marboe, Y. P. Xi, S. Y. Kai, E. Ho, E. Rose, K. Reemtsma, and D. W. King.** 1991. Role of anti-HLA antibodies in heart transplantation. *Transplantation* **51:**716–724.
97. **Takahashi, T., S. Saadi, and J. L. Platt.** 1997. Recent advances in the immunology of xenotransplantation. *Immunol. Res.* **16:**273–297.
98. **Thompson, S. C., and T. E. Mandel.** 1990. Fetal pig pancreas: preparation and assessment of tissue for transplantation, its in vivo development and function in athymic (nude) mice. *Transplantation* **49:**571–581.
99. **Tran, H. M., P. W. Nickerson, A. C. Restifo, M. A. Ivis-Woodward, A. Patel, R. D. Allen, T. B. Strom, and P. J. O'Connell.** 1997. Distinct mechanisms for the induction and maintenance of allograft tolerance with CTLA4-Ig treatment. *J. Immunol.* **159:**2232–2239.
100. **Vella, J. P., M. Spadafora-Ferreira, B. Murphy, S. I. Alexander, W. Harmon, C. B. Carpenter, and M. H. Sayegh.** 1997. Indirect allorecognition of major histocompatibility complex allopeptides in human renal transplant recipients with chronic graft dysfunction. *Transplantation* **64:**795–800.
101. **Von Willebrand, E., E. Pettersson, J. Ahonen and P. Hayry.** 1986. CMV infection, class II antigen expression, and human kidney allograft rejection. *Transplantation* **42:**364–367.
102. **Weber, D. A., N. K. Terrell, J. Zhang, et al.** 1991. Requirement for peptide in alloreactive $CD4^+$ T cell recognition of class II MHC molecules. *J. Immunol.* **154:**5153–5164.
103. **Xiao, F., A. S. Chong, P. Foster, H. Sankary, L. McChesney, G. Koukoulis, J. Yang, D. Frieders, and J. W. Williams.** 1994. Leflunomide controls rejection in hamster to rat cardiac xenografts. *Transplantation* **58:**828–834.
104. **Yamada, K., D. H. Sachs, and H. DerSimonian.** 1995. Human anti-porcine xenogeneic T cell response: evidence for allelic specificity of mixed leukocyte reaction and for both direct and indirect pathways of recognition. *J. Immunol.* **155:**5249–5256.
105. **Yamada, K., J. D. Seebach, H. DerSimonian, and D. H. Sachs.** 1996. Human anti-pig T-cell mediated cytotoxicity. *Xenotransplantation* **3:**179–187.
106. **Zinkernagel, R. M.** 1996. Immunology taught by viruses. *Science* **271:**173–178.

Section IV

ZOONOSIS IN XENOTRANSPLANTATION

Xenotransplantation
Edited by Jeffrey L. Platt

Chapter 10

Xenotransplantation as a Vector for Infection

Marian G. Michaels

Transmission of infections from donor organs, tissues, or cells is well recognized as a cause of disease after allotransplantation (24, 31). However, in the early days of allotransplantation, it was not readily apparent that microbes, asymptomatic within a donor, could cause disease in the new recipient. Only after careful epidemiologic evaluation, clinical trials, and experience did transplant physicians learn this to be the case (24, 31). Similar issues regarding transmission of infections from the donor to the recipient arise with the use of animal organs or tissues through xenotransplantation (8, 56, 62). Concern that these procedures could lead to novel infections, xenozoonoses, has led to public debate on whether the field of xenotransplantation should be permitted to progress. This chapter reviews the issue of xenotransplantation as a vector for infection to humans and considers potential mechanisms for disease, screening systems, and evaluations that need to be carried out to identify these risks as the field moves forward. Knowledge of donor-associated infections after allotransplantation and of zoonotic infections is used to help estimate the potential risk of xenotransplantation.

DONOR-ASSOCIATED INFECTIONS AFTER ALLOTRANSPLANTATION

Despite major advances in allotransplantation, infections remain a major cause of morbidity and mortality. The need for immunosuppressive treatment to prevent rejection of the new organ or tissue is the major risk for infections. It is likely that immunosuppression will also be required to prevent rejection of tissues and organs from disparate species after xenotransplantation and thus will remain as a risk factor for infections. The sources of infection after allotransplantation are multiple and include the recipient's endogenous flora, the environment, and microbes harbored within the donated organ, tissues, or cells (24, 31). The types of microorganisms from human donor organs are often predictable. In general, these infectious agents are maintained in a quiescent or intracellular state, without outward signs of disease in the donor. In this fashion they are carried to the new host within the donor organ

Marian G. Michaels • Division of Allergy, Immunology, and Infectious Diseases, University of Pittsburgh School of Medicine, and The Children's Hospital of Pittsburgh, Pittsburgh, PA 15213.

or the accompanying hematopoietic cells (24, 31, 56, 62). Examples include blood-borne pathogens such as hepatitis B virus (HBV), hepatitis C virus (HCV), and retroviruses, along with some herpesviruses and parasites. Similar classes of organisms are of concern with animal organ xenotransplantation and are worth examining more fully. Human herpesviruses, in particular, human cytomegalovirus (HCMV) and Epstein-Barr virus (EBV), are major causes of donor-associated infections after allotransplantation. Transmission from donors was first suspected on the basis of epidemiologic studies and later confirmed with molecular techniques (7, 12). Both HCMV and EBV cause more severe disease in naive hosts who undergo primary infection after transplantation (32, 73). While seronegative recipients of organs from seropositive donors are at highest risk, patients with previous HCMV or EBV infection can also be reinfected with donor strains (7, 12). This lack of complete protection from previous infection may have an impact on the chance of infection with analogous animal viruses after xenotransplantation. An important concept recognized from allotransplantation is that not all herpesviruses harbored by the donor are transmissible. Herpes simplex virus (HSV) and varicella-zoster virus (VZV) establish latency in sensory ganglia and are unlikely to be present in blood or organs unless a primary infection goes undetected at the time of donor harvest (15). Accordingly, they are at extremely low risk of transmission via a transplant. Donor transmission of blood-borne pathogens such as HBV, HCV, and human immunodeficiency virus (HIV) has unintentionally occurred after allotransplantation (16, 68, 75). This occurred most often in the era before universal donor screening for those specific viruses (16, 68). However, even in more recent times when good screening mechanisms have been implemented, infected donors occasionally remain undetected. Transmission of HIV from a single donor to all four recipients of his organs and three of four bone-graft recipients despite negative HIV screening was described by the Centers for Disease Control and Prevention (75). It was concluded that the donor's death must have been early after his own HIV infection, before an immunologic response could be detected. This highlights the need to remain cognizant of the limitations inherent with any screening test, whether it be for allotransplantation or xenotransplantation. Other types of microbial agents can be transmitted with human donor tissues. Parasites such as *Toxoplasma gondii* can be transmitted with any organ that harbors latent toxoplasma cysts; however, because *T. gondii* has tropism for cardiac muscle, heart transplant recipients are at highest risk (50, 51, 63, 83). This protozoan whose definitive hosts are members of the feline family can infect many other mammals, including humans, and animals considered as sources of tissue and organs for xenotransplantation (61, 72). Prevention of disease from human donors has relied on protocols for donor screening, recipient prophylaxis, and post-transplant surveillance. Protocols must be periodically reviewed and revised in response to ever-expanding knowledge about transmissible agents. Similarly, protocols for xenotransplant screening and surveillance will help in preventing and monitoring infections.

Occasionally, acute viremia or bacteremia goes unrecognized in the donor and is transmitted with the new organ or tissues to the newly immunosuppressed host (79). In addition, bacterial or fungal infections in the airway of the donor can lead to disease after lung or heart–lung transplantation, and histoplasmosis has been transmitted with cadaveric kidneys (24, 58, 82). These types of acute donor-associated infections will theoretically be less of a risk after xenotransplantation as source animals can be maintained under optimal healthy conditions and surgery would be performed on an elective schedule rather than under the current time pressures of allotransplantation.

EXPERIENCES WITH INFECTIONS AFTER XENOTRANSPLANTATION

Even though the modern era of xenotransplantation is relatively young, infections have been known to occur. Most of the documented infections were derived from either the recipient's endogenous flora or the surrounding environment and thus were not directly dependent on whether the donor source was a human or an animal. However, the amount of immunosuppression required to prevent rejection of non-human organs may have increased the risk for infections. This was likely the circumstance for the first baboon-to-human liver xenotransplant recipient who received aggressive immunosuppression (76). The patient developed disseminated aspergillosis, caused by an environmental pathogen, that proved fatal 70 days after transplantation (76). A second recipient of a baboon liver xenotransplant succumbed to multiorgan failure 26 days after transplantation largely due to sepsis from endogenous intra-abdominal bacteria (78). Significant problems with infection were also noted in two xenotransplant series from 1964 reporting on six chimpanzee and baboon kidney transplants, respectively (71, 77). Sepsis contributed to the early deaths of five of six patients in each series. It is likely that these infectious processes, which involved bacteria harbored on human skin or within human urinary and gastrointestinal tracts, could be attributed to surgical complications rather than from the transplanted animal organ per se. Another series reporting results of four patients in hepatic coma who underwent ex vivo pig liver perfusion found only one episode of sepsis that was noted to have started before the time of ex vivo perfusion. In this series only one patient survived longer than 24 h; he underwent four pig liver perfusion attempts followed by a human liver allotransplantation without documented infections during 18 months of follow-up (10). Likewise, no systemic infections were recognized in a newborn who survived for 20 days following a baboon heart transplant (4). These reports on human clinical trials of xenotransplantation identified infections that were caused by immunosuppression and surgical complications; however, survival times were generally short and appropriate methods to evaluate transmission of animal organisms were often lacking.

In an attempt to minimize the risk of xenozoonoses and to learn how to evaluate animal-associated infections after xenotransplantation, more extensive protocols began to be developed in the early and mid-1990s that continue to be expanded upon today (8, 20, 56, 59, 61, 62). These will be discussed in more detail later in the chapter.

POTENTIAL FOR XENOZOONOSES

Several methods can be considered that would allow for the transmission of a microbial agent from an animal xenotransplant source to a human recipient. First, it is important to consider whether a potential pathogen is present in the animal. If yes, similar to what was found with human donors, it is fundamental to know that the microorganism is specifically present in the tissue or accompanying cells being transplanted. For example, a number of organisms that are known to be transmissible from animals to humans under normal circumstances, zoonoses, inhabit the oropharynx or gastrointestinal flora of an animal and as such are unlikely to be present in transplanted tissues or cells (8, 56, 62). Accordingly, these are less of a problem. Instead, it is necessary to focus on microbial agents that are present in the animal tissues and consider the evidence for them being pathogenic to humans even if they are not currently recognized as zoonoses. In this fashion an algorithm can be followed (Fig. 1).

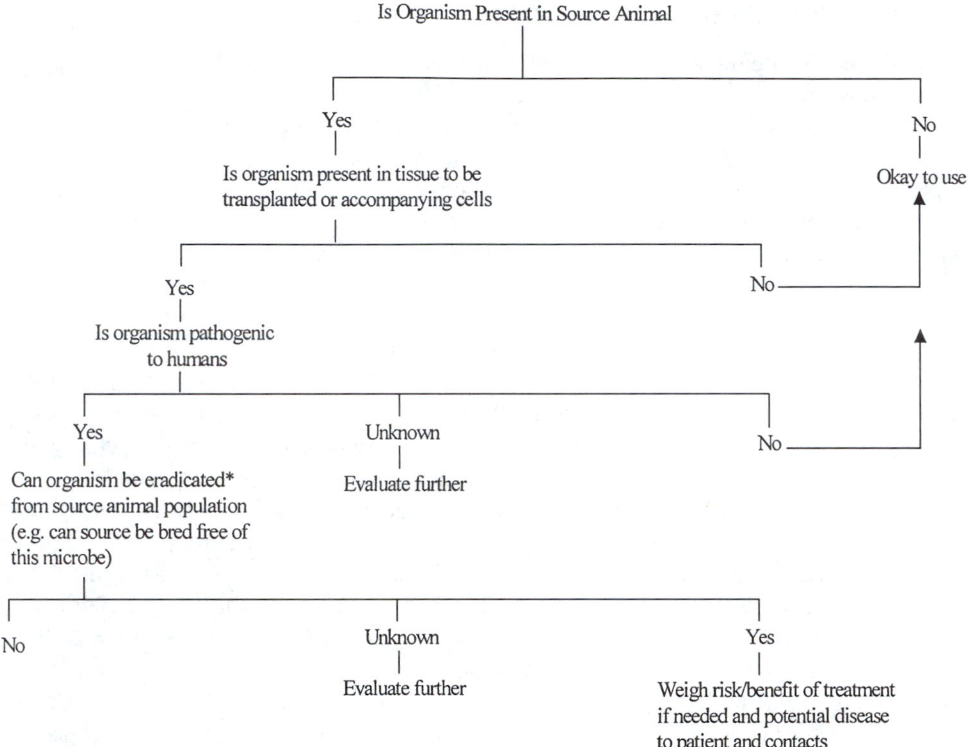

Figure 1. Algorithm to determine whether to use infected animal tissue in transplantation.

Several mechanisms for xenozoonoses have been put forth (56, 62). An organism, such as *T. gondii*, could be infectious for both the source animal and the human recipient. As noted earlier, toxoplasmosis is a high risk for a heart transplant recipient who is naive to this parasite and receives an organ from a seropositive donor whose heart asymptomatically harbors the latent cysts of *T. gondii* (63, 83). This risk would be similar regardless of the species of the heart donor. Animal viruses that are similar to analogous human viruses, even if not currently known zoonoses, might be able to gain access to human cells through transplantation. This has been postulated for primate herpesviruses such as CMV and EBV (20, 56, 62). It is possible that some animal organisms would be harmless in a healthy person but could cause disease after xenotransplantation because of the immunosuppressed environment. Another concern revolves around the potential for a crossover of genetic material to occur between an animal virus and a human virus, leading to a more virulent recombinant organism. In addition, even if it is possible that a latent animal virus present in the source animal tissue is not transmissible to humans, it may cause disease by reactivation within the animal organ, leading to graft failure. This has been postulated for porcine CMV (20, 56).

Some microbes, particularly viruses, are considered to be "species specific." If this is the case, it is possible that xenotransplantation carries less risk of donor-transmitted infections than does allotransplantation. However, examples exist that show that species specificity can be relative and that some viruses of a non-human donor may still infect the new host species. This may be particularly true for viruses belonging to a more closely related species such as the baboon but is not proven. Some herpesviruses have been shown to cross species barriers. The herpesvirus of macaques, cercopithecine herpesvirus 1 (B virus), provides a dramatic example of a virus being relatively benign in its natural host while causing severe disease in a new host. Cercopithecine herpesvirus is analogous to human HSV and causes self-limited, recurrent lesions in a monkey's oral pharynx, conjunctiva, or genital region (3, 11, 30, 33). Inadvertent inoculation of infectious monkey secretions via a bite, scratch, or splash can on rare occasions lead to an ascending myelitis that is almost always fatal without prompt aggressive therapy (3, 11, 30, 33). Proof that the virus is able to adapt to the human environment was found in the secondary transmission from an index patient to his wife who was applying creams to the wound without wearing gloves (30). It is this ability of a virus to be relatively benign in one species yet cause more severe disease in another species and to be transmissible to others that underlies some of the anxiety among critics of xenotransplantation (8, 19, 38, 42, 56, 62). While it could be argued that cercopithecine herpesvirus is unlikely to be transmissible via xenotransplantation since it is an alpha-herpesvirus that resides in nerve endings, not blood cells or organs, it has such a high case fatality rate that it would be an unacceptable risk. However, for many reasons, including size, macaques are not considered source animals for xenotransplantation. Baboons and swine have been used as source animals and do have viruses analogous to HSV, simian agent 8 (SA8) and pseudorabies, respectively (30, 53, 61). Unlike herpes B virus, SA8 has not been documented to cause disease in humans or other species. Pseudorabies has been shown to cause fatal disease when species lines are broached from accidental or experimental transmission to sheep, dogs, and cattle but has never been proven to be infectious to primates (53). However, three immunocompetent humans who presented with transient fever, weakness, and neurologic complaints were found to serologically test positive for pseudorabies between 5 and 15 months after the onset of clinical symptoms, suggesting transmission between swine and humans (66). Repeat testing was seronegative 2 to 12 months later, and the potential mechanism of transmission was not elucidated.

Baboon and swine populations also have a high prevalence of infection with their own β- and γ-herpesviruses (17, 18). Unlike α-herpesviruses, these viruses are latent in cells that could accompany transplanted tissues and organs. In addition, the analogous herpesviruses of humans are well established as causes of donor-transmitted disease after allotransplantation. Accordingly, the ability of these herpesviruses to traverse species barriers is of practical concern for xenotransplantation and requires in-depth analysis.

Several findings suggest that it is possible to have transmission of CMV or EBV between disparate species. It has long been recognized that the Towne strain of human CMV can replicate in cultures of chimpanzee skin fibroblasts (69). Of greater significance is that non-human primate CMV has been implicated as the cause of neurologic disease in two humans (9, 35, 48, 49). The Colburn strain of CMV has substantial homology with African green monkey CMV (strain GR2757) and was reported to be isolated from the brain biopsy of a boy with encephalopathy (35). Martin et al. also repeatedly isolated another African green monkey-like CMV from a woman suffering from chronic fatigue syndrome (48, 49). These findings suggest the possibility of simian CMV crossing over to humans. Detracting from this evidence was that contact between African green monkeys and these individuals was not reported. More directly related to xenotransplantation, we have shown baboon

CMV to replicate in human foreskin fibroblasts in vitro with growth characteristics similar to human CMV (57). Recent data from my laboratory also suggest that baboon CMV has been transmitted to a recipient of a baboon liver, but disease pathogenesis is being further evaluated (Michaels et al. unpublished data). Baboons are less likely to be used as xenotransplant sources in the future; accordingly, it is important to evaluate disease risk with porcine CMV. Similar to human CMV in pregnant women, porcine CMV can cause fetal disease (17). Preliminary studies of swine CMV have not been able to show growth in human cell lines; however, more work needs to be performed (20). Fewer studies are available for γ-herpesviruses such as EBV. Human EBV can infect marmoset lymphocytes in vitro (17, 64). Interestingly, serologic tests against human anti-EBV antigens have variable cross-reactivity with the analogous baboon virus *Herpesvirus papio* that may be related to variations in conservation of different areas of γ-herpesviruses (18). Molecular techniques to differentiate human from baboon herpesviruses are not currently available, hampering studies on transmissibility. In addition, little is known about the presence or absence of swine γ-herpesviruses. Further study is also required to determine whether swine or baboon herpesviruses can adapt in vivo to a human environment or recombine with human viruses.

Hepatitis viruses have been associated with donor transmission after allotransplantation. Some of these viruses appear to be species specific and that, in fact, was the underlying reason for performing baboon liver xenotransplant procedures in two individuals dying from end-stage HBV liver disease (60, 76, 78). However, related strains of hepatitis E virus have been recently found in both humans and swine, bringing up new concerns for potential xenozoonoses (54, 55).

Retroviruses have likewise been transmitted by human donors to other humans and are often found to be relatively species restricted. However, evidence exists for transmission of retroviruses between related primate species (5, 23, 43, 44, 65). Simian immunodeficiency virus (SIV) is another example of a virus that can be more virulent after crossing species lines. The virus appears to be asymptomatic in its natural host, such as the African green monkey, but can lead rapidly to a fatal AIDS-like disease in macaques (5, 65). Transmission across species lines is variable; inoculation of SIV into baboons elicited undetectable or only low-level antibody production with self-limited lymphadenopathy, whereas the same strain inoculated into macaques progressed to rapid severe disease (44, 65). SIV is genetically similar to HIV type 2 and can infect human lymphocytes and macrophages in vitro (5). Probable transmission was documented in two humans who worked with SIV-infected material (43, 44). One person gradually lost antibody against SIV/HIV-2 over 2 years while the second individual who remained seropositive had ongoing active infection, with SIV isolated from peripheral blood cells (43). Recent reports have identified a chimpanzee SIV strain that is believed to be the origin of the human AIDS epidemic (23). While SIV is unlikely to be in baboon populations, it is known to be infectious to humans, and the highly related virus, HIV-2, is pathogenic. Accordingly, if used, baboon source animals should be screened and excluded if found to be positive.

Other types of retroviruses are also of concern for xenotransplantation with non-human primates. Simian T lymphotropic virus (STLV) is an oncogenic retrovirus that is commonly found in non-human primates, including baboons, and carries sequence homology with regions of human T lymphotropic virus, type 1 (34). Accordingly, they should be excluded from source animals. Foamy viruses are the third class of retroviruses, *Spumaviridae*. There is a high seroprevalence rate in adult non-human primates, but foamy viruses have not been associated with a disease state (21, 80). Recent data have demonstrated simian foamy virus in several animal care workers, showing that, similar to SIV, this virus can be transmitted from non-human primate to humans (2, 74). In the most thoroughly evaluated case, asymptomatic infection persisted over 16 to 20 years; no evidence of transmission to spouse or child was demonstrated (74). Evidence of foamy virus DNA was found in the two human recipients of baboon liver transplants in conjunction with baboon cells (1). However, foamy virus was never isolated and serologic studies remained negative after xenotransplantation, making it difficult to determine whether true infection occurred. The risk of transmission from an infected primate source to humans appears to be real, but the clinical implications are not known.

Less information is available on swine exogenous retroviruses, although some pig retroviruses can reactivate after radiation exposure and might likewise reactivate when exposed to immunosuppressive drugs even if they prove to not be infectious to human cells (22). Concern has been raised regarding endogenous retroviruses of both baboons and pigs. As the name implies, these viruses are incorporated into the genomic structure of the animal. Thus far, all swine strains have been shown to carry porcine endogenous retroviruses (PoERV). Although these viruses have been recognized for decades, it was only with the resurgence of interest in clinical xenotransplantation that virologists have begun to do more in-depth studies of PoERV and baboon endogenous retroviruses. In vitro studies have shown both to infect human cell lines (36, 46, 47, 67, 81). Baboon endogenous retrovirus was transiently found in a human with AIDS who underwent a baboon bone marrow transplant (59). Of note, it was only found in concert with baboon mitochondria, suggesting that it represented transient chimerism rather than true infection of human cells. No evidence of PoERV was found in 10 patients who had undergone porcine fetal islet transplants (29). Accordingly, the potential impact of these retroviruses after xenotransplantation is still unclear. It is possible to screen for and exclude source animals with evidence of known exogenous retroviruses, but this is not possible with endogenous retroviruses. Further studies are required to determine their transmissibility and disease potential.

Transmission of other viruses may occur after xenotransplantation. Acute viremia can lead to donor-associated infections after allotransplantation and would likewise be expected to have the same risk after xenotransplantation. Infection with adenovirus after liver transplantation can occur in this fashion (79). Adenoviruses are capable of infecting swine and primates. While not all strains of adenovirus are considered to be pathogenic in healthy hosts, the chance of disease under the influence of immunosuppression is reason for caution and evaluation of source animal blood and organ for viruses. Encephalomyocarditis virus can be transmitted from rodents to a wide range of hosts including baboons, pigs, and humans (37, 41). Symptomatic animals can be identified and thus excluded, but animals without overt symptoms might still have damaged myocardium and be unsuitable as sources for heart transplantation. For this reason it would be prudent to screen and exclude animals with positive serology. Strict attention to rearing methods and prevention of infestation with rodents is important in animal husbandry.

It is possible that viruses may cause problems aside from reactivation or acute viremia. For example, recombination might occur if dual infection is found in the same cell (13, 25, 39, 40). Recombination occurs in vitro with passage of mixed-strain human CMV isolates from transplant recipients (13). In addition, in mice, lethal recombinations have resulted from concurrent inoculation of two avirulent herpes simplex viruses (25). Dissimilar viruses can also recombine as shown by in vitro integration of reticuloendotheliosis virus (an avian retrovirus) into an avian herpesvirus (Marek disease virus) (39).

Microbial agents other than viruses may be xenogeneic. Gastrointestinal parasites could be a problem if extraintestinal infection develops. For example, parasites such as *Entamoeba histolytica* and some *Schistosoma* species can cause liver abscesses. Primates and swine are susceptible to these and other gastrointestinal parasites (14, 62). Transplantation of an abscessed liver could lead to severe disease. Accordingly, animals should be screened and raised in protected environments.

Local epidemiology will influence potential pathogens. For example, baboons raised in the United States may be infected with *Babesia* species but would be unlikely to be infected with malaria or *Hepatocystis* species (52, 70). On the other hand, a large study of South African baboons found 10% to have *Hepatocystis* sp. parasites in the blood and/or liver (52). In addition, a baboon, immunosuppressed after a macaque heart xenotransplant, developed severe anemia secondary to *Hepatocystis kochi* presumably transmitted with the macaque heart (26).

T. gondii is common among commercial herds of swine, with 5 to 35% seropositivity noted (72). Serologic evidence of toxoplasmosis has also been found in captive and wild baboons, with a reported prevalence of 32% and 16%, respectively (52, 61). Although this organism is known to cause disease in susceptible humans after allotransplantation, the severe shortage of human organ donors has prevented its presence from being a basis for exclusion. Instead, prophylaxis strategies have been used by some centers in high-risk recipients (63, 83). However, because of the additional bone marrow toxicity of these drugs and the experimental nature of xenotransplantation, it is recommended that this organism be excluded from potential animal sources. Raising animals in protected environments should also prevent source animal infections with *T. gondii*. *Mycobacterium* species can infect and cause disease in many mammals. In particular, Old World primates, including baboons, are very susceptible to infection with *Mycobacterium tuberculosis* (usually from a human source). Often no apparent clinical symptoms are noted until disseminated end-stage disease (6). Swine are also at risk for being infected with *M. tuberculosis* and *Mycobacterium bovis*. Serial tuberculin skin testing of animals and human caregivers should be a routine part of animal husbandry.

PRETRANSPLANT CONSIDERATIONS OF THE SOURCE ANIMAL

Eliminating adventitious microbial agents by raising source animals under strict gnotobiotic conditions would help abolish many xenogeneic concerns. Germ-free environments have been used successfully to rear small laboratory animals and some farm animals. Pigs have been reared under these germ-free experimental conditions, by taking advantage of their short, predictable gestational period, large number of offspring, and their independence during infancy. However, these rearing conditions become more difficult when the pigs reach several months of age because of increased waste production. Also swine raised under gnotobiotic conditions lack microbial agents in their gastrointestinal tract that help with digestion of food; accordingly, these animals are less robust than animals not raised under such strict conditions (20, 56, 62). Germ-free environments are not suitable for nonhuman primates. For this reason, rearing animals under controlled environments in which specific pathogens are eliminated from the initial population and maintained free of those organisms is attractive for all potential animal sources (20, 56, 62, 84). Developing and maintaining specific-pathogen–free environments for baboons would still be a difficult undertaking but has been successfully performed for macaques (45). Difficulties arise because primates have a variable gestational period, usually produce a single offspring per pregnancy, and are dependent during infancy. For these reasons it would take a prolonged time to generate a baboon colony of sufficient size to supply donors and replenish itself (30). This costly venture might be justified if xenotransplantation proves to be a viable alternative to allotransplantation and more disparate animals are unable to be used because of rejection. However, much concern exists for the possibility of emerging pathogens that could not be screened out of the population initially. Therefore, strict, careful screening programs are warranted for all source animals and potential recipients. Once a colony is established, strict controls must be maintained as unwanted microbes from outside animals or human caretakers can contaminate herds (20, 45).

Decisions about screening methods and organisms to be screened for must be considered prospectively. Microbial agents were classified as absolute contraindications, relative contraindications, permissible, or indeterminate groups in the development of a screening method for source animals to be used in baboon bone marrow transplantation into a human with AIDS (59). Microbes that were known to be zoonotic specifically from baboons or hazardous to humans, even if they were not commonly found in baboons raised in the United States, were considered to be absolute contraindications. In particular, organisms that could be secondarily transmitted from an infected recipient to close contacts were placed in this category. Examples included SIV, STLV, filoviruses, *T. gondii*, *M. tuberculosis*, and cercopithecine herpesvirus (B virus). Baboons that tested negative were maintained in quarantined areas and retested over time to decrease the risk of a false negative test. Relative contraindications included organisms that were hypothesized to be transmissible but were unproven or have unclear consequence. At the time the procedure was performed, baboon herpesviruses and foamy virus were included in this category. The source animal was negative for all organisms classified as absolute or relative contraindications, with the exception of *H. papio*. Treatable infectious agents were permissible if they could be identified and eradicated successfully before harvest, such as *Babesia* species or gastrointestinal pathogens, although none of these were found. Finally, a category called "unavoidable" was created that included baboon endogenous virus and all the organisms that have yet to be recognized, and thus were considered to have an indeterminate risk to the patient or close contacts (59).

As noted above, swine have been reared in controlled environments more easily than primates. Similar types of categories can be designed for microbial agents of swine as suggested by several investigators (20, 84). Ten newborn piglets bred and born in specific-pathogen–free environments (free of brucellosis, pseudorabies virus, atrophic rhinitis, and *Mycoplasma hyopneumoniae*) were screened (84). Skin, urine, feces, and nasal swabs were cultured for bacteria and examined for fungi and parasites. Blood was cultured for bacteria and viruses and tested by commercial laboratory tests for antibody against human CMV, HBV, HCV, HIV, *Treponema pallidum*, and *T. gondii*. Testing was performed within the first 2 months of life, again between 16 and 30 weeks, and again at necropsy. Although no animal was found to have serious pathogens that were considered a risk for xenozoonoses, 2 of the 10 piglets had a false positive ELISA test for HIV. More specific testing was negative, but this finding again highlights the limitations that can occur with using tests developed for human specimens and human organisms.

A serologic survey was performed of 36 baboons raised in captivity in the United States from a single baboon colony. Paired serum samples were sent to two laboratories for testing for retroviruses, herpesviruses, and hepatitis A and B viruses (61). Significant discordance was found between laboratories when testing for EBV. Both laboratories relied on cross-reactivity of *H. papio* with human EBV; however, the laboratory using a test designed to detect EBV viral capsid antigen found a high prevalence compared to the laboratory using antibody directed against EBV nuclear antigen. This difference may be due to conservation of the viral capsid antigen in γ-herpesviruses of different species compared to more divergence in the region coding for EBV nuclear antigen (61). This again highlights the need for research and development of new diagnostic tests (8, 27, 28, 56, 62, 70).

SURVEILLANCE AFTER XENOTRANSPLANTATION

While raising animals in controlled environments and screening animals before using their tissues or cells will do much to decrease the threat of xenozoonoses, some risk will still exist. Accordingly, surveillance of individuals after xenotransplantation will be critical. This will help define the true risks of xenotransplant-associated infections to the recipient and help ascertain whether a risk exists for secondary transmission of infections to close contacts. Because the field is new, it has the luxury of developing these procedures prospectively. Samples from the recipient and transplanted tissues should be serially collected and cultured and/or assayed by current diagnostic techniques for microbes that were known to be harbored within the source animal, such as endogenous viruses. As important, serial collections of specimens (tissue, cells, and plasma) must be archived for future investigation. This is necessary because the current knowledge of infections is not static, and by having archived samples, testing can be performed for newly recognized agents. A central repository for archived specimens as well as a central registry of infectious disease surveillance results from individuals who undergo xenotransplantation would be ideal (19, 38, 42, 56). Finally, discussions should be held with candidates of xenotransplant procedures so that they understand the potential for infections with the use of any biologic agent. At the current time, when the full risks of xenotransplant infections remain ill defined, it is prudent to counsel candidates about methods to avoid the spread of potentially infectious secretions.

POTENTIAL BENEFITS AND OTHER INFECTIOUS DISEASE ISSUES

Xenotransplantation may have positive implications for decreasing the risk of some infections after transplantation. For example, acute donor-transmitted infections may be avoided by adequately maintaining healthy source animals in clean environments. Also the screening out of many potential latent viruses from a source animal colony will eliminate their risks. Patients may also be at less risk for infection because of the ability to schedule elective procedures as opposed to the current method of performing emergency surgery when a donor organ becomes available. In addition, a potential benefit may be realized if animal organs are resistant to human infections. This was the rationale for baboon liver xenotransplantation for two patients with chronic hepatitis B infection (60, 76, 78) and the use of baboon bone marrow to reconstitute the immune system of a person with advanced HIV infection (39). The potential benefits need to be studied and considered with caution as the field moves forward. Finally, studies need to be conducted to determine whether latent organisms within the human recipient will be harmful to the tissues from the new host.

REFERENCES

1. **Allan, J. S., S. R. Broussard, M. G. Michaels, T. E. Starzl, K. L. Leighton, E. M. Whitehead, A. G. Comuzzie, R. E. Lanford, M. M. Leland, W. M. Switzer, and W. Heneine.** 1998. Amplification of simian retroviral sequences from human recipients of baboon liver transplants. *AIDS Res. Hum. Retrov.* **14:**821–824.
2. **Anonymous.** 1997. Nonhuman primate spumavirus infections among persons with occupational exposure—United States, 1996. *JAMA* **277:**783–785.
3. **Artenstein, A. W., C. B. Hicks, B. S. Goodwin, Jr., and J. K. Hilliard.** 1991. Human infection with B virus following a needle stick injury. *Rev. Infect. Dis.* **13:**288–291.
4. **Bailey, L. L., S. L. Nehlsen-Cannarella, W. Concepcion, and W. B. Jolley.** 1985. Baboon-to-human xenotransplantation in a neonate. *JAMA* **254:**3321–3329.
5. **Benveniste, R. E., W. R. Morton, E. A. Clark, C. C. Tsai, H. D. Ochs, J. M. Ward, L. Kuller, W. B. Knott, R. W. Hill, M. J. Gale, et al.** 1988. Inoculation of baboons and macaques with SIV/mne, a primate lentivirus closely related to HIV 2. *Virology* **2:**2091–2101.
6. **Cappucci, D. T.** 1972. Tuberculosis from man to primates. *Am. Rev. Respir. Dis.* **106:**819–823.
7. **Cen, H., M. C. Breinig, R. W. Atchinson, M. Ho, and J. L. C. McKnight.** 1991. Epstein-Barr virus transmission via the donor organs in solid organ transplantation: polymerase chain reaction and restriction fragment length polymorphism analysis of IR2, IR3 and IR4. *Virology* **65:**976.
8. **Chapman, L. E., T. M. Folks, D. R. Salomon, A. P. Patterson, T. E. Eggerman, and P. D. Noguchi.** 1995. Xenotransplantation and xenogeneic infections. *N. Engl. J. Med.* **333:**1498.
9. **Charamella, L. J., R. B. Reynolds, L. T. Ch'ien, and C. A. Alford, Jr.** 1973. Biologic characterization of an unusual human cytomegalovirus isolated from the brain. Abstr. V 373. *Ann. Meetings Amer. Soc. Med.* **256.**
10. **Chari, R. S., B. H. Collins, J. C. Magee, M. DiMaio, A. D. Kirk, R. C. Harland, R. L. McCann, J. L. Platt, and W. C. Meyers.** 1994. Brief report: treatment of hepatic failure with ex vivo pig-liver perfusion followed by liver transplantation. *N. Engl. J. Med.* **331:**234–237.
11. **Chellman, G. J., V. S. Lukas, E. M. Eugui, K. P. Altera, S. J. Almqist, and J. K. Hilliard.** 1992. Activation of B virus in chronically immunosuppressed cynomolgus monkeys. *Lab. Anim. Sci.* **42:**146–151.
12. **Chou, S.** 1986. Acquisition of donor strains of cytomegalovirus by renal-transplant recipients. *N. Engl. J. Med.* **314:**1418.
13. **Chou, S.** 1989. Reactivation and recombination of multiple cytomegalovirus strains from individual organ donors. *J. Infect. Dis.* **160:**11–15.
14. **Cooper, D. K. C., Y. Ye, L. L. Rolf, Jr., and N. Zuhdi.** 1991. The pig as a potential organ donor for man, p. 481–499. *In* D. K. C. Cooper, K. Kemp, K. Reemtsma, and D. J. G. White (ed.), *Xenotransplantation: The Transplantation of Organs and Tissues Between Species.* Springer-Verlag, Berlin, Germany.
15. **Dummer, J. S., J. Armstrong, J. Somers, S. Kusne, B. J. Carpenter, J. T. Rosenthal, and M. Ho.** 1987. Transmission of infection with herpes simplex by renal transplantation. *J. Infect. Dis.* **155:**202.
16. **Dummer, J. S., S. Erb, M. Breinig, M. Ho, C. R. Rinaldo, Jr., P. Gupta, M. V. Ragni, A. Tzakis, L. Makowka, D. Van Thiel, and T. E. Starzl.** 1989. Infection with human immunodeficiency virus in the Pittsburgh transplant population. *Transplantation* **47:**134.
17. **Edington, N., A. E. Wrathall and J. T. Done.** 1988. Porcine cytomegalovirus (PCMV) in early gestation. *Vet. Micro.* **17:**117–128.
18. **Falk, L., F. Deinhardt, M. Nonoyama, L. G. Wolfe, and C. Bergholz.** 1976. Properties of a baboon lymphotropic herpesvirus related to Epstein-Barr virus. *Int. J. Cancer* **18:**798–807.
19. **Federal Register.** 1996. Draft Public Health Service guideline on infectious disease issues in xenotransplantation. *Fed. Regist.* September 23, **61:**49920–49932.
20. **Fishman, J. A.** 1994. Miniature swine as organ donors for man: strategies for prevention of xenotransplant-associated infections. *Xenotransplantation* **1:**47–57.
21. **Flugel, R. M.** 1991. Spumaviruses: a group of complex retroviruses. *Acquired Immune Defic. Syndromes* **4:**739–750.
22. **Frazier, M. E.** 1985. Evidence for retrovirus in miniature swine with radiation-induced leukemia or metaplasia. *Arch. Virol.* **83:**83–97.
23. **Gao, F., E. Bailes, D. L. Robertson, Y. Chen, C. M. Rodenburg, S. F. Michael, L. B. Cummins, L. O. Arthur, M. Peeters, G. M. Shaw, P. M. Sharp, and B. H. Hahn.** 1999. Origin of HIV-1 in the chimpanzee *Pan troglodytes troglodytes. Nature* **397:**436–441.

24. **Green, M., and M. G. Michaels.** 1997. Infections in solid organ transplant recipients, p. 626–634. *In* S. S. Long, L. Pickering, and C. Prober (ed.), *Principles and Practice of Pediatric Infectious Diseases*. Churchill Livingstone Inc., New York, N.Y.
25. **Halliburton, I. W., R. E. Randall, R. A. Killington, and D. H. Watson.** 1977. Some properties of recombinants between type 1 and type 2 herpes simplex viruses. *J. Gen. Virol.* **36:**471–484.
26. **Henderson, J. D., Jr.** 1992. Diagnostic exercise: anemia in a baboon. *Lab. Anim. Sci.* **42:**514–515.
27. **Heneine, W.** 1996. Strategies for diagnosis of xenotransplant-associated retroviral infections. *Mol. Diag.* **1:**255–257.
28. **Heneine, W., and W. M. Switzer.** 1996. Highly sensitive and specific polymerase chain reaction assays for detection of baboon and pig cells following xenotransplantation in humans. *Transplantation* **62:**1360–1362.
29. **Heneine, W., A. Tibell, W. M. Switzer, P. Sandstrom, G. V. Rosales, A. Mathews, O. Korsgren, L. E. Chapman, T. M. Folks, and C. G. Groth.** 1998. No evidence of infection with porcine endogenous retrovirus in recipients of porcine islet-cell xenografts. *Lancet* **352:**695–699.
30. **Hilliard, J. K., D. Black, and R. Eberle.** 1989. Simian alphaherpesviruses and their relation to the human herpes simplex viruses. *Arch. Virol.* **109:**83–102.
31. **Ho, M., and J. S. Dummer.** 1990. Risk factors and approaches to infections in transplant recipients. *In* G. C. Mandell, G. R. Douglas, Jr., and J. E. Bennet (ed.), *Principles and Practice of Infectious Diseases*, 2nd ed. Churchill Livingstone, New York, N.Y.
32. **Ho, M., G. Miller, R. W. Atchison, M. K. Breinig, J. S. Dummer, W. Andiman, T. E. Starzl, R. Eastman, B. P. Griffith, R. L. Hardesty, et al.** 1985. Epstein-Barr virus infections and DNA hybridization studies in post-transplantation lymphoma and lymphoproliferative lesions: the role of primary infection. *J. Infect. Dis.* **152:**876.
33. **Holmes, G. P., L. E. Chapman, J. A. Stewart, S. E. Straus, J. K. Hilliard, and D. S. Davenport.** 1995. Guidelines for the prevention and treatment of B-virus infections in exposed persons. *Clin. Infect. Dis.* **20:**421–439.
34. **Homma, T., P. J. Kanki, N. W. King, Jr., R. D. Hunt, M. J. O'Connell, N. L. Letvin, M. D. Daniel, R. C. Desrosiers, C. S. Yang, and M. Essex.** 1984. Lymphoma in macaques: association with virus of HTLV family. *Science* **225:**716–718.
35. **Huang, E., B. Kilpatrick, A. Lakeman, and C. A. Alford.** 1978. Genetic analysis of a cytomegalovirus-like agent isolated from human brain. *J. Virol.* **26:**718–723.
36. **Huang, L., J. Silberman, H. Rothschild, and J. C. Cohen.** 1989. Replication of baboon endogenous virus in human cells. *J. Biol. Chem.* **264:**8811–8814.
37. **Hubbard, G. B., K. F. Soike, T. M. Butler, K. D. Carey, H. Davis, and W. I. Butcher.** 1992. An encephalomyocarditis virus epizootic in a baboon colony. *Lab. Anim. Sci.* **42:**233–239.
38. **Institute of Medicine.** 1996. *Xenotransplantation: Science, Ethics and Public Policy*. National Academy Press, Washington, D.C.
39. **Isfort, R., D. Jones, R. Kost, R. Witter, and H. Kung.** 1992. Retrovirus insertion into herpesvirus in vitro and in vivo. *Proc. Natl. Acad. Sci. USA* **89:**991–995.
40. **Javier, R. T., F. Sedarati, and J. G. Stevens.** 1986. Two avirulent herpes simplex viruses generate lethal recombinants in vivo. *Science* **234:**746–748.
41. **Kalter, S. S., and R. L. Heberling.** 1990. Primate viral diseases in perspective. *Med. Primatol.* **19:**519–535.
42. **Kennedy, I., and Advisory Group on Ethics of Xenotransplantation.** 1996. *Animal Tissue Into Humans*. ISBN 011 321866 4. Department of Health, Publications Center, London, U.K.
43. **Khabbaz, R. F., W. Heneine, and J. R. George.** 1994. Brief report. Infection of a laboratory worker with simian immunodeficiency virus. *N. Engl. J. Med.* **330:**172–177.
44. **Khabbaz, R. F., T. Rowe, M. Murphey-Corb, W. M. Heneine, C. A. Schable, J. R. George, C. P. Pau, B. S. Parekh, M. D. Lairmore, J. W. Curran, et al.** 1992. Simian immunodeficiency virus needle stick accident in a laboratory worker. *Lancet* **340:**271–273.
45. **Lerche, N. W., J. L. Yee, and M. B. Jennings.** 1994. Establishing specific retrovirus-free breeding colonies of macaques. *Lab. Anim. Sci.* **44:**217–221.
46. **Le Tissuer, P., J. P. Stoye, Y. Takeuchi, C. Patience, and R. A. Weiss.** 1997. Two sets of human-tropic pig retrovirus. *Nature* **389:**681–682.
47. **Martin, U., V. Kiessig, J. H. Blusch, A. Haverich, K. von der Helm, T. Herden, and G. Steinhoff.** 1998. Expression of pig endogenous retrovirus by primary porcine endothelial cells and infection of human cells. *Lancet* **352:**692–694.

48. **Martin, W. J., K. Ahmed, L. C. Zeng, J. Olsen, J. G. Seward, and J. S. Seehrai.** 1995. African green monkey origin of the atypical cytopathic 'stealth virus' isolated from a patient with chronic fatigue syndrome. *Clin. Diag. Virol.* **4:**93–103.
49. **Martin, W. J., L. C. Zeng, K. Ahmed, and M. Roy.** 1994. Cytomegalovirus-related sequence in an atypical cytopathic virus repeatedly isolated from a patient with chronic fatigue syndrome. *Am. J. Pathol.* **145:**440–451.
50. **Mason, J. C., K. S. Ordelheide, G. M. Grames, T. V. Threasher, R. D. Harris, R. H. Dang Bui, and M. C. T. Mackett.** 1987. Toxoplasmosis in two renal transplant recipients from a single donor. *Transplantation* **44:**588.
51. **Mayes, J. T., A. R. O'Connor, W. Castellani, and W. Carey.** 1995. Transmission of *Toxoplasma gondii* infection by liver transplantation. *Clin. Infect. Dis.* **21:**511.
52. **McConnell, E. E., P. A. Basson, V. De Vos, B. J. Myers, and R. E. Kuntz.** 1974. A survey of diseases among 100 free-ranging baboons from the Kruger national park, Onderstepoort. *J. Vet. Res.* **41:**97–167.
53. **Melby, E. C., and N. J. Altman (ed.).** 1976. *Handbook of Laboratory Animal Science*, Vol. III, P. 49. CRC Press, Boca Raton, Fla.
54. **Meng, X. J., P. G. Halbur, M. S. Shapiro, S. Govindarajan, J. D. Bruna, I. K. Mushahwar, R. H. Purcell, and S. U. Emerson.** 1998. Genetic and experimental evidence for cross-species infection by swine hepatitis E virus. *J. Virol.* **72:**9714–9721.
55. **Meng, X. J., R. H. Purcell, P. G. Halbur, J. R. Lehman, D. M. Webb, T. S. Tsareva, J. S. Haynes, B. J. Thacker, and S. U. Emerson.** 1997. A novel virus in swine is closely related to the human hepatitis E virus. *Proc. Natl. Acad. Sci. USA* **94:**9860–9865.
56. **Michaels, M. G.** 1997. Infectious concerns of cross-species transplantation: xenozoonoses. *World J. Surgery* **21:**968–974.
57. **Michaels, M. G., D. Alcendor, K. St. George, C. R. Rinaldo, Jr., G. Ehrlich, and H. G. Becich.** 1997. Distinguishing baboon CMV from human CMV: importance for xenotransplantation. *J. Infect. Dis.* **176:**1476–1483.
58. **Michaels, M. G., and M. D. Green.** 1997. Infectious complications of heart and lung transplantation in children, p. 27–45. *In* K. L. Franco (ed.), *Pediatric Cardiopulmonary Transplantation*. Futura Publishing Company Inc., New York, N.Y.
59. **Michaels, M. G., J. Hilliard, S. Deeks, P. Gupta, W, Heneine, D. Pardi, C. Kaufman, C. Rinaldo, K. St. George, L. Chapman, T. Folks, Y. Colson, P. Volberding, and S. T. Ildstad.** 1997. Baboon bone marrow xenotransplant in a patient with advanced HIV: a model for the evaluation of potential xenozoonoses. *Proc. Inst. Hum. Virol. Annu. Meet., J. Acquired Immune Defic. Syndr. Hum. Retrovirol.*, Abstr. 11, p. 3.
60. **Michaels, M. G., R. Lanford, A. J. Demetris, D. Chavez, K. Brasky, J. Fung, and T. E. Starzl.** 1996. Lack of susceptibility of baboons to infection with hepatitis B virus. *Transplantation* **61:**350–351.
61. **Michaels, M. G., J. McMichael, K. Brasky, S. Kalter, R. L. Peters, T. E. Starzl, and R. L. Simmons.** 1994. Screening donors for xenotransplantation: the potential for xenozoonoses. *Transplantation* **57:**1462.
62. **Michaels, M. G., and R. L. Simmons.** 1994. Xenotransplant-associated zoonoses. *Transplantation* **57:**1.
63. **Michaels, M. G., E. T. Wald, F. J. Fricker, P. J. del Nido, and J. Armitage.** 1992. Toxoplasmosis in pediatric recipients of heart transplants. *Clin. Infect. Dis.* **14:**847.
64. **Miller, G.** 1990. Epstein-Barr virus: biology, pathogenesis, and medical aspects, p. 1921. *In* B. N. Fields and D. M. Knipe (ed.), *Virology*, 2nd ed. Raven Press, New York, N.Y.
65. **Morton, W. R., L. Kuller, R. E. Benveniste, E. A. Clark, C. C. Tsai, M. J. Gale, M. E. Thouless, J. Overbaugh, and M. G. Katze.** 1989. Transmission of the SIV in macaques and baboons. *Med. Primatol.* **18:**237–245.
66. **Mravak, S., U. Bienzle, H. Feldmeier, H. Hampl, and K. Habermehl.** 1987. Pseudorabies in man. *Lancet* **1:**501.
67. **Patience, C., Y. Takeuchi, and R. A. Weiss.** 1997. Infection of human cells by an endogenous retrovirus of pigs. *Nature Med.* **3:**282–286.
68. **Pereira, B. J. G., E. L. Milford, R. L. Kirkman, and A. S. Levey.** 1991. Transmission of hepatitis C virus by organ transplantation. *N. Engl. J. Med.* **325:**454.
69. **Perot, K., C. M. Walker, and R. R. Spaete.** 1992. Primary chimpanzee skin fibroblast cells are fully permissive for human cytomegalovirus replication. *J. Gen. Virol.* **73:**3281–3284.
70. **Persing, D. H.** 1996. Nucleic acid-based pathogen discovery techniques. Potential application to xenozoonoses. *Molec. Diagn.* **1:**243.

71. **Reemtsma, K., B. H. McCracken, J. U. Schlegel, M. A. Pearl, C. W. Pearce, C. W. DeWitt, P. E. Smith, R. L. Hewitt, R. L. Flinner, and O. Creech, Jr.** 1964. Renal heterotransplantation in man. *Ann. Surg.* **160:**384–410.

72. **Remington, J. S., R. McLeod, and G. Desmonts.** 1995. Toxoplasmosis, p. 140–267. *In* J. S. Remington and J. O. Klein (ed.), *Infectious Diseases of the Fetus and Newborn Infant*, 4th ed. W. B. Saunders Co., Philadelphia, Pa.

73. **Rubin, R. H.** 1990. Impact of cytomegalovirus infection on organ transplant recipients. *Rev. Infect. Dis.* **12**(Suppl. 7)**:**S754–S766.

74. **Schweizer, M., V. Falcone, J. Gange, R. Turek, and D. Neumann-Haefelin.** 1997. Simian foamy virus isolated from an accidentally infected human individual. *J. Virol.* **71:**4821–4824.

75. **Simonds, R. J., S. D. Holmberg, R. L. Hurwitz, T. R. Coleman, S. Bottenfield, L. J. Conley, S. H. Kohlenberg, K. G. Castro, B. A. Dahan, C. A. Schable, M. A. Rayfield, and M. F. Rogers.** 1992. Transmission of human immunodeficiency virus type I from a seronegative organ and tissue donor. *N. Engl. J. Med.* **326:**726.

76. **Starzl, T. E., J. Fung, A. Tzakis, S. Todo, A. J. Demetris, I. R. Marino, H. Doyle, A. Zeevi, V. Warty, M. Michaels, S. Kusne, W. A. Rudert, and M. Trucco.** 1993. Baboon-to-human liver transplantation. *Lancet* **341:**65–71.

77. **Starzl, T. E., T. L. Marchioro, G. N. Peters, C. H. Kirkpatrick, W. E. C. Wilson, K. A. Porter, D. Rifkind, D. A. Ogden, C. R. Hitchcock, and W. R. Waddell.** 1964. Renal heterotransplantation from baboon to man: experience with 6 cases. *Transplantation* **2:**752–776.

78. **Starzl, T. E., A. Tzakis, J. J. Fung, S. Todo, A. J. Demetris, R. Manez, I. R. Marino, L. Valdivia, and N. Murase.** 1994. Prospects of clinical xenotransplantation. *Transplant. Proc.* **26:**1082–1088.

79. **Varki, N. M., S. Bhuta, T. Drake, and D. D. Porter.** 1990. Adenovirus hepatitis in two successive liver transplants in a child. *Arch. Pathol. Lab. Med.* **114:**106.

80. **Weiss, R. A.** 1988. Foamy retroviruses: a virus in search of a disease. *Nature* **33:**497.

81. **Wilson, C. A., S. Wong, J. Muller, C. E. Davidson, T. M. Rose, and P. Burd.** 1998. Type C retrovirus released from primary peripheral blood mononuclear cells infects human cells. *J. Virol.* **72:**3082–3087.

82. **Wong, S. Y., and D. M. Allen.** 1992. Transmission of disseminated histoplasmosis via cadaveric renal transplantation: case report. *Clin. Infect. Dis.* **14:**232.

83. **Wreghitt, T. G., M. Hakim, J. J. Gray, A. H. Balfour, P. G. I. Stovin, S. Stewart, J. Scott, and J. Wallwork.** 1989. Toxoplasmosis in heart and heart and lung transplant recipients. *J. Clin. Pathol.* **42:**194.

84. **Ye, Y., M. Niekrasz, S. Kosanke, R. Welsh, H. D. Jordan, J. C. Fox, W. C. Edwards, C. Maxwell, and D. K. C. Cooper.** 1994. The pig as a potential organ donor for man. *Transplantation* **57:**694–703.

Xenotransplantation
Edited by Jeffrey L. Platt

Chapter 11

Zoonosis as a Risk to the Xenograft Recipient and to Society: Theoretical Issues

Louisa E. Chapman

BACKGROUND: XENOTRANSPLANTATION AT THE CUSP OF THE 21ST CENTURY

During the latter half of the 20th century, the availability of allotransplantation has increased both the number of people benefiting from life-saving transplantation procedures and the number of potential beneficiaries on waiting lists (58). This visible success of allotransplantation, combined with its equally visible limitations, has encouraged interest in xenotransplantation—the therapeutic use of living animal tissue in humans (49).

Until recently, the most visible aspect of xenotransplantation, and that which has largely shaped public perception, has been intermittent attempts at whole-organ transplantation, such as the transplantation of a baboon heart into an infant ("Baby Fae") in 1984 (7) or of baboon livers into an HIV-infected patient dying of hepatitis B in 1992 (53). These well-publicized incidents were typical of most of the U.S. clinical experience with xenotransplantation prior to the past decade. Recipients could be expected to remain hospitalized and to survive no longer than weeks following the procedure.

The second example above was inspired by the recognition that baboons are refractory to infection with HIV-1 and hepatitis B virus (HBV), both of which cause persistent destructive infections in humans. This species differential also motivated the transplantation of baboon bone marrow into a human infected with HIV-1 in an attempt to reconstitute the patient's immune system (40). This latter type of experiment is more typical of most recent and proposed xenotransplantation clinical trials.

While successful whole organ xenotransplantation is still viewed as a potential solution to the human donor organ shortage, in recent years the majority of proposed clinical xenotransplantation trials used avascular cellular preparations. In the United States, current or proposed clinical trials in xenotransplantation use porcine neurologic, pancreatic, and hepatic cells to treat degenerative neurologic disorders (such as Parkinson's disease), diabetes, and hepatic failure (15, 18, 24); bovine adrenal preparations to ameliorate intractable pain

Louisa E. Chapman • Retrovirus Diseases Branch, Division of AIDS, STD, and TB Laboratory Research, National Center for Infectious Diseases, Centers for Disease Control and Prevention, Atlanta, GA 30333.

in cancer patients (49); and baboon hearts as bridges for pediatric patients with heart failure (41). Except for heart transplants, these applications propose to use cellular rather than whole organ xenografts. As a result, increasing numbers of xenograft recipients are both leaving the hospital and surviving for months to years after receiving cellular transplants that function for prolonged periods.

PUBLIC HEALTH CONCERNS RAISED BY XENOTRANSPLANTATION

The use of living animal tissue for therapeutic purposes in humans has raised concerns that xenotransplantation clinical trials may pose a presently unquantifiable but undeniable risk to the public health (14). Allotransplantation is known to transmit infections endemic in humans from donors to recipients (21). Xenotransplantation has the potential to introduce new infections to the human community by infecting human recipients with agents that were not previously endemic in human populations (xenogeneic infections). A reasonable basis for these concerns is supported by a history of both individual and epidemic human infections caused by zoonotic infections (diseases transmitted between humans and animals under natural conditions). At least two major human pandemics have been attributed to zoonotic viruses: the 1918 "Spanish" influenza pandemic, attributed to infection of humans with a swine influenza virus (62), and the current HIV/AIDS pandemic, believed to have originated with the infection of humans by a simian immunodeficiency virus (SIV) endemic to chimpanzees (52). Both associations have been further supported by recent scientific work (23, 31).

By juxtaposing animal tissue and its microbiologic flora with humans in ways that bypass most or all of the normal host-defense systems, xenotransplantation creates intimate and prolonged contact that may facilitate transmission of infections (13). Manipulations intended to prevent xenograft rejection may also facilitate the transmission of agents that rarely or never infect humans under natural circumstances (63). Therefore, xenotransplantation clinical trials combine a potential benefit for individual recipients with a potential, presently unquantifiable, risk to the human community (6, 14). This latter aspect arguably takes xenotransplantation out of the realm of a private decision between the health care provider and the individual patient and into a more public realm (6, 14).

Developing Public Policy

The absence of an adequate scientific base to support policy development has resulted in often sharply conflicting conclusions about whether it is appropriate to proceed with clinical trials (12). Scientists have proffered widely varying opinions on the extent to which xenotransplantation clinical trials threaten to introduce new infections into the human community. Observers at one extreme conclude that the risk of introducing new infections to the human community is too great, and the potential for benefit is too unclear. These observers argue that the only responsible stance is to impose a complete moratorium on clinical xenotransplantation until there is sufficient knowledge to assess these risks. Observers on the other extreme argue that in the absence of data to support these fears, restrictions that slow or halt the progress of xenotransplantation research would unnecessarily impede progress in an area that promises unmeasurable relief to human suffering. Other observers note that both the risks and the benefits associated with clinical xenotransplantation remain theoretical at present. These observers argue that the only way to clarify these issues is to allow limited clinical trials to go forward while carefully monitoring both safety and efficacy. Advocates of this approach argue that these trials can be accompanied by safeguards stringent enough to adequately protect the public. This diversity of opinion is reflected in guidance documents on xenotransplantation developed (or under development) by a number of national and international organizations (1, 8, 19, 20, 30, 33, 44, 59, 61, 66).

Cautious Progress: Monitoring for Xenogeneic Infections

The U.S. Public Health Service (PHS) has adopted a stance of cautious progress, allowing limited numbers of regulated xenotransplantation clinical trials to proceed under carefully monitored conditions, an approach outlined in the PHS Guideline on Infectious Disease Issues in Xenotransplantation (19, 59). In addition to the importance of including experts in human and veterinary infectious diseases and microbiology on the xenotransplant team, this guideline emphasizes the importance of the informed consent and education processes and adequate protocol review. Because of the public health concerns raised by the potential for secondary transmission of xenogeneic infections, these consent and education processes must extend beyond the individual recipient to include close contacts and health care workers. Xenotransplantation clinical trials in the United States are regulated by the Food and Drug Administration (FDA) (59). Particular emphasis is given to the importance of safety monitoring, which is built around two key concepts: pretransplantation screening and post-transplantation surveillance (19, 59). The goal of pretransplant screening is to eliminate recognized zoonotic infectious agents, as well as agents with suspected or unexplored zoonotic potential, from the xenograft prior to transplantation. As such, it is nested in animal-husbandry techniques that limit and define the life-long exposure history of the source animals (19, 59).

Critics of this approach point out that knowledge of xenotransplant source-animal microbiology is incomplete. Pretransplant screening can dependably eliminate only those agents for which adequate diagnostic assays exist (4). The PHS guideline acknowledges the limitations of pretransplantation screening and thus also recommends post-transplantation surveillance. Post-transplantation surveillance is intended to identify infectious agents that were either not detectable in the xenograft (e.g., prions) or not removable from the xenograft (e.g., endogenous retroviruses). At present, for example, FDA requires that all U.S. recipients of porcine xenograft be monitored for porcine endogenous retrovirus (PERV) infections.

Life-long surveillance for clinical episodes compatible with xenogeneic infections is the major post-transplantation tool available to detect infections by agents that are not presently identifiable pretransplant (19, 59). The development of national or international registries would amplify the ability to recognize significant events by enabling epidemiologic surveillance of populations of xenograft recipients (64). Laboratory-based surveillance for endogenous retroviruses and other identifiable agents that cannot be removed from the xenograft can augment clinical surveillance. Laboratory-based studies of xenograft survivors will also increase our ability to quantify xenotransplant-associated risks and thereby expand our capacity to make science-based assessments of appropriate public policy.

This approach of cautious progress, with monitored clinical trials, has been criticized for relying on a system of safeguards primarily organized around rapid identification and containment of xenogeneic infections that have already occurred in individual human recipients (4). Critics have argued that our ability to confidently detect xenogeneic infections in a xenograft recipient prior to transmission to others is too limited to merit public confidence.

ADVANCES IN SCIENCE: ENDOGENOUS RETROVIRUSES

There have been substantial advances in the scientific understanding of infectious disease issues in xenotransplantation during the past few years. The most active research has focused on endogenous retroviruses. All xenografts from any species can be expected to contain species-specific endogenous retroviruses. All studied mammals contain multiple endogenous retroviral sequences as part of their genomes. The origin of these genetically transmitted endogenous retroviruses is unclear. Since all retroviruses intercalate into the genome of the infected cell, endogenous retroviruses are thought to represent the germline fixation of previously infectious (or "exogenous") retroviruses (11). Most endogenous retroviral sequences are defective. However, some endogenous retroviral sequences can express replication-competent virus. While these are usually incapable of forming an active infection in their host species, they can infect cells from other species in vitro (so-called xenotropic endogenous retroviruses).

Both pigs and baboons have been shown to have endogenous retroviruses that are capable of infecting human cells in vitro, raising concerns that transplantation of porcine or baboon xenografts into humans may enable these endogenous retroviruses to infect humans in vivo (34, 35, 47, 65). Multiple pig cell types have been shown to express replication-competent PERV, including spleen, kidney, heart, aortic endothelium, hepatocyte, skin, lung, and pancreatic islet cells. Three PERV variants with distinct envelope sequences (PERV-A, -B, and -C) have been partially characterized and demonstrated to differ in infectivity for human cells in vitro (2, 34, 35, 47, 54, 65).

Diagnostic tools for PERV and baboon endogenous retrovirus (BaEV) have been developed (2, 26, 27, 36, 55) and used to investigate endogenous retrovirus infection in recipients of baboon and porcine xenografts (29, 40, 46). These include Western blot serology to detect antibodies to PERV and BaEV (36). However, assays for serologic reactivity may be less reliable in the xenotransplant setting, where many recipients will be immunocompromised. Thus, molecular approaches are important in this patient population (26, 27, 55). Researchers have developed polymerase chain reaction (PCR) assays to detect both BaEV and PERV DNA as well as reverse transcriptase–PCR (RT–PCR) assays to assess evidence of viral expression (55). PCR assays specific for mitochondrial DNA from pigs and baboons have also been developed to enable assessment of the presence of microchimerism (the persistent presence of source animal cells in the human recipient). These assays are used in tandem with assays for PERV and BaEV DNA to distinguish endogenous retrovirus infection of the recipient from persistent microchimerism. Positive PCR signals for PERV accompanied by positive signals for porcine mitochondrial DNA suggest microchimerism. Endogenous retrovirus infection of human tissue should result in persistent detection of PERV in the absence of, or at levels disproportionate to, detection of porcine mitochondrial DNA (26, 27, 55). Prolonged xenograft survival, however, may necessitate quantification of the presence of porcine mitochondrial DNA relative to that of PERV DNA to discriminate microchimerism from infection.

Retrospective Studies of Xenograft Survivors

Persons who have undergone xenotransplantation are being retrospectively studied for evidence of in vivo endogenous retroviral infections. In an HIV-1–infected recipient of baboon bone marrow, PCR signals for both BaEV and baboon mitochondrial DNA were detectable at 5 days post transplant in peripheral blood lymphocytes from the recipient, indicating microchimerism. Thirteen days after the transplant, baboon mitochondrial DNA was persistently identifiable in the recipient, but BaEV DNA was no longer detectable; thereafter, neither signal was detected (40). The inability to detect BaEV at 13 days after transplant, despite the persistence of microchimerism with baboon tissue, can be explained by the difference in the quantity of cellular DNA and the limits of detection of the assays. Baboon mitochondrial DNA is present in thousands of copies per cell, while BaEV is present in at most hundreds of copies per cell. Thus, at low levels of microchimerism, BaEV would be expected to be undetectable while baboon mitochondrial DNA would remain identifiable.

No evidence of PERV infection was found in two renal dialysis patients whose blood was extracorporally perfused through porcine kidneys. Serial blood samples collected from these two patients were tested for pig DNA (porcine mitochondrial cytochrome oxidase subunit II [COII] and beta globin) and PERV DNA by nested PCR assays. The serum was also tested for neutralizing antibodies to two distinct PERV isolates. No evidence of pig or PERV DNA was found, even as early as 6 h after perfusion, and neutralizing antibodies were not identified in the plasma of either patient (46). These patients underwent only short-term extracorporeal exposure to pig tissue and were not immunosuppressed. As a result, they probably represent the lower end of risk for PERV infection among exposed persons.

Evidence of PERV infection was also absent in 10 diabetic patients, who had each received 200,000 to 1,000,000 pig fetal islet cells between 1990 and 1993 (9, 22, 29, 51, 57). Eight patients had evidence of persistent pig tissue for at least 2 to 3 days after xenograft receipt. Prolonged xenograft survival (more than 6 months) was documented in five patients (29, 57). However, markers of PERV infection were not detected in any patient, despite extended exposure to implanted pig cells and concomitant immunosuppressive therapy. Markers of PERV expression, including viral RNA and RT, were undetectable in sera collected both early (day 3 to day 180) and late (4 to 7 years) after xenotransplantation. Western blot analysis for PERV-reactive antibodies was also consistently negative (29).

Defining the Level of Risk Associated with Porcine Xenograft Exposure

Defining the overall risks of PERV infection for xenograft recipients is complex. Based on in vitro culture dynamics and characteristics, many retrovirologists anticipate that in vivo PERV infection of humans is likely to be a low-frequency event. However, some also believe that in vivo infection is almost inevitable given enough opportunities for infection. The studies described above offer limited reassurance. However, the extent to which the results of these or any individual studies can be generalized to other types of exposures is limited.

The risk that any xenograft recipient may become infected with PERV is likely a function of multiple factors associated with the source animal, the xenotransplantation technique, the characteristics of the human recipient, and the level of PERV expression by the transplanted cells. Galactose-α-1-3-galactose (α-Gal) terminal sugar residues are present on the cell surfaces of most mammals but absent in humans and Old World primates. As a result, humans have circulating IgG specific for α-Gal. Preexisting α-Gal–specific antibodies in humans bind to α-Gal moieties on the surface of xenografts. This results in complement activation, destroying the vascular endothelium of porcine xenograft within minutes of implantation (49). Pigs have been transgenically engineered to circumvent hyperacute rejection (HAR) and thus to facilitate graft survival. However, this barrier to porcine xenograft acceptance may also provide humans with a barrier to infection with porcine retroviruses.

Retroviruses budding from normal pig cells bear surface α-Gal residues, rendering them susceptible to lysis by the α-Gal–specific antibody and complement found in normal human sera. The sensitivity of pig-cell–derived PERV to inactivation and lysis by human sera has been demonstrated, and a single passage of PERV through human cells has been shown to cause the virus to become resistant to inactivation by normal human sera (47). Thus, the modification enacted to circumvent HAR of the xenograft may compromise lytic complement clearance of PERV and thereby facilitate PERV infection of human cells (45, 47, 54, 60, 63). As a result of this, recipients of xenografts from nontransgenic pigs, the only population studied and reported to date, likely represent the lowest end of a spectrum of risk for PERV infection (29, 46). In addition, no attempts were made to remove preformed xenoantibodies or to block complement activation before any of these reported patients received porcine xenografts. Risks will need to be independently assessed for alternative xenograft applications, including the use of xenografts procured from transgenic pigs (29, 54).

Reasoning by Analogy: Hypotheses about the Nature and Significance of Xenogeneic Infections

Although in vivo PERV infection of humans has not been identified to date, prudence dictates that clinical xenotransplantation protocols should anticipate the potential for such infection when developing plans for post-transplantation infection control. Some researchers have noted that consensus sequences of PERV virions are closely related to gibbon ape leukemia virus (GaLV) and feline leukemia virus (FeLV). These researchers have reasoned that infections with FeLV, which have been extensively studied and well characterized, is an appropriate model for speculation about the nature of putative PERV infections in humans (45). Abortive infection with subsequent recovery is the most frequent outcome of feline infection with FeLV. The minority of cats that develop persistent infection have high levels of plasma viremia and shed the virus in saliva and other body fluids. This model suggests that hepatitis B virus or cytomegalovirus infections may provide more appropriate models for infection control practices following human exposure to PERV than do infections with human retroviruses (HIV, HTLV) in which saliva poses negligible transmission risk (45, 50). The utility of transient peritransplant prophylactic intervention with antiretroviral pharmaceuticals may also be an appropriate avenue for research (45, 50).

The identification of microchimeric baboon cells in which simian foamy virus (SFV) and BaEV persisted in widely dispersed anatomic sites of baboon liver recipients weeks after transplantation confirms that xenografts can result in prolonged exposure to infectious agents carried with them (5). Studies of workers occupationally exposed to baboons confirm the ability of baboon SFV to infect humans and suggest that at least 2% of persons exposed to SFV-infected xenografts will acquire persistent SFV infections (28). Given that humans have been infected with SFV of baboon origin following transient occupational exposures, it is highly likely that this more intimate ongoing exposure would result in infection.

Demonstrating the presence or absence of xenogeneic infections in humans may be easier than determining the significance of any such infections. Rare zoonotic infection in humans can serve as a surrogate for xenogeneic infections and provide a basis for reasoning by analogy about the significance of purported xenogeneic infections. For example, the absence of recognized disease attributable to foamy virus in infected animals from any species, including the small numbers of SFV-infected humans studied to date, combined with the absence of identified secondary transmission among humans, has led some experts to argue that foamy virus infections in humans are insignificant to human health. However, observations on SFV-infected humans are too limited to confirm that these infections will remain persistently asymptomatic. Thus, the high prevalence of SFV infections in all endemic species for spumaviruses, including non-human primates, likely precludes the availability of foamy-virus–free animals as xenograft sources in the near future.

Defining Significant Exposures

The presence or absence of archived biologic material has often been the limiting factor in historic public health investigations. For example, a laboratory worker whose employer had regularly collected and archived sera was found to be infected with SIV. Investigators were able to retrospectively test banked sera and thereby to identify a narrow window of seroconversion that corresponded to a specific risk factor: a time frame when the worker, who regularly handled the blood of SIV-infected macaque monkeys without wearing gloves, had experienced a severe dermatitis of the hands and arms (32). Thus, the availability of stored sera allowed the investigators to identify the specific exposure that placed the worker at risk of infection. In contrast, an investigation of four workers infected with SFV documented durations of infection ranging from 2 to 20 years. However, the sparse availability of stored sera allowed documentation of a window of seroconversion for only one worker, and this based on sera collected more than a decade apart (28). This inability to pinpoint a narrow window of seroconversion for any of these four SFV-infected workers prevented the association of these SFV infections with any specific types of exposures. Thus, maintenance of archives of biologic specimens obtained from the xenograft source animals and human recipients will be important to ensure the availability of biologic materials for public health investigations, if such investigations become necessary (19, 59).

ADVANCES IN UNDERSTANDING: SYNTHESES AND REVIEWS

The accumulation of new knowledge combined with critical reviews and synthesis of existing data has broadened our understanding, facilitating the development of new consensuses while raising doubts about some assumed truisms. Critical review of data addressing the evolutionary history of recognized retroviruses raises questions about the assumption that phylogenetic proximity predicts the risk of cross-species transmission (11, 45, 50, 56, 60). Reviews of the microbial flora of pigs and primates have facilitated decision making on appropriate husbandry, quarantine, and screening of source animals (10, 38, 39, 42, 48). The recent identification of newly recognized infectious agents that infect species considered potential sources for xenografts (e.g., persistent asymptomatic hepatitis E virus infections of pigs with associated human infections, circovirus infections associated with wasting syndromes of pigs, and fatal nipahvirus infections of pigs and humans in Malaysia) confirms the importance of careful attention to animal-husbandry methods, active herd surveillance, and pretransplant screening for specific infectious agents (3, 25, 37, 38, 43). Reviews of historic developments in xenotransplantation (16) coupled with critiques of developing public policy and procedures have furthered efforts at consensus development (17). All of this has allowed public policy development to move along the spectrum from reasoned speculation toward a science-based approach.

REFERENCES

1. **Advisory Group on the Ethics of Xenotransplantation.** 1997. *Animal Tissues into Humans.* Stationery Office, London, United Kingdom.
2. **Akiyoshi, D. E., M. Denaro, H. Zhu, J. L. Greenstein, P. Banerjee, and J. A. Fishman.** 1998. Identification of a full length cDNA for an endogenous retrovirus of miniature swine. *J. Virol.* **72:**4503–4507.
3. **Allan, G. M., F. McNeilly, S. Kennedy, B. Daft, E. G. Clarke, J. A. Ellis, D. M. Haines, B. M. Meehan, and B. M. Adair.** 1998. Isolation of porcine circovirus-like viruses from pigs with a wasting disease in the USA and Europe. *J. Vet. Diagn. Invest.* **10:**3–10.
4. **Allan, J. S.** 1996. Xenotransplantation at a crossroads: prevention vs progress. *Nature Med.* **2:**18–21.
5. **Allan, J. S., S. R. Broussard, M. G. Michaels, T. E. Starzl, K. L. Leighton, E. M. Whitehead, A. G. Comuzzie, R. E. Lanford, M. M. Leland, W. M. Switzer, and W. Heneine.** 1998. Amplification of simian retroviral sequences from human recipients of baboon liver transplants. *AIDS Res. Hum. Retroviruses* **14:**821–824.
6. **Bach, F. H., J. A. Fishman, N. Daniels, J. Proimos, B. Anderson, C. B. Carpenter, L. Forrow, S. C. Robson, and H. V. Fineberg.** 1998. Uncertainty in xenotransplantation: individual benefit versus collective risk. *Nature Med.* **4:**141–144.
7. **Bailey, L. L., S. L. Nehlsen-Cannarella, W. Concepcion, and W. B. Jolley.** 1985. Baboon-to-human cardiac xenotransplantation in a neonate. *JAMA* **254:**3321–3329.
8. **Bellucci, S., A. Bondolfi, B. Husing, and A. Ruegsegger.** 1998. The Swiss technology assessment (TA) project on xenotransplantation. *Ann. N. Y. Acad. Sci.* **862:**155–165.
9. **Bjöersdorff, A., O. Korsgen, R. Feinstein, A. Andersson, J. Tollemar, A.-S. Malmborg, A. Ehrnst, and C. G. Groth.** 1995. Microbiological characterization of porcine fetal islet-like cell clusters for intended clinical xenografting. *Xenotransplantation* **2:**26–31.
10. **Borie, D. C., D. V. Cramer, L. Phan-Thanh, J. C. Vaillant, J. L. Bequet, L. Makowka, and L. Hannoun.** 1998. Microbiological hazards related to xenotransplantation of porcine organs into man. *Infect. Control Hosp. Epidemiol.* **19:**355–365.
11. **Brown, J., A. L. Matthews, P. A. Sandstrom, and L. E. Chapman.** 1998. Xenotransplantation and the risk of retroviral zoonosis. *Trends Microbiol.* **6:**411–415.
12. **Chapman, L. E.** 1999. Speculation, stringent reasoning, and science. *Bull. W. H. O.* **77:**68–70.
13. **Chapman, L. E., and J. A. Fishman.** 1997. Xenotransplantation and infectious diseases, p. 736–748. *In* D. K. C. Cooper, E. Kemp, J. L. Platt, and D. J. White (ed.), *Xenotransplantation: The Transplantation of Organs and Tissues Between Species.* Springer-Verlag, Berlin, Germany.
14. **Chapman, L. E., T. M. Folks, D. R. Salomon, A. P. Patterson, T. E. Eggerman, and P. D. Noguichi.** 1995. Xenotransplantation and xenogeneic infections. *N. Engl. J. Med.* **333:**1498–1501.
15. **Chari, R. S., B. H. Collins, J. C. Magee, J. M. DiMaio, A. D. Kirk, R. C. Harland, R. L. McCann, J. L. Platt, and W. C. Meyers.** 1994. Brief report: treatment of hepatic failure with ex vivo pig-liver perfusion followed by liver transplantation. *N. Engl. J. Med.* **331:**234–237.
16. **Daar, A. S.** 1998. Analysis of factors for the prediction of the response to xenotransplantation. *Ann. N. Y. Acad. Sci.* **862:**222–233.
17. **Daar, A. S.** 1999. Animal-to-human transplants—a solution or a new problem? *Bull. W. H. O.* **77:**54–61.
18. **Deacon, T., J. Schumacher, J. Dinsmore, C. Thomas, P. Palmer, S. Kott, A. Edge, D. Penney, S. Kassissieh, P. Dempsey, and O. Isacon.** 1997. Histological evidence of fetal pig neural cell survival after transplantation into a patient with Parkinson's disease. *Nature Med* **3:**350–353.
19. **DHHS Interagency Working Group on Xenotransplantation.** 1998. The draft US Public Health Service guideline on infectious disease issues in xenotransplantation. *Ann. N. Y. Acad. Sci.* **862:**166–170.
20. **De Sola, C.** 1998. Current developments on xenotransplantation in the Council of Europe. *Ann. N. Y. Acad. Sci.* **862:**211–213.
21. **Eastlund, T.** 1995. Infectious disease transmission through cell, tissue, and organ transplantation: reducing the risk through donor selection. *Cell Transplant.* **4:**455–477.

22. **Galili, U., A. Tibell, B. Samuelsson, L. Rydberg, and C. G. Groth.** 1995. Increased anti-gal activity in diabetic patients transplanted with fetal porcine islet cell clusters. *Transplantation* **59:**1549–1556.
23. **Geo, F., E. Bailes, D. L. Robertson, Y. L. Chen, C. M. Rodenburg, S. F. Micheal, L. B. Cummins, L. O. Arthur, M. Peeters, G. M. Shaw, P. M. Sharp, and B. H. Hahn.** 1999. Origin of HIV-1 in the chimpanzee *Pan troglodytes. Nature* **397:**436–441.
24. **Groth, C. G., O. Korsgren, A. Tibell, J. Tollemar, E. Moller, J. Bolinder, J. Ostman, F. P. Reinholt, C. Hellerstrom, and A. Andersson.** 1994. Transplantation of porcine fetal pancreas to diabetic patients. *Lancet* **344:**1402–1404.
25. **Hamel, A. L., L. L. Lin, and G. P. Naylar.** 1998. Nucleotide sequence of porcine circovirus associated with postweaning multisystemic wasting syndrome in pigs. *J. Virol.* **72:**5262–5267.
26. **Heneine, W.** 1996. Strategies for diagnosis of xenotransplant-associated retroviral infections. *Mol. Diagn.* **1:**255–260.
27. **Heneine, W., and W. M. Switzer.** 1996. Highly sensitive and specific polymerase chain reaction assays for detection of baboon and pig cells following xenotransplantation in humans. *Transplantation* **62:**1360–1362.
28. **Heneine, W., W. M. Switzer, P. Sandstrom, J. Brown, S. Vedapuri, C. A. Schable, A. S. Khan, N. W. Lerche, M. Schweizer, D. Neumann-Haefelin, L. E. Chapman, and T. M. Folks.** 1998. Identification of a human population infected with simian foamy viruses. *Nature Med.* **4:**391–392.
29. **Heneine, W., A. Tibell, W. M. Switzer, P. A. Sandstrom, G. Vazaquez-Rosales, A. Mathews, O. Korsgren, L. E. Chapman, T. M. Folks, and C. G. Groth.** 1998. No evidence of infection with porcine endogenous retrovirus in recipients of porcine islet-cell xenografts. *Lancet* **352:**695–699.
30. **Institute of Medicine.** 1996. *Xenotransplantation: Science, Ethics, and Public Policy.* National Academy Press, Washington, D.C.
31. **Ito, T., J. N. S. S. Couceiro, S. Kelm, L. G. Baum, S. Krauss, M. R. Castrucci, I. Donatelli, H. Kida, J. C. Paulson, R. G. Webster, and Y. Kawaoka.** 1998. Molecular basis for the generation in pigs of influenza A viruses with pandemic potential. *J. Virol.* **72:**7367–7373.
32. **Khabbaz, R. F., W. Heneine, J. R. George, B. Parekh, T. Rowe, T. Woods, W. M. Switzer, H. M. McClure, M. Murphey-Corb, and T. M. Folks.** 1994. Brief report: infection of a laboratory worker with simian immunodeficiency virus. *N. Engl. J. Med.* **330:**172–177.
33. **La Prairie, A. J. P., and D. R. Brodie.** 1998. Public confidence and government regulation. *Ann. N. Y. Acad. Sci.* **862:**171–176.
34. **Le Tissier, P., J. P. Stoye, Y. Yasuhiro, C. Patience, and R. A. Weiss.** 1997. Two sets of human-tropic pig retrovirus. *Nature* **389:**681–682.
35. **Martin, U., V. Kiessig, J. H. Blusch, A. Haverich, K. von der Helm, T. Herden, and G. Steinhoff.** 1998. Expression of pig endogenous retrovirus by primary porcine endothelial cells and infection of human cells. *Lancet* **352:**692–694.
36. **Matthews, A. L., J. Brown, W. Switzer, T. M. Folks, W. Heneine, and P. A. Sandstrom.** 1999. Development and validation of a Western immunoblot assay for detection of antibodies to porcine endogenous retrovirus. *Transplantation* **67:**939–943.
37. **Meng, X. J., P. G. Halbur, M. S. Shapiro, S. Govindarajan, J. D. Bruna, I. K. Mushahwar, R. H. Purcell, and S. U. Emerson.** 1998. Genetic and experimental evidence for cross-species infection by swine hepatitis E. virus. *J. Virol.* **72:**9714–9721.
38. **Meng, X. J., R. H. Purcell, P. G. Halbur, J. R. Lehman, D. M. Webb, T. S. Tsareva, J. S. Haynes, B. J. Thacker, and S. U. Emerson.** 1997. A novel virus in swine is closely related to the human hepatitis E. virus. *Proc. Natl. Acad. Sci. USA* **94:**9860–9865.
39. **Michaels, M. G.** 1997. Infectious concerns of cross-species transplantation: xenozoonoses. *World J. Surg.* **21:**968–974.
40. **Michaels, M., J. Hilliard, S. Deeks, P. Gupta, W. Heneine, D. Pardi, C. Kaufman, C. Rinaldo, K. St. George, L. Chapman, T. Folks, Y. Colson, P. Volberding, and S. Ildstat.** 1996. Baboon bone marrow xenotransplant in a patient with advanced HIV: a model for the evaluation of potential xenozoonoses. Institute of Human Virology Abstract #11. *J. Acquir. Immune Defic. Syndr. Hum. Retrovirol.* **14:**S3.
41. **Michler, R.** 1996. Xenotransplantation: risks, clinical potential, and future prospects. *Emerg. Infect. Dis.* **2:**64–70.
42. **Morgan, F.** 1997. Babe the magnificent organ donor? The perils and promises surrounding xenotransplantation. *J. Contemp. Health Law Policy* **14:**127–160.

43. **Naylar, G. P., A. Hamel, and L. Lin.** 1997. Detection and characterization of porcine circovirus associated with postweaning multisystemic wasting syndrome in pigs. *Canad. Vet. J.* **38:**385–386.
44. **Organization for Economic Co-operation and Development.** 1998. Policy consideration on international issues in transplantation biotechnology including the use of non-human cells, tissues, and organs. Report by Elettra Ronchi, Organization for Economic Co-operation and Development, Paris, France.
45. **Onions, D., D. Galbraith, D. Hart, C. Mahoney, and K. Smith.** 1998. Endogenous retroviruses and the safety of porcine xenotransplantation. *Trends Microbiol.* **6:**430–431.
46. **Patience, C., G. S. Patton, Y. Takeuchi, R. A. Weiss, M. O. McClure, L. Rydberg, and M. E. Breimer.** 1998. No evidence of pig DNA or retroviral infection in patients with short-term extracorporeal connection to pig kidneys. *Lancet* **352:**699–701.
47. **Patience, C., Y. Takeuchi, and R. A. Weiss.** 1997. Infection of human cells by an endogenous retrovirus of pigs. *Nature Med.* **3:**282–286.
48. **Patience, C., Y. Takeuchi, and R. A. Weiss.** 1998. Zoonosis in xenotransplantation. *Curr. Opin. Immunol.* **10:**539–542.
49. **Patterson, A. P., E. Bloom, and L. E. Chapman.** 1999. Clinical trials in xenotransplantation: the public health promises and challenges of an emerging technology. *J. Irish Coll. Phys. Surg.* **28:**222–227.
50. **Sandstrom, P. A., and L. E. Chapman.** 1998. Author's response. [letter]. *Trends Microbiol.* **6:**432.
51. **Satake, M., et al.** 1994. Kinetics and character of xenoantibody formation in diabetic patients transplanted with fetal porcine islet cells clusters. *Xenotransplantation* **1:**24.
52. **Sharp, P. M., D. L. Robertson, and B. H. Hahn.** 1995. Cross species transmission and recombination of 'AIDS' viruses. *Phil. Trans. R. Soc. London–Series B: Biol. Sci.* **349:**41–47.
53. **Starzl, T. E., J. Fung, A. Tzakis, S. Todo, A. J. Demetris, I. R. Marino, H. Doyle, A. Seevi, V. Warty, M., Michaels, et al.** 1993 Baboon-to-human liver transplantation. *Lancet* **341:**65–71.
54. **Stoye, J.** 1998. No clear answers on safety of pigs as tissue donor source. *Lancet* **352:**666–667.
55. **Switzer, W. M., V. Shanmugan, and W. Heneine.** 1999. Polymerase chain reaction assays for the diagnosis of infection with the porcine endogenous retrovirus and the detection of pig cells in human and nonhuman recipients of pig xenografts. *Transplantation* **68:**183–188.
56. **Takeuchi, Y.** 1998. Retroviral time travel. *Trends Microbiol.* **6:**430.
57. **Tibell, A., F. P. Reinholt, O. Korsgren, A. Andersson, C. Hellerstrom, E. Moller, and C. G. Groth.** 1994. Morphological identification of porcine islet cells three weeks after transplantation to a diabetic patient. *Transplant. Proc.* **26:**1121.
58. **United Network for Organ Sharing.** 1997 *Data Highlights from the 1997 Annual Report: the U.S. Scientific Registry of Transplant Recipients and the Organ Procurement and Transplantation Network—Transplant Data: 1988–1996.* U. S. Department of Health and Human Services, Rockville, Md.
59. **U. S. Public Health Service.** 1996. Draft guideline on infectious disease issues in xenotransplantation. *Fed. Reg.* **61:**49920–49932.
60. **Van der Kuyl, A. C., and J. Goudsmit.** 1998. Xenotransplantation: about baboon hearts and pig livers. *Trends Microbiol.* **6:**431–432.
61. **Van Rongen, E.** 1998. Xenotransplantation: perspective for the Netherlands. *Ann. N. Y. Acad. Sci.* **862:**177–183.
62. **Webster, R. G., G. B. Sharp, and E. C. Claas.** 1995. Interspecies transmission of influenza viruses. *Am. J. Respir. Crit. Care. Med.* **152:**S25–S30.
63. **Weiss, R.** 1998. Commentary: transgenic pigs and virus adaptation. *Nature* **391:**327–328.
64. **Whitehead, J., A. P. Patterson, and A. Moulton.** 1998. Development of databases and registries: international issues. *Ann. N. Y. Acad. Sci.* **862:**217–221.
65. **Wilson, C. A., S. Wong, J. Muller, C. E. Davidson, T. M. Rose, and P. Burd.** 1998. Type C retrovirus released from porcine primary peripheral blood mononuclear cells infects human cells. *J. Virol.* **72:**3082–3087.
66. **World Health Organization.** 1998. *Xenotransplantation: Guidance on Infectious Disease Prevention and Management.* World Health Organization, Geneva, Switzerland.

Xenotransplantation
Edited by Jeffrey L. Platt

Chapter 12

Zoonotic Agents in Swine-to-Human Xenotransplants

Peter J. Matthews

In human allotransplantation, an area of concern is the diseases that may be transmitted to the recipient via the donor's organs and tissues. Reported transmission of disease by infected human allografts includes human immunodeficiency virus (HIV), Epstein-Barr virus, herpes simplex virus, hepatitis C virus, and *Toxoplasma gondii* (4, 12, 16, 33, 39, 41). The history of human donors regarding infectious disease is difficult to assess. Despite the use of sophisticated screening techniques to detect infectious agents in donors, the risk of disease transmission via allografts still remains. In xenotransplantation, where swine are used as donors, there is also a risk that disease may be transmitted to the human recipient via the donor's organs and tissues.

Infectious agents that have the potential to be transmitted via swine xenografts fall into three categories:

1. **Traditional zoonotic organisms.** These are agents that can cause infectious disease in both swine and humans. Their transmission from swine to human under natural conditions has been documented or they have the potential to be transmitted to humans.
2. **Swine-specific organisms.** These are organisms that can cause infectious disease in swine, but currently there is no evidence that they are zoonotic.
3. **Undiscovered swine-specific organisms.** These are organisms yet to emerge.

All three categories will be discussed, but the emphasis will be on the traditional zoonotic organisms. Risk of disease transmission via xenografts and the public health aspects of porcine xenotransplantation will be discussed.

The literature that describes the traditional zoonotic diseases is extensive. It addresses the history, occurrence, etiology, epidemiology, mode of transmission, animal infection, diagnosis, prevention and control, human infection, and public health aspects of each specific disease. This information will be cited for those readers who wish to obtain a broad overview of each specific zoonosis. The intention in this chapter is to narrow the scope of the review to

Peter J. Matthews • 10046 161st St., Chippewa Falls, WI 54729.

describe the occurrence, the epidemiology, and the clinical signs of the traditional zoonotic diseases in the pig. The knowledge of the epidemiology, especially mode of transmission, in the pig itself is essential for the design of facilities and the establishment of biosafety and disease control programs that will minimize the risk of transmitting infectious disease agents via swine xenografts. For example, a review of the epidemiology of toxoplasmosis in swine reveals the following. The definitive host for the protozoan *T. gondii* is the cat (including wild *Felidae*). Cats are the only animals that excrete sporulated oocysts of *T. gondii* in their feces. Mammals (including swine) and birds are intermediate hosts and become infected by ingestion of feed and water contaminated with oocysts. In the intermediate host the organism forms cysts in the tissues. Tissue cysts are found mainly in the central nervous system and cardiac and skeletal muscles, and they remain viable for many years. Swine may ingest tissue cysts by killing and eating infected animals such as rodents, by cannibalism, by tail and ear biting, or by consumption of raw garbage. Transplacental infection can occur when susceptible sows or gilts are infected during pregnancy. Therefore, to maintain swine free of *T. gondii*, facilities should be built to exclude cats, other mammals, and birds that are a potential source of infection. The biosafety program should include storage of swine feed to prevent contamination by cats and intermediate hosts and an aggressive pest control program. Because transplacental infection does occur, pregnant females that are used for the derivation of specific-pathogen–free swine by hysterectomy or hysterotomy should be free of *T. gondii*.

TRADITIONAL ZOONOTIC ORGANISMS

Bacterial Diseases

Disease

Anthrax (23, 57, 58).

Agent. *Bacillus anthracis.*

Occurrence. Anthrax has been reported in the Middle East, Africa, Central and South America, and other areas of the world. In the United States, it is most commonly reported in the southern Mississippi River valley, but the disease has been reported in nearly every state. The incidence is low and sporadic but presents a local problem in areas of alkaline soil subject to periods of drought and flooding.

Epidemiology. Most animals are infected while grazing in areas that have previously experienced anthrax. After flooding, low-lying areas can become contaminated with spores. The most common source of infection for cattle, sheep, and horses is by ingestion of water and hay contaminated with spores. Infection of swine in this manner is possible. However, because of the small number of spores likely to be picked up and the greater degree of resistance in swine to anthrax, it rarely occurs. Anthrax in swine generally occurs following ingestion of inadequately processed infective foodstuffs of animal origin, such as blood and bone meal. Swine may also become infected by eating carcasses of animals that have died of anthrax.

Clinical Signs. Three forms of disease are recognized in animals: peracute, acute/subacute, and chronic. The chronic form is most commonly reported in swine. In this form of the disease, ingested organisms become localized in the lymph nodes of the pharyngeal area. The resulting tissue edema is responsible for the typical clinical signs of chronic anthrax, i.e., cervical edema, dyspnea, and serosanguinous discharge from the mouth. Other common clinical signs are general depression, anorexia, and vomiting. Death follows in many of the swine within 24 h after the cervical edema is noticed. However, some swine may recover even in the absence of treatment and may remain carriers of *B. anthracis*. In some cases the organism may pass into the intestinal tract. Clinical signs are not as obvious as those in the pharyngeal form of the disease. In severe cases vomiting, anorexia, and bloody diarrhea may be observed. Death may follow in the most severely affected animals, but recovery occurs in many affected with milder disease. If organisms gain entrance to the general circulation from the pharyngeal or intestinal sites, septicemic anthrax occurs. However, the septicemic form of the disease is rarely seen in swine.

Disease

Brucellosis (9, 30, 35).

Agent. *Brucella* species. There are six species of *Brucella*: *B. melitensis*, *B. abortus*, *B. suis*, *B. neotomae*, *B. ovis*, and *B. canis*.

Occurrence. Brucellosis occurs in most countries where swine exist in the feral or domestic state. Britain and Scandinavia are free.

Epidemiology. *B. suis* is the only *Brucella* species that causes generalized infection leading to reproductive failure in swine. Infection with other species is almost always subclinical, and the organisms are localized in the lymph nodes at the site of entry. *B. suis* is divided into five biotypes. Swine are the most common host for biotypes 1 and 3, and they are worldwide in distribution. There are few known reservoirs of *B. suis* infection other than infected domestic swine. Only the European hare (*Lepus capinensis*) and feral swine have been established as potential reservoir hosts. As early as 1954 the European hare was incriminated as a natural host for *B. suis* biotype 2 and was apparently responsible for periodic outbreaks of swine brucellosis in Europe. Feral swine in the southeastern United States were found to have a high rate of serologic reactors and *B. suis* was isolated from selected animals.

B. suis biotype 4 is responsible for enzootic disease in reindeer and caribou, and biotype 5 causes murine brucellosis. Apparently these two biotypes are not pathogenic for swine. Most *B. suis* infections are a result of direct association with infected swine. The most important routes of infection are through the alimentary and genital tracts. Swine may eat food or drink fluids contaminated with discharges from infected swine. Infection may also occur when aborted fetuses and/or fetal membranes are consumed. Suckling pigs can be infected by nursing infected dams. Brucellosis is a venereal disease of swine, and sows and gilts can be infected when bred by boars with genital infection or by artificial insemination with semen containing *B. suis*.

Clinical Signs. The majority of affected herds may have no recognizable signs. The classical signs of infection with *B. suis* are abortion, infertility, orchitis, posterior paralysis, and lameness. These signs may be transient, and death rarely occurs. Abortions may occur at any time during gestation and are usually a result of time of exposure rather than time of gestation.

Disease

Campylobacteriosis (46, 60).

Agent. *Campylobacter jejuni* and *Campylobacter coli*.

Occurrence. Worldwide.

Epidemiology. *C. jejuni* and *C. coli* are commensals commonly found in the gastrointestinal tract of swine. As with most intestinal organisms transmission is by the fecal-oral route. Asymptomatic carriers can shed the organisms in their feces for prolonged periods and can contaminate food, water, and the environment. *C. jejuni* is also a commensal in the gastrointestinal tract of wild and domestic ruminants, dogs, cats, fowl, and rodents. Therefore, they have the potential to be a source of infection for swine.

Clinical Signs. Diarrhea has been reported in various animal hosts including dogs, cats, calves, sheep, ferrets, mink, and several species of laboratory animals. However, infections in swine most commonly result in the asymptomatic carrier state.

Disease

Erysipelas (61, 62).

Agent. *Erysipelothrix rhusiopathiae.*

Occurrence. Swine erysipelas (SE) occurs in most parts of the world where domestic swine are produced. It is a ubiquitous organism that has been isolated from many species of mammals, birds, reptiles, amphibians, and fish.

Epidemiology. Domestic swine are probably the most important reservoir. It is estimated that 30 to 50% of healthy swine harbor the organism in their tonsils and other lymphoid tissue. These animals can discharge the organism in their feces and oronasal secretions and are an important source of infection. Swine affected with acute erysipelas shed large amounts of the organism in their feces, urine, saliva, and nasal secretions. Besides direct transmission from pig to pig, indirect transmission can also occur when soil, bedding, feed, and water are contaminated by infected pigs. The organism has been isolated from at least 50 species of wild mammals, of which nearly half were rodents, and from over 30 species of wild birds. Therefore, wild animals and particularly rodents may serve as a source of infection for susceptible swine. The organism has been isolated from cattle, sheep, horses, poultry, dogs, and cats, and these animals may provide an additional potential reservoir of infection. It causes polyarthritis in sheep and lambs and an acute fatal septicemic disease in turkeys, ducks, and occasionally other birds. *E. rhusiopathiae* has been found in reptiles, amphibians, and the surface slime of fish. The presence in the surface slime of fish creates a possible source of infection for swine when improperly processed fish meal is used in feed. Transmission of SE by various species of biting flies and ticks has been demonstrated. The significance of this mode of transmission has not been established.

Clinical Signs. The disease can take three forms: acute, subacute, and chronic. In the acute form of the disease sudden death may occur. Other pigs in the herd may appear visibly sick, and some may subsequently die. Temperatures of 104 to 108°F (40 to 42°C) and over are common. Some pigs may appear normal but have temperatures around 106°F (41°C). Temperatures in surviving pigs usually return to normal in 5 to 7 days. Animals are often found withdrawn from the herd and lying down. They resent being disturbed, and when approached, they get up and move away. This is usually accompanied by squealing, and when walking, they manifest a stiff, stilted gait. If left alone, they will soon lie down. Most affected animals are depressed and inappetant. Older animals may be constipated, but diarrhea can occur in younger animals. Abortion may occur in females with acute or subacute SE. Two to 3 days after exposure to *E. rhusiopathiae* cutaneous urticarial, or "diamond-skin" lesions appear. They may be few in number or so numerous they are difficult to count. Individual lesions may assume a characteristic rhomboid shape. In the acute fatal disease, dark purplish discoloration often occurs over the belly, ears, tail, thighs, and jowls. In pigs with subacute SE, signs are less severe than manifested in the acute form of the disease. Animals do not appear as sick. Temperatures may not be as high, and appetite may not be affected. A few skin lesions may occur, but they may be easily overlooked. Chronic SE may follow acute, subacute disease or subclinical infection. The most common sign of chronic SE is arthritis. As early as three weeks after infection animals may manifest varying degrees of stiffness and enlargement in one or more of the joints. The hock, stifle, elbow, and carpal joints are most commonly affected. Signs of cardiac insufficiency, due to vegetative proliferative granular growths on the heart valves, is a less common finding.

Disease

Leptospirosis (15, 49, 56).

Agent. *Leptospira* species. The species found in warm-blooded animals are *L. interrogans*, *L. weilii*, *L. borgpetersenii*, *L. noguchi*, and *L. santarosae*. As an aid to epidemiologic studies the species are subdivided into serogroups and further divided into serovars. There are now 23 serogroups containing 212 serovars. The serovars that are important as pathogens of swine are *pomona*, *bratislava*, *tarrasovi*, *muenchen*, *sejroe*, *canicola*, *grippotyphosa*, *icterohaemorrhagiae*, and *hardjo*.

Occurrence. Leptospirosis is a complex disease affecting most species of warm-blooded animals. It has been reported in swine from all parts of the world.

Epidemiology. The epidemiology of swine leptospirosis is complicated since swine can be infected by any of the pathogenic serovars. However, each serovar tends to be maintained in specific maintenance hosts. *Pomona* is a common swine-maintained serovar. It has been the cause of widespread clinical disease in pigs in North and South America, Australia, New Zealand, parts of Asia, and eastern and central Europe. *Bratislava* and *muenchen* are also swine-maintained serovars. *Bratislava* is now recognized as the most common swine-maintained serovar. Other species of animals recognized as maintenance hosts for specific serovars are the dog *canicola*, the brown rat (*Rattus norvegicus*) *icterohaemorrhagiae*, cattle *hardjo*, and wildlife *L. grippotyphosa* and *L. sejroe*. *Pomona* leptospires have a particular affinity for the kidneys of infected pigs, where they persist, multiply, and are voided in the urine. This characteristic is important in the transmission of infection. Infection can be introduced into a herd or group of pigs by three possible routes: introduction of infected pigs, exposure to a contaminated environment, or contact with an infected animal vector. Carrier pigs are probably the most common route of introduction, with infected replacement gilts or boars being one of the most important means of introducing infection. *Bratislava* infection is characterized by rapid transmission from pig to pig and a prolonged renal carrier state. It has been isolated from the genital tract of boars and sows, and venereal transmission is thought to have an important role in its spread.

Clinical Signs. Abortions late in pregnancy, stillbirths, weak pigs, and infertility are the signs most often associated with leptospirosis in a herd. In some pigs infections may be inapparent. In herds where the disease is endemic, acute leptospirosis is rare. In natural infections only a few animals are affected at one time, and there is transient fever, anorexia, and listlessness that may easily be missed. There have been a few reports of jaundice and hemoglobinuria in piglets under 3 months of age infected with strains of the *icterohaemorrhagiae* serogroup. Infections with *bratislava* are associated with infertility in breeding females, i.e., increased farrowing rates and reduced number of live pigs farrowed per sow.

Disease

Melioidosis (18, 52).

Agent. *Pseudomonas pseudomallei.*

Occurrence. Tropical and subtropical regions such as Asia and northern Australia.

Epidemiology. The organism is present in water and soil. Contaminated water and soil are the source of infection for swine.

Clinical Signs. Infection is often clinically inapparent. However, clinical signs that have been reported due to infection with *P. pseudomallei* include rectal temperatures of 104 to 108°F (40–42°C), unsteady gait, lameness, nasal discharge, subcutaneous swelling of the limbs, and abortion. Death may occur, but it is rare in adult animals. Large abscesses in the lungs, liver, spleen, kidney, and mesenteric and subcutaneous lymph nodes are features of the disease.

Disease

Pasteurellosis (10, 43).

Agent. *Pasteurella multocida* (toxigenic strains).

Occurrence. The disease has been recognized in most areas of the world where swine are produced.

Epidemiology. This is a complex disease, and numerous factors are involved in its spread. Severity of disease is associated with intensive methods of swine production. It is most severe when stocking density is high and buildings are continuously occupied and poorly ventilated. Some pigs may have subclinical disease and carry toxigenic strains of *P. multocida* in the tonsil and upper respiratory tract. The main method of spread is by introduction of carrier pigs into a susceptible herd or group. Transmission can occur by direct contact, infected droplets produced by sneezing, and the fecal-oral route. Infected carrier sows can infect their offspring. Toxigenic strains of *Pasteurella* have been isolated from cattle, goats, rabbits, dogs, cats, rats, and sheep. These species have to be considered as a potential source of infection for swine.

Clinical Signs. Toxigenic strains of *P. multocida* alone or in combination with other organisms, e.g., *Bordetella bronchiseptica*, cause shrinkage or total disappearance of the nasal turbinate bones. Clinical signs are not usually seen in pigs until they are 4 to 12 weeks of age or later. Severity of signs is dependent on the amount of toxin absorbed by the animal. The disease can be subclinical or very slight; in severe outbreaks sneezing, snuffling, snorting, nose bleeding, snout deviation, and growth retardation can be observed. Mucopurulent material and turbinate debris may be expelled during violent sneezing. The most characteristic sign of the disease is the facial distortion due to disturbance of normal bone development in the nose.

Disease

Salmonellosis (40, 59, 63).

Agent. *Salmonella* species.

Occurrence. Worldwide. The organism has been isolated from all vertebrates in which it has been sought.

Epidemiology. There are over 2,000 serologically distinct serotypes usually named by the geographic site of first isolation. Swine can be infected by a wide variety of serotypes, but clinical disease caused by serotypes other than *S. choleraesuis* or *S. typhimurium* is rare. For these latter serotypes the infected pig is the major source of new infections. Disease spread is fecal-oral, and pigs with acute disease shed large numbers of organisms in their feces. Transmission by aerosol may also be possible as the disease has been experimentally reproduced by intranasal inoculation, and pneumonia is often a clinical sign in the septicemic form of the disease. The carrier state occurs after clinically apparent disease and animals may become carriers for life. Because shedding in carrier animals is usually sporadic, repeated fecal cultures are often necessary to isolate the organism.

For serotypes other than *S. choleraesuis* and *S. typhimurium* the source of infection is feed or water contaminated by birds, rodents, or other livestock. Feeds containing animal protein may also be a source of infection. The result of transmission from these sources, in most instances, is a clinically inapparent infection with the establishment of the carrier state. However, stresses such as transportation, intercurrent disease, high pig density, commingling of pigs of different ages and origins, etc., may result in the normally nonpathogenic serotypes causing clinical disease.

Clinical Signs. Pigs are anorexic, reluctant to move, and febrile, with temperatures of 105 to 107°F (40.5–41.6°C), and often a shallow moist cough is present. The first indications of disease may be finding several dead pigs with purple extremities and abdomens. In the septicemic disease diarrhea is usually not seen until 3 to 4 days after onset. In most outbreaks morbidity is high, and mortality is usually less than 10%. Pneumonia is often a prominent clinical sign, especially with infection by *S. choleraesuis*.

Disease

Streptococcosis (2, 17, 45).

Agent. *Streptococcus suis*.

Occurrence. Europe, Far East, Australia, New Zealand, Brazil, and the United States.

Epidemiology. Infection is usually introduced into a herd or group by healthy carrier pigs. Organisms are present in the tonsil and nasal cavities and can exist there even in the presence of circulating antibody. Sows and gilts infect their offspring early in life by the respiratory route. Disease caused by *S. suis* is more prevalent in modern, intensive, complete confinement systems with high population density.

Clinical Signs. In peracute cases sudden death may occur without clinical signs. However, the predominant clinical signs are due to meningitis. In most cases a progression of anorexia, depression, fever, incoordination, paralysis, paddling, opisthotonos, tremors, and convulsions develops. Blindness, deafness, and lameness can also be seen. Septicemia can be followed by suppurative arthritis without the signs of meningitis. Occasionally seen are vegetative valvular endocarditis and hemorrhagic necrotizing myocarditis. Also a fibrinous bronchopneumonia has been reported.

Disease

Tuberculosis (53, 54, 55).

Agent. *Mycobacterium tuberculosis*, *M. bovis*, and the *M. avium* complex (*M. avium–M. intracellulare*).

Occurrence. Swine are susceptible to infection by all three agents. However, the agent most commonly associated with infections in swine is *M. avium*. Isolates of *M. avium* from tuberculous lesions in swine have been reported from Australia, Brazil, Denmark, France, Germany, Hungary, Japan, South Africa, and the United States. These reports indicate the worldwide distribution of tuberculosis in swine due to *M. avium*.

Epidemiology. The occurrence of tuberculosis in swine is related to the opportunity for direct or indirect contact with tuberculous cattle, humans, and fowl. The bovine tubercle bacillus is not a frequent cause of swine tuberculosis where the disease in cattle is controlled by programs of eradication. *M. bovis* may be transmitted to swine by the feeding of unpasteurized milk and dairy by-products. Feces of infected cattle may contain viable tubercle bacilli. Where swine and cattle are maintained in a common area this is an obvious source of infection for swine. Outbreaks of tuberculosis in swine have resulted from the feeding of improperly cooked offal from slaughterhouses or uncooked garbage. In Denmark tuberculosis in a swine feeding establishment was traced to improperly cooked offal from a poultry plant. In the United States an epizootic of tuberculosis in a herd of swine due to feeding improperly cooked offal from tuberculous cattle has been described. In 1939, it was reported that of 264 garbage-fed swine, 75 (28.4%) were found to have tuberculous lesions at slaughter. From 47 of the pigs tubercle bacilli were isolated, of which 35 were avian type and 12 were human type. It was concluded that garbage may contain the offal of tuberculous chickens and material from tuberculous human patients that is not properly disposed of. Infection in swine usually occurs by ingestion, as it was found that the primary disease complex involved the alimentary tract in 97.3% of 1,000 carcasses with tuberculous lesions; a pulmonary route of infection was noted in only 2.7%, as indicated by involvement of the bronchial lymph nodes. Wild birds may be a source of avian tuberculosis in swine. Tuberculosis due to *M. avium* has been found in various wild birds, some of which frequent feed lots. Tuberculosis was found in starlings on a swine farm with a high incidence of tuberculosis. Sawdust and wood shavings have also been incriminated as a source of infection for swine. It was reported that the same serovars of avian tubercle bacilli as found in swine could be isolated from sawdust. These workers also reported that sawdust could contain infectious mycobacteria even after 4 years of storage. A report from Arizona described a herd in which the source of infection with *M. avium* was sawdust and wood shavings. At slaughter or necropsy tuberculous lesions are not always grossly visible. Avian tubercle bacilli have been isolated from tonsils and lymph nodes of apparently normal swine as well as from grossly normal lymph nodes of carcasses passed for human consumption.

Clinical Signs. Generally the tuberculous lesions are limited to small foci in the lymph nodes of the cervical and mesenteric regions, and clinical signs due to infection are not apparent. Generalized tuberculosis in swine is not commonly seen, and when it does occur, it is usually a result of infection with *M. bovis*. However, generalized infection due to *M. avium* has been reported. Clinical signs are those usually associated with a generalized infectious disease process.

Disease

Yersiniosis (25, 51).

Agent. *Yersinia* species. *Y. pseudotuberculosis* subsp. *pseudotuberculosis*, *Y. pseudotuberculosis* subsp. *pestis*, *Y. enterocolitica*, *Y. intermedia*, *Y. fredikensia*, and *Y. kristensenii*.

Occurrence. The infection is distributed worldwide in pigs.

Epidemiology. Although a number of species of *Yersinia* have been isolated from pigs, clinical disease has only been associated with *Y. pseudotuberculosis* subsp. *pseudotuberculosis* and *Y. enterocolitica*. *Y. enterocolitica* is found throughout the world and has been frequently isolated from healthy warm-blooded and cold-blooded animals, from foods, including both meat and milk products, and from the environment, including soil and water.

In pigs, in addition to being a fecal commensal, *Y. entercolitica* also inhabits the oral cavity, especially the tongue and tonsils. The bacterium is widespread among herds of pigs, and newborn piglets are easily colonized and become long-term intestinal carriers. The organism can be shed in the feces for 30 weeks following infection, and it appears that transmission from pig to pig is via fecal contamination of the facilities, food, or water. In the United States *Y. enterocolitica* is more commonly isolated from pigs than is *Y. pseudotuberculosis*. However, in Europe and Japan, *Y. pseudotuberculosis* subsp. *pseudotuberculosis* is isolated from pigs more frequently than in America. It is also commonly found in rodents and birds, which probably represent a source of infection in pigs.

Clinical Signs. Infection in pigs is usually inapparent. *Y. enterocolitica* was isolated from pigs in outbreaks of diarrhea. Mild fever was present, and feces were blackish in color and did not contain blood or mucus. The organism has been isolated from the rectal mucosa in cases of rectal stricture. An outbreak described in Japan was associated with *Y. pseudotuberculosis* subsp. *pseudotuberculosis*. Clinical signs included anorexia, blood-stained diarrhea, and edema of the eyelids, lower part of the face, and dependent parts of the abdomen. Lesions associated with infection with *Y. enterocolitica* are confined to the large and small intestines. Lesions in *Y. pseudotuberculosis* subsp. *pseudotuberculosis* infection are more generalized, with the occurrence of granulomatous lesions in the lung, liver, spleen, and mesenteric lymph nodes.

Viral Diseases

Disease

Encephalomyocarditis (24, 65).

Agent. Encephalomyocarditis virus (EMCV).

Occurrence. Clinical outbreaks of EMCV in swine were first encountered in Panama in 1958 and in Florida in 1960. Since then, sporadic outbreaks have been reported in Australia, Brazil, Cuba, Italy, New Zealand, South Africa, and North America.

Epidemiology. The epidemiology of EMCV is not well understood because of lack of experimental data. The EMCV group is regarded as a rodent virus, although it naturally infects a wide range of vertebrate species. The host range includes chimpanzees, monkeys, elephants, lions, squirrels, mongooses, raccoons, and swine, the domestic animal most susceptible to clinical disease. Rats and mice are believed to be the principal reservoirs of the virus. EMCV antibodies have been demonstrated in sera from wild rats trapped in several areas of the United States and Canada. Experimentally infected rodents excreted the virus in their feces and urine, and high levels of EMCV were found in their tissues. The virus has been isolated from dried feces and from the intestines of rats and mice captured on farms where disease in pigs had previously occurred. Even though the virus has been isolated from mosquitoes and from ticks, there is no evidence that arthropod vectors can transmit EMCV to swine.

The most important sources of infection for swine appear to be feed or water contaminated with feces and urine of infected rats or other rodents, and diseased carcasses. Infected carcasses contain high levels of virus. Lion deaths at a zoo were found to be due to their having been fed carcasses of African elephants that had died of EMCV infection. Pig-to-pig transmission has been questioned because sentinel pigs failed to become infected after contact with experimentally infected pigs showing clinical signs of disease. However, since infected pigs have been shown to excrete virus for a short period, pig-to-pig transmission is a possibility. EMCV antibodies have been detected in swine without clinical disease.

Clinical Signs. EMCV infection in young pigs is characterized by acute disease with sudden deaths due to myocardial failure. Other signs include anorexia, listlessness, trembling, paralysis, and dyspnea. Severity of the disease appears to vary, depending on virus strain and age of pigs at the time of infection. Mortality approaching 100% is usually confined to pigs of preweaning age. Infections in weaned pigs to adults are usually subclinical although some mortality may be seen even in adult pigs. In breeding females the first clinical signs noted may be anorexia and fever. Such sows will show late-term abortions (107 to 111 days of gestation) and low farrowing rates. After the abortions the numbers of mummified and stillborn piglets increase along with preweaning mortality. These reproductive problems may last for 2 to 3 months and are observed in sows of all parities.

Disease

Japanese B encephalitis (JE) (5, 21).

Agent. Japanese B virus.

Occurrence. The disease is the most common mosquito-borne disease of the central nervous system (CNS) in Japan, China, and other Western Pacific countries. The disease has been reported in Japan, far eastern Soviet Union, Korea, China, Taiwan, the Philippines, Indonesia, Singapore, Malaysia, Hong Kong, Vietnam, Laos, Bangladesh, Nepal, Thailand, Burma, Sri Lanka, India, and the Pacific Islands.

Epidemiology. The pig is considered the most important amplifying host for the JE virus (JEV). In nature, infection is maintained cyclically by vector mosquitoes (mainly *Culex tritaeniorhynchus*), birds, and mammals. Other mosquito species may assume the role of vector, depending on the local ecology. In enzootic areas, pigs are found in high concentration and are favored feeding sources of mosquitoes. Consistent development of viremia in susceptible pigs ensures a continuous supply of infected mosquitoes.

In Japan and Korea the mosquito season starts in late June, whereas in tropical areas of Southeast Asia the pig–mosquito cycle may continue throughout the year. In temperate zones, reservoirs of infection allow JEV to survive the winter. Chickens and wild birds, especially herons and egrets, are viremic throughout the year. The virus has been isolated from snakes, and bats are also potential reservoirs of infection. JEV may also be carried by cold-blooded vertebrates throughout the winter.

Clinical Signs. Young piglets may occasionally show clinical signs, but illness is not a feature of JE infection in adults. However, when infected pregnant sows and gilts come to term, their offspring may show varying degrees of abnormality. Litters may contain weak piglets, with signs of CNS involvement, stillborn pigs, mummified fetuses, and apparently normal piglets. Subcutaneous edema and hydrocephalus may be evident in some piglets. Infertility in boars in summer appears to be associated with JE infection. Infected boars develop edematous and congested testicles and a reduced libido, and the virus is excreted in their semen.

Disease

Rabies (1, 6, 38).

Agent. Rabies virus.

Occurrence. Confirmed cases of porcine rabies have been reported in 25 different countries on five continents. The United Kingdom, Australia, New Zealand, Sweden, and Portugal remain free of rabies.

Epidemiology. The disease has been said to exist in two epidemiologic forms. The urban type, spread mainly by dogs, and the wildlife type, seen principally in skunks, foxes, wolves, jackals, and bats. In the United States in 1964, 75% of the rabies was in wildlife and less than 10% in dogs. This trend has continued, as in 1989, 88.4% of recorded rabies cases were in wildlife and only 2.7% in dogs. This increased percentage of rabies in wild animals has put farm animals at a greater risk of exposure. The true incidence of rabies in swine is difficult to assess. In the United States over a 17-year period from 1938 to 1955, 854 cases were reported, which represented 6.6% of the cases reported in all farm animals.

Clinical Signs. Typically there is sudden onset, loss of coordination, dullness, prostration, and death. Excessive salivation, rapid chewing movements, and clonic muscular spasms may also be seen. Death will likely ensue within 72 h after clinical signs appear. The furious form of rabies does not appear to be common in infected pigs. Only one case of the furious form of rabies in a pig has been documented, but this pattern of behavior occurred in only one of 17 affected pigs. There is a wide variation in the incubation period. In an outbreak of rabies in swine where the exposure time from rabid foxes was documented, incubation periods of 9, 56, and 123 days were reported.

Disease

Swine influenza (SI) (13, 47).

Agent. Influenza A viruses.

Occurrence. SI and type A have been reported in most parts of the world where swine are found.

Epidemiology. Most SI is caused by H1N1 viruses; H3N2 viruses are responsible to a lesser extent, but significant disease due to this strain has been reported in England and Europe. Until recently it was thought that H1N1 was the only strain of swine flu present in the United States. However, the H3N2 strain of the swine flu virus has now been isolated from swine in North Carolina, Iowa, and Minnesota (37). Serologic surveillance studies showed that about 25 to 30% of 6- to 7-month-old pigs going to slaughter in the United States have SI antibodies. Adult swine that have been used for breeding purposes and then slaughtered have a higher rate (about 45%).

The primary route of transmission is pig to pig by the nasopharyngeal route. During the acute febrile stage of the disease nasal secretions are laden with virus, providing an abundant source of infectious material. The first appearance of clinical SI in a swine population is commonly associated with movement of animals, e.g., introduction of breeding stock. After the initial infection of a breeding herd it is likely that the virus will become established in the herd and may be responsible for episodes of classical acute SI, or by interaction with copathogens may cause pneumonia in nursery, grower, and finishing pigs. Even though acute SI occurs more commonly from late summer into the winter, especially in the North Central United States, infection and disease are present throughout the year. Swine influenza virus (SIV) has been recovered from pigs with respiratory disease without the typical signs of classical swine flu and also has been recovered from pigs with no clinical signs of disease. There are no data that support or reject the existence of the carrier state in swine. Evidence accumulated in recent years indicates that H1N1 viruses have the capacity to move among species, particularly swine, ducks, turkeys, and humans. Pigs can be infected with viruses from birds and humans. Transmission of H3N2 virus from humans to swine has been reported.

Clinical Signs. In acute classical SI, onset is sudden and most animals in the herd appear affected at the same time. There is anorexia, inactivity, prostration, huddling, and piling. Fever is in the range of 105 to 107°F (40.5 to 41.7°C). There is open-mouthed, labored breathing, and this may be accentuated when the animals are forced to move. Movement is also accompanied by severe paroxysms of coughing. Conjunctivitis, rhinitis, nasal discharge, and sneezing may also be seen. Recovery is as rapid as onset and usually begins about 5 to 7 days after onset. Morbidity is nearly 100% and mortality is generally less than 1%. Abortions, stillbirths, infertility, and small weak litters have been reported in association with acute SI. SIV usually in association with other viral or bacterial pathogens has been implicated in outbreaks of respiratory disease in nursery, grower, and finishing pigs. The clinical signs associated with these cases are not those usually seen in acute classical SI.

Disease

Vesicular diseases (3, 22, 44).

Agents. Foot-and-mouth disease virus (FMDV), vesicular stomatitis virus (VSV).

Occurrence. Sporadic outbreaks of foot-and-mouth disease (FMD) occur in Europe. FMD is endemic in South America, Asia, and Africa. North and Central America, New Zealand, Panama, Scandinavia, Japan, and the Caribbean Basin are free of FMDV. Outbreaks of vesicular stomatitis (VS) have only been reported in North, Central, and South America.

Epidemiology. The main species affected with FMDV are swine, cattle, sheep, and goats. Transmission occurs by aerosol, contact, and fomites. Swine produce aerosols up to 1,000 times greater in viral concentration than do cattle. Aerosols can be carried by air currents over long distances. High humidity, cloud cover, and moderate temperatures favor airborne spread. Carrier states in cattle, sheep, goats, and African buffalo have been demonstrated. A carrier state for FMDV in swine has not been described.

VSV affects swine, horses, cattle, and many species of wildlife, including rodents. It is not a highly contagious disease, and the origin of outbreaks and means of spread are not thoroughly understood. VS is endemic in the coastal regions of the Carolinas and Georgia and in Central and South America, infecting horses, cattle, feral swine, raccoons, and deer. Two strains of VSV, VS New Jersey and VS Indiana, have caused periodic epizootics in the United States. VS occurs in the United States at about 10- to 15-year-intervals, and outbreaks typically begin during warm weather and end in the fall with the onset of cold weather and a killing frost. However, during the 1982 and 1983 VS epizootic, clinical cases in Colorado continued throughout the winter months. In the tropical regions of Mexico and Central America VS is enzootic and appears annually. In these areas a high proportion of humans and domestic and wild animals are seropositive. The seasonal occurrence and geographic distribution of VS have led to the hypothesis that insects may be important in transmitting the VSV. Transmission may occur by direct contact (biting) and fomites. The carrier state has not been demonstrated in any of the affected species.

Clinical Signs. The clinical signs of FMD and VS in swine are essentially identical. Within 1 to 5 days after exposure body temperature rises sharply to 105°F (40.5°C) or higher. Areas of epithelium become blanched, followed by formation of vesicles. Vesicles may be found on the snout extending into the nares and on the lips, tongue, and hard and soft palate. Lesions also occur on the soft tissues of the feet and around the soft tissues of the dew claws as well as other areas in the skin. Nursing sows may have vesicles on the teats. The fluid-filled vesicles rupture rapidly (usually 6 to 24 h after formation), leaving irregular erosions that may coalesce. Epithelium is lost and lesions become eroded, hyperemic, and hemorrhagic. In young animals infected with FMDV, myocardial necrosis may occur, and mortality may reach 50% or higher. FMD is highly contagious, infecting virtually 100% of the susceptible animals. For VS in a given herd of swine, morbidity can be variable. In general, VS is not considered to be a highly contagious disease in swine. Low mortality is usually seen with vesicular diseases (<5%).

Fungal Diseases

Disease

Ringworm (42, 50).

Agent. *Microsporum nanum* and *Trychophyton verrucosum.*

Occurrence. Worldwide.

Epidemiology. *M. nanum* and *T. verrucosum* are the most common agents causing ringworm in swine, although *M. canis*, *M. gypseum*, and *T. mentagrophytes* have also been reported as causing disease in swine. Transmission is by direct contact or fomites.

Clinical Signs. Ringworm may affect any age pig. Lesions start as small (2 cm) red to brownish circular lesions that spread concentrically and later are covered with a thin, dark, crusty scab. Lesions may occur anywhere on the body, especially behind the ears. There is minimal hair loss, and pruritus is not a feature of the disease in swine. Sows sometimes develop chronic infections behind the ears. The disease is usually self-limiting in 2 to 3 months but may persist 6 months without treatment.

Protozoal Diseases

Disease

Cryptosporidiosis (27, 37).

Agent. *Cryptosporidium parvum.*

Occurrence. Worldwide.

Epidemiology. Cryptosporidia parasitize the intestinal tracts of various vertebrate species, including swine. Porcine cryptosporidiosis is caused by *C. parvum*. A similar species, *C. muris*, infects the gastric glands of mice, rats, cats, and calves but is not known to infect swine. *C. parvum* is prevalent particularly in neonates of ruminant species and is ubiquitous in the intestinal tracts of beef and dairy calves. About 25% of diarrheic calves 5 days to 1 month old are infected with *C. parvum*. Subclinical or clinical infections have also been reported in cats, dogs, horses, chickens, turkeys, geese, reptiles, rodents, rabbits, non-human primates, and exotic and wild animals. Transmission occurs when pigs ingest feed or water contaminated with feces containing oocysts.

Clinical Signs. Most cases of porcine cryptosporidiosis are asymptomatic. When clinical disease does occur, signs consist of nonhemorrhagic diarrhea and unthriftiness. Most cases are seen in 6- to 12-week-old pigs, although infections have been reported in nursing and market age pigs. Coinfections with agents such as *Salmonella* species, *Escherichia coli*, or viral pathogens can exacerbate the disease.

Disease

Toxoplasmosis (11, 28).

Agent. *Toxoplasma gondii.*

Occurrence. *T. gondii* is prevalent in pigs in most countries of the world.

Epidemiology. *T. gondii* is transmitted via three primary ways: fecal-oral, carnivorism, and congenital. Cats, including wild *Felidae*, are the only definitive hosts of *T. gondii. Felidae* excrete *T. gondii* oocysts in their feces. Mammals, including swine, and birds are intermediate hosts. Swine become infected by ingestion of feed, water, or soil contaminated by oocysts. After ingestion the oocysts rupture, releasing sporozoites. Multiplication occurs in the intestine and associated lymph nodes, and the organisms are spread to the rest of the body via blood and lymph and eventually encyst in the central nervous system, skeletal and cardiac muscles, and liver. The cysts survive in tissues as long as the host lives. Swine can also become infected by consuming the tissues of infected rodents and other wild animals and birds. Cannibalism and tail and ear biting can also be a source of infection. Congenital infection can occur when a susceptible animal is infected during pregnancy.

Clinical Signs. Most *T. gondii* infections in pigs are subclinical. Abortions due to *T. gondii* are uncommon. Transplacentally infected pigs may be born premature, dead, or weak, or die soon after birth. Pigs that are infected postnatally may develop diarrhea, incoordination, tremors, or cough. Experimental studies indicate that transplacental infections are difficult to produce in swine.

Disease Caused by Nematodes

Disease

Ascariasis (7).

Agent. *Ascaris suum.*

Occurrence. *A. suum* is cosmopolitan in distribution. It is the most common gastrointestinal worm parasite in pigs.

Epidemiology. The life cycle is direct. Adult worms in the intestine lay eggs that are passed out in the feces. Eggs become infective in 21 to 30 days and may remain infective for 7 years or longer in protected areas and lots. When ingested infective eggs hatch in the digestive tract, larvae are liberated and penetrate the intestinal wall and generally pass by the hepatic portal system to the liver. However, a few may "wander" through other organs or tissues. They leave the liver and migrate to the lungs. Larvae are coughed up, swallowed, and become egg-producing adults. Female ascarids lay hundreds of thousands to nearly 2 million eggs per day. The eggs are sticky and can be transported by cockroaches and other arthropods, birds, workers' boots, etc.

Clinical Signs. Migration of larvae through the lungs may cause a verminous pneumonia. Pigs cough and may breathe with difficulty. Adult worms compete with the host for nutrients and interfere with absorption of nutrients, resulting in reduced weight gain and feed efficiency. They may occlude and rupture the small intestine. In addition, adults may migrate into and occlude the common bile duct, resulting in icterus.

Disease

Trichinellosis (8, 26).

Agent. *Trichinella spiralis.*

Occurrence. *T. spiralis*, a ubiquitous parasite, has been found in more than 100 species of mammals and has a worldwide distribution.

Epidemiology. Swine become infected by ingestion of skeletal muscle containing the infective larvae of *Trichinella*. After ingestion, larvae are liberated from the cysts and after four molts become adults. The males die after mating, and the females penetrate the wall of the small intestine and enter the lymph spaces where they deposit larvae. Larvae are carried by the blood to the skeletal muscle where they penetrate the sarcolemma and become encysted. The encysted larvae can be viable for up to 11 years.

Historically, meat scraps in garbage have been an important source of swine infection. Where garbage cooking regulations are not enforced, meat scraps still pose a threat for introduction of the parasite to swine. Swine can also become infected by ingestion of carcasses of infected farm cats, rats, or other wild animals. Although less often considered, cannibalism among swine can be an important mode of transmission.

Clinical Signs. Pigs infected with *Trichinella* do not usually have clinical signs of disease. Even in heavy infections, signs are nonspecific. Infected pigs generally appear healthy and act normally.

Risk of Transmission of Traditional Zoonotic Diseases via Porcine Xenografts

The risk of disease transmission from swine to human via xenografts will be minimized by establishing specific-pathogen–free donor source herds, maintaining them in barrier facilities, instituting biosafety measures to prevent infection with specific pathogens, and establishing procedures to control the diseases present in the herds. The surveillance of source herds and donors by observation and serological, microbiological, and parasitological monitoring on a regularly scheduled basis will further enhance the safety of porcine xenografts. The facilities and biosafety measures currently being used in developed nations to produce specific-pathogen–free seed stock could also be used to produce donors free of many of the traditional zoonotic disease organisms. This level of isolation would be adequate to produce donors free of the specific pathogens that cause anthrax, brucellosis, leptospirosis, melioidiosis, toxoplasmosis, trichinosis, tuberculosis, encephalomyocarditis, Japanese encephalitis, rabies, swine influenza, vesicular diseases, and ascariasis. The knowledge and technology are available to produce donor swine of a microbiological quality comparable to laboratory animals such as rats and mice (19). However, this would require such measures as positive pressure HEPA filtered air, sterilization of feed and water, and gowns and masks for animal care personnel. Such measures would have to be taken to produce donors free of such ubiquitous organisms as *Campylobacter* spp., *Cryptosporidium* spp., *E. rhusiopathiae, Salmonella* spp., *Streptococcus suis*, and *Yersinia* spp. This level of isolation may not be necessary. In the infected clinically healthy pig these organisms have a predilection for and appear to be confined to certain tissues in the body, i.e., in the gastrointestinal tract, *Campylobacter* spp., *Cryptosporidia* spp., *Salmonella* spp., and *Yersinia* spp.; in tonsil and upper respiratory tract, *E. rhusiopathiae* and *Streptococcus suis*. Therefore, as only clinically healthy swine will be used as donors, even though they may be infected, the risk of transmission of these organisms via whole organ and tissue xenografts is probably minimal. The use of vaccines to protect donors against possible acute outbreaks of erysipelas and salmonellosis could further minimize the risk of transmission via xenografts.

SWINE-SPECIFIC ORGANISMS

Table 1 presents a list of swine-specific organisms. As previously stated, there is no evidence that these organisms have been transmitted from swine to man under "field" conditions. The effect that swine-specific organisms may have if directly implanted, via xenografts, into immunocompromised human recipients is not known.

Information on swine-specific organisms in Table 1 can be found in the 7th edition of *Diseases of Swine*. For those organisms noted in bold, the literature cited updates the information found in *Diseases of Swine* or provides new information.

Risk of Transmission of Swine-Specific Organisms via Porcine Xenografts

Facilities and procedures used to produce donors free of the traditional zoonotic organisms should also be adequate to produce donors free of a number of swine-specific organisms, i.e., (i) bacterial agents: *Actinobacillus pleuropneumoniae* and *Serpulina* spp. (specifically *S. hyodysenteriae*, the cause of swine dysentery); (ii) viral agents: African swine fever virus, bovine viral diarrhea virus, hog cholera virus, porcine epidemic diarrhea, porcine paramyxovirus, porcine reproductive and respiratory syndrome virus, pseudorabies virus, and transmissible gastroenteritis virus; (iii) protozoal agents: *Babesia* spp.; and (iv) internal and external parasites.

Ubiquitous swine-specific organisms that are widespread in the domestic pig population include (i) the bacteria: *Actinobacillus suis*, *Actinomyces pyogenes*, *Bordetella bronchiseptica*, *Chlamydia psittaci*, *Clostridia* spp., *Eperythrozoon suis*, *Escherichia coli*, *Eubacterium (Corynebacterium) suis*, *Haemophilus parasuis*, *Mycoplasma* spp., *Serpulina* spp., *Staphylococcus* spp., and *Streptococcus* spp.; (ii) the viruses: hemagglutinating encephalomyelitis virus, porcine adenovirus, pig endogenous retroviruses, porcine circovirus, porcine cytomegalovirus, porcine enteroviruses, porcine parvovirus, porcine respiratory coronavirus, rotavirus and reovirus, swine hepatitis E virus, and swine pox virus; and (iii) the protozoa: *Eimeria* spp. and *Isospora* spp.

B. bronchiseptica, *E. coli*, *H. parasuis*, porcine enteroviruses, porcine parvovirus, and porcine rotavirus have been responsible for losses of economic significance to the swine industry. Facilities, biosafety measures, and management practices used for commercial swine production in the United States are not adequate for consistently maintaining herds free of these specific pathogens. Therefore, the emphasis was placed on controlling these diseases through vaccination, use of antimicrobials and management techniques such as all-in all-out, early weaning of piglets, and geographical separation of sites for the different phases of swine production.

As described for the traditional zoonotic organisms, for those swine-specific organisms that are sequestered in tissues such as gastrointestinal tract, tonsil, and upper respiratory tract of clinically healthy donors, the risk of being transmitted via xenografts is probably minimal. Also for certain swine-specific organisms where no carrier state exists, pigs that have mounted a protective immune response from natural infection or vaccination may have "cleared" the organisms from their organs or tissues.

Swine-specific viruses that present the greatest risk of being transmitted via xenografts are porcine cytomegalovirus (PCMV) and the pig endogenous retroviruses (PERV). PCMV is widespread in domestic swine throughout the world. It appears to be host specific as it has failed to replicate in rabbits, mice, hamsters, chick embryos, or cattle. PCMV is a member of the family *Herpesviridae*, and like most of the herpesviruses, it has the ability to induce

Table 1. Swine-specific organisms[a]

Bacteria
Actinobacillus pleuropneumoniae
Escherichia coli
Actinobacillus suis
Eubacterium (Corynebacterium) suis
Actinomyces pyogenes
Haemophilus parasuis
Bordetella bronchiseptica
Mycoplasma spp.
Chlamydia psittaci
Serpulina spp.
Clostridium spp.
Staphylococcus spp.
Eperythrozoon suis
Streptococcus spp.
Lawsonia intracellularis (31, 32)
Viruses
African swine fever virus
Porcine paramyxovirus
Bovine viral diarrhea virus
Porcine parvovirus
Hemagglutinating encephalomyelitis virus
Porcine respiratory coronavirus
Hog cholera virus
Pseudorabies virus
Porcine adenovirus
Rotavirus and reovirus
Porcine cytomegalovirus
Swine pox virus
Porcine enteroviruses
Transmissible gastroenteritis virus
Porcine epidemic diarrhea virus
Pig endogenous retroviruses (see chapter 13)
Porcine circovirus (20)
Porcine reproductive and respiratory syndrome virus (65)
Swine hepatitis E virus (33, 34)
Protozoa
Babesia perroncitoi
Eimeria spp.
Babesia trautmanni
Isospora suis
Nematodes[b]
Hyostrongylus rubidus (red stomach worm)
Stephanuris dentatus (kidney worm)
Metastrongylus spp. (lungworms)
Strongyloides ransomi (intestinal threadworm)
Oesophagostomum spp. (nodular worm)
Trichuris suis (whipworm)
External parasites[c]
Demodex phyloides (demodectic mange mite)
Sarcoptes scabiei var. *suis* (sarcoptic mange mite)
Haematopinus suis (hog louse)

[a] For those organisms noted in bold, the literature cited updates the information found in *Diseases of Swine*, 7th ed.

[b] The above are the most important nematodes of swine. Other less common internal parasites are described in the 7th edition of *Diseases of Swine*.

[c] Fleas, flies, and ticks are important external parasites, not only for the discomfort they cause swine by irritation and biting, but as biological and mechanical vectors of disease.

latency and be vertically transmitted by passing the placental barrier and infecting pigs in utero. In latent infections viral genomes become incorporated into the host DNA, but there is no synthesis of virus. Stress factors or experimental immunosuppression will initiate synthesis of the virus, and excretion occurs even in the presence of circulating antibody. Transplacental infections in fetal or neonatal pig result in dissemination of virus to the cells of the reticuloendothelial system. Piglets may be born dead or die soon after birth without signs of disease. Others may be stunted and pale due to anemia. Virus has been recovered from nasal and ocular secretions and cervical fluids of pregnant sows exposed to PCMV for the first time. The virus has also been isolated from the testes and epididymus of boars. In most herds where the disease is endemic, clinical signs are not apparent. Initial infection occurs in most pigs at about 3 weeks of age, and the viremia results in dissemination of the virus to epithelial sites in the body, e.g., harderian glands, nasal mucosa, and tubules of the kidney. For a short time after infection virus is transmitted via the nasal route and through contamination of the environment with urine. PCMV has been isolated from lung macrophages of recovered pigs that are no longer shedding virus.

No attempts have been made to establish commercial herds free of the virus. However, surgical derivation of pigs negative for PCMV should be possible, but because transplacental infection can occur, progeny should be monitored serologically for at least 2 to 3 months post surgery. Currently the only option available to minimize the risk of transmission of PCMV via xenografts is to test each individual donor or xenograft for the presence of virus.

Of all the known swine-specific viruses, pig endogenous retroviruses (PERV) generate the greatest concern. The PERV are complements of viral genomes that are integrated into the cell genomes of the pig. They persist in swine primarily through vertical transmission in germ cells. Since the PERV genomes are coded in the genomic DNA of pigs, all tissues in a xenograft may potentially express PERV. All swine tested to date have been PERV positive. Derivation of donors free of PERV is not possible as the procedures normally employed to derive swine free of specific pathogens, i.e., hysterectomy, hysterotomy, segregated early weaning, or test and remove, will not prevent vertical transmission.

Hemagglutinating encephalomyelitis virus, porcine adenovirus, porcine circovirus, porcine enteroviruses, reovirus, swine hepatitis E virus, and swine pox virus are ubiquitous and distributed worldwide in the swine population. These viruses are "unknown quantities" regarding their potential for transmission via xenografts.

UNDISCOVERED SWINE-SPECIFIC ORGANISMS

It is unrealistic to believe that all swine-associated microbes have been"discovered." A recent publication describing the detection of two "new" porcine herpes viruses (14) and the 1997 report of the isolation of the swine hepatitis E virus (34) underscore this fact. There is no doubt that other swine-associated organisms will emerge that will have the potential to be transmitted via swine xenografts.

Public Health Aspects of Porcine Xenotransplantation

Matthews and Beran have discussed public health aspects of porcine xenotransplantation (29). They reviewed the history of the use of animal products in humans and found there were few reported complications from the use of these products.

They also reported on investigations regarding the transmission of animal-specific viruses to humans. They cited the most famous case of incidental transmission of an animal-derived organism when over 1 million people received Salk poliovirus vaccine and/or adenovirus vaccine contaminated with simian virus 40 (SV40). A study of SV40-contaminated vaccine recipients detected no alteration in morbidity or mortality and no increased incidence of leukemia. Because the PERV are oncogenic viruses, they reviewed a number of studies that were designed to determine if animal oncoviruses had zoonotic potential. One of the studies described the inadvertent injection of U.S. military personnel with avian leukosis virus (ALV), which was a contaminant of a yellow fever virus vaccine. A third or more of World War II veterans received the yellow fever vaccine that was produced using chick embryos. There is little doubt that most, if not all, of the vaccine was contaminated with ALV. A follow-up study has not revealed the occurrence of higher than normal rate of cancers in recipients of the vaccine. Serological studies on sera from recipients of yellow fever vaccine have shown no evidence of antibodies against ALV. In two other studies involving bovine leukemia virus and feline leukemia virus, no correlation was found between the risk of human cancer and association with cattle or cats. The two cases of direct transmission of non-human viruses into the human population could be compared to what might occur in xenotransplantation. However, a direct comparison is not possible, as those who were vaccinated were not receiving immunosuppressive drugs.

The results of these studies are encouraging, but they cannot be used to assess the infectious disease risk associated with porcine xenografts. The true risk of infection for recipients of xenografts and the public health aspects associated with xenotransplantation can only be determined by retrospective studies. The risk of disease transmission via swine xenografts can be minimized by addressing the following critical control points: (i) monitoring the health of swine from conception to donation; (ii) pretransplant communication to recipients, family, and the surgical and medical care personnel to explain the possibility of xenograft-transmitted infections and the wider implications for infection of family and friends; (iii) pretransplant serological screening of recipients for antibodies against zoonotic agents; (iv) post-transplant surveillance of recipients and contacts for evidence of clinical disease, making every effort to arrive at a definitive diagnosis of clinical disease in recipients and contacts; and (v) specifically monitoring the recipient for evidence of PERV infection.

Disease transmission via swine xenografts and the possible implications for public health should not be taken lightly. However, the view held by some that porcine xenotransplantation may lead to the next AIDS-like epidemic (48) is extreme. This "doomsday" theory is often voiced by those who oppose the use of xenotransplantation. The ability to monitor swine donors from conception to donation, pretransplant communication, and post-transplant monitoring of recipients and their contacts will minimize the risk of disease transmission to recipients and protect the public's health.

The following poem sums up my thoughts on the safety of porcine xenotransplantation.

The Choice

My kidneys were failing, my heart was no good,
I needed to get transplants as quick as I could.
The surgeon said in his best bedside voice,
"Allo or xeno, you make the choice."
"I'll take the xeno," I said with a grin,
"Because I know where the pigs have been."

Peter J. Matthews
Jan. 22, 1998

REFERENCES

1. **Beran, G. W.** 1994. Rabies and infections by rabies related viruses, p. 307–358. *In* G. W. Beran (ed. in chief), Section B. *Handbook of Zoonoses*, 2nd ed. CRC Press Inc., Boca Raton, Fla.
2. **Blackmore, D. K., and S. G. Fenwick.** 1994. Streptococcal infections, p. 167–180. *In* G. W. Beran (ed. in chief), Section B. *Handbook of Zoonoses*, 2nd ed. CRC Press Inc., Boca Raton, Fla.
3. **Callis, J. J., and D. A. Gregg.** 1994. Foot-and-mouth disease, p. 453–462. *In* G. W. Beran (ed. in chief), Section B. *Handbook of Zoonoses*, 2nd ed. CRC Press Inc., Boca Raton, Fla.
4. **Cen, H., M. C. Breinig, R. W. Atchison, M. Ho, and J. L. C. McKnight.** 1991. Epstein-Barr virus transmission via the donor organs in solid organ transplantation: polymerase chain reaction and restriction fragment length polymorphism analysis of IR2, IR3, and IR4. *J. Virol.* **65:**976–980.
5. **Chu, R. M., and H. S. Joo.** 1992. Japanese B encephalitis, p. 286–292. *In* A. D. Leman, B. E. Straw, W. L. Mengeling, S. D'Allaire, and D. J. Taylor (ed.), *Diseases of Swine*, 7th ed. Iowa State University Press, Ames, Iowa.
6. **Clark, K. A.** 1995. Rabies, p. 106–109. *In Zoonosis Updates from the Journal of the American Veterinary Medical Association*, 2nd ed. American Veterinary Medical Association, Schaumburg, Ill.
7. **Corwin, R. M., and T. B. Stewart.** 1992. *Ascaris suum*, p. 722–724. *In* A. D. Leman, B. E. Straw, W. L. Mengeling, S. D'Allaire, and D. J. Taylor (ed.), *Diseases of Swine*, 7th ed. Iowa State University Press, Ames, Iowa.
8. **Corwin, R. M., and T. B. Stewart.** 1992. *Trichinella spiralis*, p. 724–726. *In* A. D. Leman, B. E. Straw, W. L. Mengeling, S. D'Allaire, and D. J. Taylor (ed.), *Diseases of Swine*, 7th ed. Iowa State University Press, Ames, Iowa.
9. **Currier, R. W.** 1995. Brucellosis, p. 31–33. *In Zoonosis Updates from the Journal of the American Veterinary Medical Association*, 2nd ed. American Veterinary Medical Association, Schaumburg, Ill.
10. **Dejong, M. F.** 1992. (Progressive) atrophic rhinitis, p. 414–435. *In* A. D. Leman, B. E. Straw, W. L. Mengeling, S. D'Allaire, and D. J. Taylor (ed.), *Diseases of Swine*, 7th ed. Iowa State University Press, Ames, Iowa.
11. **Dubey, J. P.** 1995. Toxoplasmosis, p. 144–149. *In Zoonosis Updates from the Journal of the American Veterinary Medical Association*, 2nd ed. American Veterinary Medical Association, Schaumburg, Ill.
12. **Dummer, J. S., J. Armstrong, J. Somerson, S. Kusne, B. J. Carpenter, J. T. Rosenthal, and M. Ho.** 1987. Transmission of infection with herpes simplex virus by rentransplantation, *J. Infect. Dis.* **155:**202–206.
13. **Easterday, B. C., and V. S. Hinshaw.** 1994. Swine influenza, p. 349–357. *In* A. D. Leman, B. E. Straw, W. L. Mengeling, S. D'Allaire, and D. J. Taylor (ed.), *Diseases of Swine*, 7th ed. Iowa State University Press, Ames, Iowa.
14. **Ehlers, B., S. Ulrich, and M. Goltz.** 1999. Detection of two novel porcine herpesviruses with high similarity to gammaherpesviruses. *J. Gen. Virol.* **80**(Pt 4)**:**971–978.
15. **Ellis, W. A.** 1992. Leptospirosis, p. 529–536. *In* A. D. Leman, B. E. Straw, W. L. Mengeling, S. D'Allaire, and D. J. Taylor (ed.), *Diseases of Swine*, 7th ed. Iowa State University Press, Ames, Iowa.
16. **Erice, A., F. S. Rhame, R. C. Heusssner, D. L. Dunne, and H. H. Balfour, Jr.** 1991. Human immunodeficiency virus infection in patients with solid organ transplants: report of five cases and review. *Rev. Infect. Dis.* **13:**537–547.
17. **Erickson, E. D.** 1995. Streptococcosis, p. 128–130. *In Zoonosis Updates from the Journal of the American Veterinary Medical Association*, 2nd ed. American Veterinary Medical Association, Schaumburg, Ill.
18. **Groves, G. G., and K. S. Harrington.** 1994. Glanders and melioidosis, p.149–166. *In* G. W. Beran (ed. in chief), Section A. *Handbook of Zoonoses*, 2nd ed. CRC Press Inc., Boca Raton, Fla.
19. **Hansen, A. K., H. Farlov, and P. Bollen.** 1997. Microbiological monitoring of laboratory pigs. *Lab. Anim.* **31:**193–200.
20. **Harding, J. C. S., E. G. Clark, J. H. Strokappe, P. I. Wilson, and J. A. Ellis.** 1998. Post weaning multisystemic wasting syndrome: epidemiology and clinical presentation. *Swine Health Prod.* **6:**249–254.
21. **Hoke, C. H., Jr., and J. B. Gingrich.** 1994. Japanese encephalitis, p. 59–70. *In* G. W. Beran (ed. in chief), Section B. *Handbook of Zoonoses*, 2nd ed. CRC Press Inc., Boca Raton, Fla.
22. **House, J. A., and C. A. House.** 1992. Vesicular diseases, p. 387–398. *In* A. D. Leman, B. E. Straw, W. L. Mengeling, S. D'Allaire, and D. J. Taylor (ed.), *Diseases of Swine*, 7th ed. Iowa State University Press, Ames, Iowa.
23. **Hunter, L., W. Corbett, and C. Grindem.** 1995. Anthrax, p. 12–15. *In Zoonosis Updates from the Journal*

of the American Veterinary Medical Association, 2nd ed. American Veterinary Medical Association, Schaumburg, Ill.

24. **Joo, H. S.** 1992. Encephalomyocarditis virus, p. 257–262. *In* A. D. Leman, B. E. Straw, W. L. Mengeling, S. D'Allaire, and D. J. Taylor (ed.), *Diseases of Swine*, 7th ed. Iowa State University Press, Ames, Iowa.
25. **Kapperud, G.** 1994. *Yersinia enterocolytica* infection, p. 343–354. *In* G. W. Beran (ed. in chief), Section A. *Handbook of Zoonoses*, 2nd ed. CRC Press Inc., Boca Raton, Fla.
26. **Kazacos, K. R., and K. D. Murrel.** 1995. Trichinellosis, p. 150–154. *In Zoonosis Updates from the Journal of the American Veterinary Medical Association*, 2nd ed. American Veterinary Medical Association, Schaumburg, Ill.
27. **Lindsay, D. S., B. L. Blagburn, and B. P. Stuart.** 1992. Cryptosporidiosis (*Cryptosporidium parvum*), p. 664–665. *In* A. D. Leman, B. E. Straw, W. L. Mengeling, S. D'Allaire, and D. J. Taylor (ed.), *Diseases of Swine*, 7th ed. Iowa State University Press, Ames, Iowa.
28. **Lindsay, D. S., B. L. Blagburn, and B. P. Stuart.** 1992. Toxoplasmosis (*Toxoplasma gondii*), p. 665–666. *In* A. D. Leman, B. E. Straw, W. L. Mengeling, S. D'Allaire, and D. J. Taylor (ed.), *Diseases of Swine*, 7th ed. Iowa State University Press, Ames, Iowa.
29. **Matthews, P. J., and G. W. Beran.** 1996. Assessment of public health aspects of porcine xenotransplantation, p. 163–169. *In* M. E. Tumbleson and L. B. Schook (ed.), *Advances in Swine in Biomedical Research*. Plenum Press, New York, N.Y.
30. **Mcmillen, A. P.** 1992. Brucellosis, p. 446–453. *In* A. D. Leman, B. E. Straw, W. L. Mengeling, S. D'Allaire, and D. J. Taylor (ed.), *Diseases of Swine*, 7th ed. Iowa State University Press, Ames, Iowa.
31. **McOrist, S., C. Gebhardt, R. Boid, and S. Barnes.** 1995. Characterization of *Lawsoni intracellularis* gen. nov. sp. nov., the obligately intracellular bacterium of porcine proliferative enteropathy. *Int. J. Syst. Bacteriol.* **45:**820–825.
32. **McOrist, S., S. Jasni, R. Mackie, N. MacIntyre, N. Neef, and G. Lawson.** 1993. Reproduction of porcine proliferative enteropathy with pure cultures of ileal symbiont intracellularis. *Infect. Immun.* **61:**4286–4292.
33. **Meng, X. J., P. G. Halbur, J. S. Haynes, T. S. Tsareva, J. D. Bruna, R. L. Royer, R. H. Purcell, and S. U. Emerson.** 1998. Experimental infection of pigs with a newly identified swine hepatitis E virus swine (HEV) but not with human strains of HEV. *Arch. Virol.* **143:**1405–1415.
34. **Meng, X.-J., R. H. Purcell, P. G. Halbur, J. R. Lehman, D. M. Webb, T. S. Tsareva, J. S. Haynes, B. J. Thacker, and S. U. Emerson.** 1997. A novel virus in swine closely related to the human hepatitis E virus. *Proc. Natl. Acad . Sci. USA* **94:**9860–9865.
35. **Metcalf, H. E., D. W. Luchsinger, and W. C. Ray.** 1994. Brucellosis, p. 9–40. *In* G. W. Beran (ed. in chief), Section A. *Handbook of Zoonoses*, 2nd ed. CRC Press Inc., Boca Raton, Fla.
36. **Michaels, M. G., E. T. Wald, F. J. Fricket, P. J. del Nido, and J. Armitage.** 1992. Toxoplasmosis in pediatric recipients of heart transplants. *Clin. Infect. Dis.* **14:**847–851.
37. **Moon, H. W., and D. B. Woodmansee.** 1995. Cryptosporidiosis, p. 49–53. *In Zoonosis Updates from the Journal of the American Veterinary Medical Association*, 2nd ed. American Veterinary Medical Association, Schaumburg, Ill.
38. **Morehouse, L. G.** 1992. Rabies, p. 324–330. *In* A. D. Leman, B. E. Straw, W. L. Mengeling, S. D'Allaire, and D. J. Taylor (ed.), *Diseases of Swine*, 7th ed. Iowa State University Press, Ames, Iowa.
39. **National Hog Farmer.** 1999. February 15, p. 15.
40. **Pelzer, K. D.** 1995. Salmonellosis, p. 117–127. *In Zoonosis Updates from the Journal of the American Veterinary Medical Association*, 2nd ed. American Veterinary Medical Association, Schaumburg, Ill.
41. **Pereira, B. J. G., E. L. Milford, R. L. Kirman, and A. S. Levy.** 1991. Transmission of hepatitis C virus by organ transplantation. *N. Engl. J. Med.* **325:**454–460.
42. **Pier, A. C.** 1994. Superficial mycosis (dermatophytosis), p. 475–482. *In* G. W. Beran (ed. in chief), Section A. *Handbook of Zoonoses*, 2nd ed. CRC Press Inc., Boca Raton, Fla.
43. **Pijoan, C.** 1992. Pneumonic pasteurellosis, p. 552–559. *In* A. D. Leman, B. E. Straw, W. L. Mengeling, S. D'Allaire, and D. J. Taylor (ed.), *Diseases of Swine*, 7th ed. Iowa State University Press, Ames, Iowa.
44. **Reif, S. R.** 1994. Vesicular stomatitis, p. 171–184. *In* G. W. Beran (ed. in chief), Section B. *Handbook of Zoonoses*, 2nd ed. CRC Press Inc., Boca Raton, Fla.
45. **Sanford, S. E., and R. Higgins.** 1992. Streptococcal diseases, p. 588–590. *In* A. D. Leman, B. E. Straw, W. L. Mengeling, S. D'Allaire, and D. J. Taylor (ed.), *Diseases of Swine*, 7th ed. Iowa State University Press, Ames, Iowa.

46. **Shane, S. M.** 1994. Campylobacteriosis, p. 311–320. *In* G. W. Beran (ed. in chief), Section A. *Handbook of Zoonoses*, 2nd ed. CRC Press Inc., Boca Raton, Fla.
47. **Slemons, R. D., and M. Brugh.** 1994. Influenza, p. 385–396. *In* G. W. Beran (ed. in chief), Section B. *Handbook of Zoonoses*, 2nd ed. CRC Press Inc., Boca Raton, Fla.
48. **Smith, D. M.** 1993. Endogenous retroviruses in xenografts. *N. Engl. J. Med.* **328:**142–143.
49. **Songer, J. G., and A. B. Thiermann.** 1995. Leptospirosis, p. 86–93. *In Zoonosis Updates from the Journal of the American Veterinary Medical Association*, 2nd ed. American Veterinary Medical Association, Schaumburg, Ill.
50. **Straw, B. E.** 1992. Ringworm, p. 208–209. *In* A. D. Leman, B. E. Straw, W. L. Mengeling, S. D'Allaire, and D. J. Taylor (ed.), *Diseases of Swine*, 7th ed. Iowa State University Press, Ames, Iowa.
51. **Taylor, D. J.** 1992. Infection with *Yersinia*, p. 639–641. *In* A. D. Leman, B. E. Straw, W. L. Mengeling, S. D'Allaire, and D. J. Taylor (ed.), *Diseases of Swine*, 7th ed. Iowa State University Press, Ames, Iowa.
52. **Taylor, D. J., S. E. Sandford, J. E. T. Jones, and J. A. Yager.** 1992. Melioidosis, p. 62. *In* A. D. Leman, B. E. Straw, W. L. Mengeling, S. D'Allaire, and D. J. Taylor (ed.), *Diseases of Swine*, 7th ed. Iowa State University Press, Ames, Iowa.
53. **Thoen, C. O.** 1992. Tuberculosis, p. 617–626. *In* A. D. Leman, B. E. Straw, W. L. Mengeling, S. D'Allaire, and D. J. Taylor (ed.), *Diseases of Swine*, 7th ed. Iowa State University Press, Ames, Iowa.
54. **Thoen, C. O.** 1995. Tuberculosis, p.155–158. *In Zoonosis Updates from the Journal of the American Veterinary Medical Association*, 2nd ed. American Veterinary Medical Association, Schaumburg, Ill.
55. **Thoen, C. O., and D. E. Williams.** 1994. Tuberculosis, tuberculoidosis and other bacterial infections, p. 41–60. *In* G. W. Beran (ed. in chief), Section A. *Handbook of Zoonoses*, 2nd ed. CRC Press Inc., Boca Raton, Fla.
56. **Torton, M., and R. B. Marshall.** 1994. Leptospirosis, p. 245–264. *In* G. W. Beran (ed. in chief), Section A. *Handbook of Zoonoses*, 2nd ed. CRC Press Inc., Boca Raton, Fla.
57. **Walton, J. R.** 1992. Anthrax, p. 409–413. *In* A. D. Leman, B. E. Straw, W. L. Mengeling, S. D'Allaire, and D. J. Taylor (ed.), *Diseases of Swine*, 7th ed. Iowa State University Press, Ames, Iowa.
58. **Whitford, H. W., and M. E. Hugh-Jones.** 1994. Anthrax, p. 61–82. *In* G. W. Beran (ed. in chief), Section A. *Handbook of Zoonoses*, 2nd ed. CRC Press Inc., Boca Raton, Fla.
59. **Wilcock, B. P., and K. J. Schwartz.** 1992. Salmonellosis, p. 570–583. *In* A. D. Leman, B. E. Straw, W. L. Mengeling, S. D'Allaire, and D. J. Taylor (ed.), *Diseases of Swine*, 7th ed. Iowa State University Press, Ames, Iowa.
60. **Williams, L. P., Jr.** 1995. Campylobacteriosis, p. 38–39. *In Zoonosis Updates from the Journal of the American Veterinary Medical Association*, 2nd ed. American Veterinary Medical Association, Schaumburg, Ill.
61. **Wood, R. L.** 1992. Erysipelas, p. 475–488. *In* A. D. Leman, B. E. Straw, W. L. Mengeling, S. D'Allaire, and D. J. Taylor (ed.), *Diseases of Swine*, 7th ed. Iowa State University Press, Ames, Iowa.
62. **Wood, R. L., and J. H. Steele.** 1994. *Erysipelothrix* infections, p. 83–92. *In* G. W. Beran (ed. in chief), Section A. *Handbook of Zoonoses*, 2nd ed. CRC Press Inc., Boca Raton, Fla.
63. **Wray, C.** 1994. Mammalian salmonellosis, p. 289–302. *In* G. W. Beran (ed. in chief), Section A. *Handbook of Zoonoses*, 2nd ed. CRC Press Inc., Boca Raton, Fla.
64. **Zimmerman, J., K. Jin Yoon, G. Stevenson, and S. Dee.** 1998. *PPRS Compendium.* National Pork Producers Council, Des Moines, Iowa.
65. **Zimmerman, J. L.** 1994. Encephalomyocarditis, p. 423–436. *In* G. W. Beran (ed. in chief), Section B. *Handbook of Zoonoses*, 2nd ed. CRC Press Inc., Boca Raton, Fla.

Xenotransplantation
Edited by Jeffrey L. Platt

Chapter 13

Retroviruses and Xenotransplantation

Robin A. Weiss

All transplantation procedures carry an element of risk of the unwitting transfer of infectious agents along with the organ, tissue, or tissue product. In human-to-human transplantation of allografts, there has been a history of transmissible diseases, such as Creutzfeldt-Jakob disease from pituitary extracts and corneal grafts derived from cadavers. When the recipient of the graft is immunosuppressed, the danger of disease from infection is greater, as in primary cytomegalovirus infection in recipients of allogeneic bone marrow. Thus, the concern over the transmission of animal viruses to humans (zoonosis) in xenotransplantation (11, 46) can be viewed as an extension of the need to prevent or treat infections of transplant patients more generally. Indeed, animal transplants from carefully screened, specific-pathogen–free sources should be less prone to microbial contamination than those of free-living human donors.

A new dimension, however, of xenotransplantation is the possibility that viruses that have hitherto not become adapted to human infection might cause disease not only in the transplant recipient but might also be transmitted to the community at large. It is on account of this possible, though unlikely, scenario that would-be practitioners of xenotransplantation and regulatory bodies alike wish to move forward only with great caution, so that the microbes potentially involved, and the risks they pose, can be thoroughly evaluated (4, 13, 23). Indeed, there have been calls for a moratorium on all human xenotransplantation (6, 10).

Known pathogens of animals can readily be detected by microbiologists and by veterinarians, and will be eliminated from colonies of source animals. However, it is not possible to screen for agents that are not yet discovered, though general procedures such as caesarean delivery and physical isolation of founding animals will preclude the majority of microbes that are transmitted postnatally. There are a number of porcine viruses—parvovirus, circovirus, herpesvirus, rotavirus—that ought to be excludable by appropriate screening and husbandry. Yet new microbes are coming to light all the time. In pigs, for example, several viruses have been discovered since 1997. These include a virus related to human hepatitis E virus (36) that may also infect humans (35); a torovirus (26); human-tropic pig endogenous retroviruses (28, 41); and a new epidemic in Malaysia of nipahvirus (43), which at the time of writing is causing deaths in both pigs and people.

Robin A. Weiss • Windeyer Institute of Medical Sciences, University College London, 46 Cleveland St., London W1P 6DB, United Kingdom.

When a virus crosses from its natural reservoir species to a new host, it is not easy to predict whether it will become more or less pathogenic. Yaba monkeypox virus, a relative of variola (smallpox) virus, causes severe disease in both monkeys and man. The recent outbreak of H5N1 avian influenza virus in Hong Kong killed chickens and also had a 33% human mortality but did not transmit from person to person. On the other hand, cowpox behaves in an attenuated manner in humans, which allowed the development of vaccination by Jenner 200 years ago. Most troublesome could be the viruses that are nonpathogenic in their natural animal host yet cause serious disease in humans, like the hantaviruses of rodents, such as the outbreak of Sin Nombre virus infection in the southwestern United States in 1990 (38), and the hemorrhagic viruses causing Ebola, Marburg, and Lassa fever. Herpes B virus, a relative of human herpes simplex virus, causes nothing worse than cold sores in immunocompetent monkeys but causes lethal encephalitis in humans. Simian immunodeficiency viruses (SIV) appear to have low if any pathogenicity in their natural African primate hosts but lead to fatal acquired immunodeficiency syndrome (AIDS) in Asian macaques and, sadly, in humans (29).

RETROVIRUSES

SIV is a retrovirus, and it is the retrovirus family that has engendered much of the debate on microbial risks of xenotransplantation. Pigs and primates harbor retroviruses, which are difficult to eliminate because they are vertically transmitted. Retroviruses have RNA genomes in the virus particles, or virions, and form DNA copies in the newly infected cell utilizing the viral enzyme reverse transcriptase (12). On entering the nucleus, another viral enzyme, integrase, aids the insertion of the viral DNA into host chromosomal DNA as a provirus. This is an obligatory step in the virus replication cycle. Forward transcription of viral RNA of the provirus is controlled by promoter and enhancer elements in the 5′ long terminal repeat (LTR) of the provirus. The transcripts serve as mRNA for the translation of viral proteins, and full-length transcripts are packaged into virions as progeny genomes. The DNA provirus may remain latent, and if the infected cell proliferates, it will be replicated along with the rest of host DNA during the S-phase of the cell division cycle.

Retroviruses have the general genome structure 5′ LTR-*gag-pol-env*-LTR 3′ (12). *gag* encodes core proteins; *pol*, the enzymes protease reverse transcriptase and interase; and *env*, the transmembrane (TM) and surface (SU) envelope glycoproteins. Retroviruses possessing only *gag*, *pol*, and *env* are called "simple" viruses. Some retroviruses have additional or accessory genes, such as *tat* and *rev* of HIV, and these are called "complex" retroviruses. Figure 1 shows the major subfamilies of retrovirus connected by phylogenetic relatedness.

Endogenous Retroviruses

On occasions during vertebrate evolution, retroviral genomes have integrated into germ cells, the precursors of eggs and sperm. Such proviruses can then gain a free ride to the next host generation, and thousands more, becoming genetic traits of the host. These viral genomes were first described in chickens and mice (12). Most vertebrate species harbor multiple inherited proviruses, which are called endogenous retroviruses (ERV) to distinguish them from infectiously transmitted, exogenous retroviruses. Up to 0.1% of the human genome may be of retroviral origin (42). Some human endogenous retroviral genomes

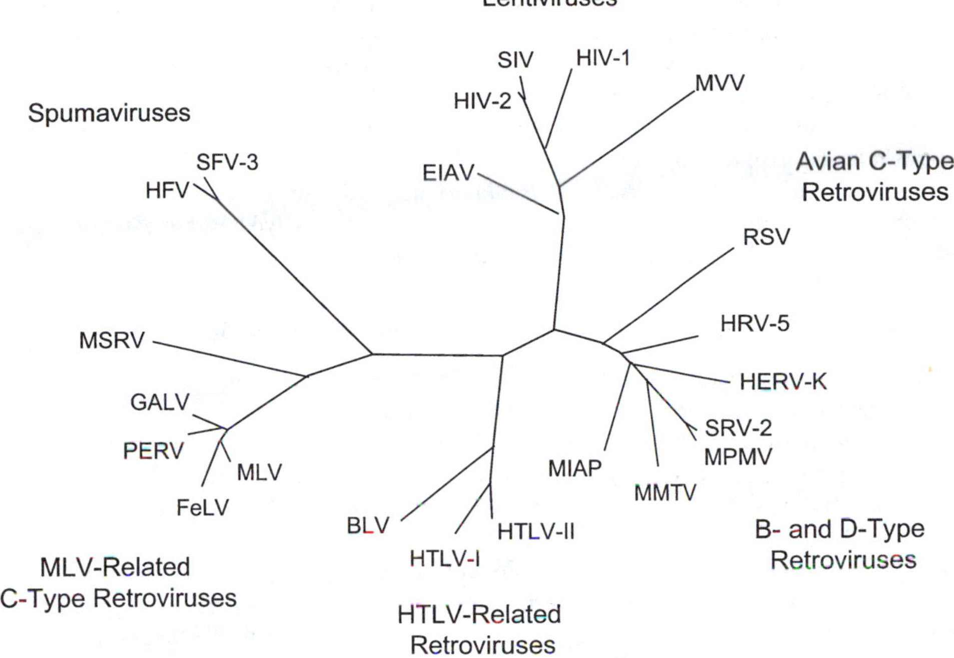

Figure 1. Unrooted phylogenetic tree showing major groups of retrovirus.

(HERV) occur as single-copy integrated elements, e.g., HERV-3, with its envelope expressed in the placenta (51), while others, e.g., HERV-K, are represented by thousands of integrated copies. Maintenance of an open reading frame over millions of years of host evolution implies selection for a useful function to the host (42, 45).

If endogenous retroviruses were pathogenic, they would be selected against during host evolution. In fact, most ERV genomes become defective over evolutionary time, with stop codons or large deletions in their genes. However, ERV proviruses of recent evolutionary origin often maintain their capacity to emerge as infectious retroviruses. Although none of the HERV genomes have been rescued in infectious form, some ERV of pigs and baboons still retain potential infectivity, including the capacity to infect human cells in culture. These inherited retroviruses in potential source animals raise questions about their potential transmission via xenotransplantation and are discussed in more detail below.

Complete ERV genomes with infectious potential do not normally cause viremia in their natural hosts. Again, host evolution has selected for genetic traits that suppress retroviral replication. One type of suppression is exemplified by the *Fv-1* locus of mice (8), which exerts a dominant, inhibitory effect on a postpenetration, preintegration step in the retroviral lifecycle of endogenous murine leukemia virus (MLV). But inbred laboratory mice, genetically selected for a high incidence of lymphoma (e.g., AKR mice), are homozygous recessive for *Fv-1* permissive alleles. Similarly, the inbred GR mouse strain, with a high incidence of mammary carcinoma, has an endogenous genome of mouse mammary tumor virus (MMTV) (12), presumably integrated into the germ line during laboratory selection from the milk-transmitted, infectious strains of MMTV.

Another means of genetic resistance to viremia by ERV is to render non-functional the cell surface receptors utilized by the retrovirus. This is achieved in two ways, by mutation of the receptors or by blocking them through the expression of endogenous viral envelope glycoproteins (12, 52). Thus, if any one or a few cells in the body become activated to produce the virus, it cannot infect neighboring cells and the infection peters out. If, however, the virus could gain access to cells of a foreign species, which has not evolved specific resistance to the retrovirus in question, it may readily infect the foreign cells. Such endogenous retroviruses, which are transmitted as Mendelian proviruses in a nonpermissive host but can infect cells of foreign species, are called xenotropic viruses (30).

Xenotropic Retroviruses and Xenotransplantation

It is noteworthy that xenotropic retroviruses have been found to infect foreign cells in the xenotransplantation setting. The endogenous retrovirus of domestic cats was first identified in a human tumor cell line and was initially thought to be a human retrovirus. Only 2 years later was it realized that the human tumor cells had been passed as a xenograft in the brain of a fetal cat (before immunodeficient mice were available) and had become contaminated by this hitherto unknown feline retrovirus (12).

Human xenografts in nude mice or mice with severe combined immunodeficiency also become infected with xenotropic endogenous murine leukemia virus (MLV-X) (1). In Balb/c mice the primary infection rate is approximately 1%, varying with the tumor type transplanted, and up to 30% of serially passaged human xenografts harbor MLV-X (C. Patience and R. A. Weiss, 1998, unpublished observations). Because host-into-graft retrovirus infection occurs so readily in experimental xenotransplantation, caution is necessary to avoid graft-into-host transmission in clinical xenotransplantation.

PRIMATE RETROVIRUSES

If monkeys or apes are to be further used as sources of tissues for humans, retroviruses must be added to the list of ethical and practical questions. It is surprising that little attempt was made to check for retroviruses other than SIV in the baboons used for liver transplantation to humans and for bone marrow to Baby Fae and to an AIDS patient (27). Only now, in the wake of the debate about pig retroviruses, are biopsy and autopsy specimens from the human recipients of baboon tissues being tested retrospectively.

Many kinds of retrovirus commonly infect various primate species (Table 1). Spumaviruses (foamy viruses) are almost universal infections of Old World monkeys and apes (12). They are not generally associated with disease, although a severe neurological disease associated with marked viral load in the brain was noted in an orangutan (34). The human foamy virus (HFV), first described in an African patient with nasopharyngeal carcinoma (1), is no longer thought to represent widespread human infection (3). HFV is very closely related in genetic sequence to a simian foamy virus strain (SFV-6) of chimpanzees, and with hindsight, the index patient may have had a zoonotic infection. Indeed, it has become apparent that humans are susceptible to SFV. Seroconversion of persistent, asymptomatic infection up to 20 years or more has been documented in staff at primate centers who have been bitten by baboons (20). SFV in humans has not spread to their spouses. An examination of recipients of blood transfusions from

Table 1. Primate retroviruses[a]

Virus			Disease	Primate host	Zoonosis to human
Group	Type	Exogenous or endogenous			
Foamy	SFV	Exo	None	OWM Apes	Yes
Lenti	SIV	Exo	AIDS	OWM Apes	Yes
HTLV	STLV	Exo	Leukemia CNS	OWM NWM Apes	Yes
D-type	SRV SMRV	Exo Endo	AIDS None	OWM NWM	? No
C-type	GALV BaEV	Exo Endo	Leukemia None	Gibbons Baboons	No No

[a]SFV, simian foamy virus; SIV, simian immunodeficiency virus; HTLV, human T-lymphotropic virus; STLV, simian T-lymphotropic virus; SRV, simian retrovirus; SMRV, squirrel monkey retrovirus; GALV, gibbon ape leukemia virus; BaEV, baboon endogenous virus; OWM, Old World monkey; NWM, New World monkey.

SFV-positive humans is under way. Thus, it is likely that SFV can be readily transmitted to humans via xenotransplantation. Although foamy viruses are usually nonpathogenic, they are highly cytopathic in culture and might be expected to cause disease in immunosuppressed individuals.

Lentiviruses were first characterized in sheep (Maedi-Visna virus, MVV), goats (caprine arthritis encephalitis virus), and horses (equine infectious anemia virus). They include the immunodeficiency viruses of primates (HIV-1, HIV-2, SIV) (29). Lentiviruses cause slow, progressive, and often fatal disease, as is so well known in human AIDS. On the other hand, some naturally infected hosts live asymptomatically with their lentivirus. MVV was transmitted from asymptomatic Karakal sheep to highly susceptible Icelandic sheep in which the virus causes progressive and fatal wasting disease and central nervous system (CNS) degeneration, but without CD4 T-cell immunodeficiency. SIVagm infection of African green monkeys, which is widespread among cervets, grivets, and other *Cercopithecus aethiops* subspecies, does not typically progress to disease. The same rude health is evident in sooty mangabey monkeys in West Africa, which sustain SIVsm infection with equivalent viral load to HIV in humans. Yet when SIVsm crosses to new hosts, to become SIVmac in macaques and HIV-2 in humans (16), it causes AIDS.

It is clear that HIV-1 and HIV-2 represent new and independent infections of humans in the 20th century. HIV-2 represents human infection by SIVsm and first arose in West Africa where the natural simian host, the sooty mangaby, occurs. Genetic sequence analysis of SIVsm and HIV-2 strains indicates that several separate transfers from monkey to human occurred (16). But unlike the human cases of foamy virus infection, HIV-2 has adopted a human-to-human mode of transmission. Not only is it endemic in West Africa, but it has also spread epidemically to India and occurs sporadically in other countries such as Portugal, where there is contact with or recent immigration from West Africa. A human case of SIVmac infection by a primate handler has been recorded (20, 25).

HIV-1 is similarly thought to have originated from a non-human primate source. Although the data are not as compelling as for the SIVsm/HIV-2 connection, owing to a lack of serological surveys in wild apes, the evidence is growing that chimpanzees may be a natural reservoir of SIVcpz from which HIV-1 diverged (15, 54). Moreover, the three main groups of HIV-1, M, N, and O, probably represent separate zoonotic transfers from chimpanzees to humans because they are as divergent from each other as they are from SIVcpz strains. It is the M group that has radiated from Africa to form the various HIV-1 subtypes (B in the United States, E in Thailand, etc.) that represent the worldwide pandemic (56).

Human T-cell lymphotropic virus type 1 (HTLV-1) causes adult T-cell leukemia and also a demyelinating CNS disease known as tropical spastic paraparesis or HTLV-associated myopathy (HAM) (12). HTLV-1 is an older infection of humans than HIV-1 or HIV-2. It is endemic in southwest Japan, West Africa, and the Caribbean and occurs sporadically elsewhere. It is readily transmitted by blood transfusion, but unlike HIV, not by acellular blood products. HTLV-2 is a related virus endemic in Native Americans and some Africans. It is associated with neurological disease but not leukemia. Many species of Asian and African Old World monkeys (macaques, baboons) harbor simian T-lymphotropic viruses (STLV) related to HTLV. Like HIV, evidence from viral genome sequence analysis indicates that humans initially acquired HTLV infection from their simian neighbors (17, 44).

D-type retroviruses represent another widespread group of primate retroviruses. Infectious simian retrovirus strains (SRV-1 to 5) cause a severe immunodeficiency syndrome in macaque monkeys. Endogenous, inherited forms of D-type retroviruses are also documented in several simian species (44). D-type viruses readily replicate in human cells in culture. One case of apparent infection of an HIV-1–positive patient in the United States was reported (9) but has not been further characterized. We have identified a novel human retrovirus, HRV-5 (19), associated with arthritis and systemic lupus erythematosus (18). HRV-5 is related to D-type retroviruses (Fig. 1), although its sequence appears too distant from SRV to be derived by recent zoonosis from monkeys.

The HERV-K human endogenous retroviruses also belong to the D-type/B-type subfamily of retroviruses (Fig. 1) (42). These genomes are also present in numerous copies in Old World monkey chromosomes and in some New World monkeys (45). None of these viruses have to date been found to be recoverable as infectious viruses, although a few have apparently nondefective, complete genomes. They appear to have co-evolved with their host species, but with a remarkable dispersion as retro-elements in the chromosomes of Old World primates soon after their separation from New World monkeys (47).

C-type retroviruses in primates are represented both as endogenous genomes and as infectious, pathogenic retroviruses. The best characterized C-type ERV is the baboon endogenous virus (BaEV) (12). This virus is produced as replication-competent particles in the full-term placenta of baboons and related geladas. Numerous defective C-type genomes are also present in the DNA of baboons and other monkeys as well as apes and humans (50).

BaEV is a xenotropic virus, being unable to reinfect baboon cells but readily infecting human cells in culture. In recent evolutionary times, BaEV has transferred from ancestral baboons to cats of the genus *Felis* and have colonized this new host's germ line. The ERV of cats (RD114) described above is closely related to BaEV (12). Both RD114 and BaEV have *gag* and *pol* genes related to other C-type viruses such as MLV, but the *env* gene appears to be a chimera between C-type and D-type retroviruses. The cytoplasmic tail of the TM protein is close in amino-acid sequence to C-type viruses, whereas the remainder of TM and the whole of the SU envelope glycoprotein, gp70, is closer to SRV. Thus BaEV is a genetically recombinant retrovirus, having a distinct phylogeny for *gag*, *pol*, and the start of *env* from the rest of *env*.

This evidence of past genetic recombination among retroviruses serves to remind us that different strains of retrovirus readily form recombinants provided they possess compatible packaging signals so that the two parental RNA transcripts become incorporated into the retroviral particles. The possibility of recombination between animal retroviruses and endogenous or infectious human retroviral genomes needs to be borne in mind in xenotransplantation. The initial infecting virus from a xenograft could lead to a recombinant virus emerging in the transplant recipient that may in turn be better adapted for onward transmission.

An infectious, pathogenic C-type retrovirus of primates is evident in the gibbon ape leukemia virus (GALV) (12, 24). GALV causes lymphoid and myeloid leukemia in Lar gibbons kept in captivity. There is no evidence to date that wild gibbons are a reservoir for this virus. Among the close relatives of GALV are endogenous genomes in southeast Asian mouse species, *Mus caroli* and *Mus cervicolor* (22, 31), and recently this type of ERV sequence has been detected in marsupials too (32). The GALV epidemic in certain gibbon colonies could be a recent outbreak of infection possibly originating from mice when gibbons were brought down from the tropical forest canopy to ground level. GALV is the C-type virus with closest sequence similarity to C-type viruses of swine.

PORCINE ENDOGENOUS RETROVIRUSES (PERV)

Because pigs are a favored species for xenotransplantation to humans, there has been renewed interest in porcine retroviruses (46). Unlike ruminants such as sheep, pigs appear to carry only one group of infectious retrovirus, the C-type retroviruses, related to MLV and GALV leukemia viruses. These viruses were originally detected in cell lines derived from porcine kidneys and from lymphoma (5, 37, 49). The C-type genomes are endogenous (7) with many genome copies in porcine DNA (28, 41). Recently, further sets of endogenous retroviral genome have been detected in porcine DNA, including those of B/D-type and other taxonomic groups (40). Since these new sequences appear to be defective, they probably pose little problem for xenotransplantation.

When the infectivity of PERV was first examined, it was found that PERV released from the PK15 kidney cell line replicated both in porcine cells (the ST-Iowa testis cell line) and in human cells (293 kidney cells and some other human cell types) (41). In fact, PK15 cells release a mixture of two PERV strains with distinct envelope sequences, designated PERV-A and PERV-B (28). The virus released by another porcine kidney cell line, MPK, was infectious for pig cells but not for human 293 cells (41), and this PERV strain is designated PERV-C. The envelope sequence of PERV-C is indistinguishable from a PERV genome originally cloned from a pig lymphoma (2).

A summary of PERV host range studies (41, 48) on cell lines in culture is shown in Table 2. PERV-A and -B are "amphotropic" in being able to propagate both on pig cells and foreign cells, whereas PERV-C behaves as an "ecotropic" virus, replicating only in porcine cells. More extensive studies using MLV vectors with a reporter gene and PERV envelopes indicated that many human cells but few simian cells are permissive for PERV-A and PERV-B entry (48). Not all human cells are fully permissive for PERV replication, yet they may take up and integrate the PERV provirus (41). Even in human cell lines such as 293 and HeLa, which are among the most permissive for PERV replication, the levels of

Table 2. Summary of PERV infection in porcine, human, and simian cells[a]

Virus	Pig ST-Iowa	Human 293	Simian
PERV-A	++	+	−
PERV-B	+	++	−
PERV-C	++	−	−

[a] ++, $>10^3$ infectious units; +, 10^1 to 10^2 infectious units; −, <10 infectious units. Cells were exposed to virus and propagated by reverse transcript activity in culture medium detected by product enhanced RT-PCR (48). Simian cells included cell lines from baboons, cynomolgus macaques, and African green monkeys.

PERV reverse transcriptase and infectious virus released are low compared with those of other human-tropic C-type viruses such as GALV or MLV-X (48).

Host range studies (Table 2) indicate that simian cell lines from African green monkeys, cynomolgus monkeys, and baboons are not susceptible to PERV-A or PERV-B infection and thus differ from human cells in this regard (48). It would, therefore, be rash to assume that any lack of evidence of PERV transfer in experimental monkeys that have received porcine xenografts should reflect the human situation.

Normal diploid human cells, such as MRC 5 fibroblasts, can also be infected with PERV-A and PERV-B (41), so the human host range is not limited to cell lines. Receptor interference studies show that PERV-A and PERV-B utilize different cell surface receptors from each other on porcine and human cells, which are also distinct from previously characterized MLV, RD114, BaEV, and GALV receptors (48). Primary, short-term cultures of porcine cells spontaneously release PERV infectious for human cells. This has been demonstrated with porcine lymphocytes (55) and aortic endothelial cells (33). It is, therefore, likely that some porcine cells or tissues xenotransplanted in vivo will also release PERV.

Southern blotting indicates that most strains of domestic pig carry multiple copies of PERV proviral genomes, dispersed among pig chromosomes, approximately 30 of PERV-A and 15 of PERV-B (28). Many of these might be defective and incapable of giving rise to infectious virus. The endogenous proviruses will need to be mapped, cloned, and sequenced to determine which are potentially infectious. Thus, it will not be simple to develop PERV-negative herds of pig, either by conventional breeding or by knockout technology.

BENEFIT VERSUS RISK IN XENOTRANSPLANTATION

There is a genuine risk that a proportion of human recipients of animal tissues will become infected by endogenous retroviruses released from those tissues. Whether the retroviruses would be pathogenic is not known, but in the immunosuppressed patient they may have the opportunity to propagate to titers capable of causing disease. Murine leukemia virus, which emerged as an unwanted, replication-competent retrovirus from supposedly sterile gene therapy vectors, has caused malignancy in monkey hosts (14). This, and the foregoing discussion of natural and experimental infection across large phylogenetic distances, shows that retroviruses are able to infect and cause disease in hosts wholly unrelated to those from which they emerge.

The limited investigations reported to date, however, show no evidence of transfer of C-type viruses such as BaEV or PERV to humans. In a study of retroviral infection of primate center staff, foamy retrovirus infection was reported, but significantly BaEV did not infect even those individuals who had suffered deep puncture wounds from baboons (20). Among 12 patients exposed to living porcine tissue, 10 diabetic patients who were transplanted with porcine islets of Langerhans, and 2 kidney dialysis patients linked extracorporeally to pig kidneys showed no evidence of PERV infection after many months when studied with sensitive detection techniques (21, 39). Novartis and the U.S. Centers for Disease Control and Prevention then investigated a larger set of 160 patients exposed to live porcine tissue with negative results (38a). Thus, the interim data indicate that PERV is not highly contagious for humans. Nevertheless, a 1% or 0.1% infection rate among xenograft recipients would still be cause for concern.

Of much greater concern would be the infectious spread of PERV from a xenograft recipient to his or her close contacts and perhaps to the population at large. Such a community risk is extremely difficult to gauge—who would have calculated that the handful of AIDS patients among gay men in the United States reported in 1981 heralded a pandemic that has now affected 50 million persons (including the 15 million who have already died as a result of HIV infection)?

It is sometimes argued (10) that there is nothing unique about xenograft procedures regarding cross-species infection. Indeed, the zoonoses discussed in this chapter illustrate that animal retroviruses have found other means of infiltrating humans. Xenotransplantation, however, could offer the otherwise improbable, extremely rare event of zoonosis much more opportunity to occur, for three distinct reasons. First, the physical barrier to cross-species infection is breached by implanting animal tissues in humans. Second, the immunosuppression necessary to prevent graft rejection may allow the virus to take and propagate in the human body. Third, genetic modification of pigs to lessen hyperacute rejection (HAR) may allow viruses to become pre-adapted in the swine for human infection.

The human complement-modulating genes bred into transgenic pigs could have a direct impact on viruses (53): CD55/Daf acts as a receptor for human picornaviruses such as ECHO and coxsackie B myocarditis viruses, and CD46 acts as a receptor for measles virus. Therefore, related viruses of pigs might adapt to utilize the human receptor homologs in transgenic pigs. Moreover, human complement acts on enveloped viruses budding from animal cells in the same way as HAR. Antibodies to αGal and other carbohydrate xenoantigens bind to virus envelopes bearing these sugar antigens, and this leads to complement inactivation, a sort of hyperacute rejection of virus. For example, PERV released by wild-type porcine cells expressing αGal is rapidly inactivated by fresh human plasma, whereas the same virus after one passage through αGal-negative human 293 cells is completely resistant (41). If the virus particles budding from transgenic porcine cells also incorporated human CD46, CD55, or CD59 into their envelopes, complement-mediated lysis may be abrogated (53). Thus, the genetic modification of pigs designed to make organ xenotransplantation possible could also result in "humanizing" porcine viruses.

Overall, the factors concerning viral zoonosis in xenotransplantation are complex, and the risks are extremely difficult to quantify. The worst-case scenario would be a major new viral pandemic like HIV/AIDS. A more realistic scenario, to my view, is that, perhaps, 1 in 1,000 xenograft recipients may pick up a porcine retrovirus, and if detected, that infection should be treatable by antiretroviral therapy. Clearly, more research is required on retroviral and other infections in relation to xenotransplantation. On account of recent studies of PERV, the reagents and tools are available to carry out that research. Ethical issues, discussed elsewhere, need to be coordinated with scientific data on safety issues.

REFERENCES

1. **Achong, B. G., P. A. Trumper, and B. C. Giovanella.** 1976. C-type virus particles in human tumours transplanted into nude mice. *Br. J. Cancer* **34:**203–206.
2. **Akiyoshi, D. E., M. Denaro, H. Zhu, J. L. Greenstein, P. Banerjee, and J. A. Fishman.** 1998. Identification of a full-length cDNA for an endogenous retrovirus of miniature swine. *J. Virol.* **72:**4503–4507.
3. **Ali, M., G. P. Taylor, R. J. Pitman, D. Parker, A. Rethwilm, R. Cheingsong-Popov, J. N. Weber, P. D. Bieniasz, J. Bradley, and M. O. McClure.** 1996. No evidence of antibody to human foamy virus in widespread human populations. *AIDS Res. Human Retrovir.* **12:**1473–1483.
4. **Allan, J. S.** 1996. Xenotransplantation at a crossroads: prevention versus progress. *Nature Med.* **2:**18–21.
5. **Armstrong, J. A., J. S. Porterfield, and A. T. De Madrid.** 1971. C-type virus particles in pig kidney cell lines. *J. Gen. Virol.* **10:**195–198.
6. **Bach, F. H., J. A. Fishman, N. Daniels, J. Proimos, B. Anderson, C. B. Carpenter, L. Farrow, S. C. Robson, and H. V. Fineberg.** 1998. Uncertainty in xenotransplantation: individual benefit versus collective risk. *Nature Med.* **4:**141–144.
7. **Benveniste, R. E., and G. J. Todaro.** 1975. Evolution of type C viral genes: preservation of ancestral murine type C viral sequences in pig cellular DNA. *Proc. Natl. Acad. Sci. USA* **72:**4090–4094.
8. **Best, S., P. Le Tissier, G. Towers, and J. P. Stoye.** 1996. Positional cloning of the mouse retrovirus restriction gene *Fv-1*. *Nature* **382:**826–829.
9. **Bohannon, R. C., L. A. Donehower, and R. J. Ford.** 1991. Isolation of a type D retrovirus from B-cell lymphomas of a patient with AIDS. *J Virol.* **65:**5663–5672.
10. **Butler, D.** 1998. Last chance to stop and think on risks of xenotransplants. *Nature* **391:**320–325.
11. **Chapman, L. E., T. M. Folks, D. R. Salomon, A. P. Patterson, T. E. Eggerman, and P. D. Noguchi.** 1995. Xenotransplantation and xenogeneic infections. *N. Engl. J. Med.* **333:**1498–1501.
12. **Coffin, J., S. H. Hughes, and H. E. Varmus.** 1997. *Retroviruses*. Cold Spring Harbor Laboratory Press, New York, N.Y.
13. **Department of Health, Advisory Group on the Ethics of Xenotransplantation.** 1997. *Animal Tissues into Humans.* HMSO, London, United Kingdom.
14. **Donahue, R. E., S. W. Kessler, D. Bodine, K. McDonagh, C. Dunbar, S. Goodman, B. Agricola, E. Byrne, M. Raffeld, R. Moen, J. Bacher, K. M. Zsebo, and A. W. Nienhuis.** 1992. Helper virus induced T cell lymphoma in nonhuman primates after retroviral mediated gene transfer. *J. Exp. Med.***176:** 1125–1135.
15. **Gao, F., E. Bailes, D. L. Robertson, Y. Chen, C. M. Rodenburg, S. F. Michael, L. B. Cummins, L. O. Arthur, M. Peeters, G. M. Shaw, P. M. Sharp, and B. H. Hahn.** 1999. Origin of HIV-1 in the chimpanzee *Pan troglodytes troglodytes*. *Nature* **397:**436–441.
16. **Gao, F., L. Yue, A. T. White, P. G. Pappas, J. Barchue, A. P. Hanson, B. M. Greene, P. M. Sharp, G. M. Shaw, and B. H. Hahn.** 1992. Human infection by genetically diverse SIVSM-related HIV-2 in west Africa. *Nature* **358:**495–499.
17. **Gessain, A., and R. Maheux.** 1999. Genetic diversity and molecular epidemiology of HTLV and related simian retroviruses, p. 281–327. *In* A. G. Dalgleish and R. A. Weiss (ed.), *HIV and the New Viruses,* 2nd ed. Academic Press, London, United Kingdom.
18. **Griffiths, D. J., S. P. Cooke, C. Herve, S. P. Rigby, E. Mallon, A. Hajeer, M. Lock, V. Emery, P. Taylor, P. Pantelidis, C. B. Bunker, R. du Bois, R. A. Weiss, and P. J. Venables.** 1999. Detection of human retrovirus 5 in patients with arthritis and systemic lupus erythematosus. *Arthritis Rheum.* **42:**448–454.
19. **Griffiths, D. J., P. J. Venables, R. A. Weiss, and M. T. Boyd.** 1997. A novel exogenous retrovirus sequence identified in humans. *J. Virol.* **71:**2866–2872.
20. **Heneine, W., W. M. Switzer, P. Sandstrom, J. Brown, S. Vedapuri, C. A. Schable, A. S. Khan, N. W. Lerche, M. Schweizer, D. Neumann-Haefelin, L. E. Chapman, and T. M. Folks.** 1998. Identification of a human population infected with simian foamy viruses. *Nature Med.* **4:**403–407.

21. **Heneine, W., A. Tibell, W. M. Switzer, P. Sandstrom, G. V. Rosales, A. Mathews, O. Korsgren, L. E. Chapman, T. M. Folks, and C. G. Groth.** 1998. No evidence of infection with porcine endogenous retrovirus in recipients of porcine islet-cell xenografts. *Lancet* **352:**695–699.
22. **Herniou, E., J. Martin, K. Miller, J. Cook, M. Wilkinson, and M. Tristem.** 1998. Retroviral diversity and distribution in vertebrates. *J. Virol.* **72:**5955–5966.
23. **Institute of Medicine.** 1996. *Xenotransplantation, Science, Ethics and Public Policy.* National Academy Press, Washington, D.C.
24. **Kawakami, T. G., L. Sun, and T. S. McDowell.** 1978. Natural transmission of gibbon leukemia virus. *J. Natl. Cancer Inst.* **61:**1113–1115.
25. **Khabbaz, R. F., W. Heneine, J. R. George, B. Parekh, T. Rowe, T. Woods, W. M. Switzer, H. M. McClure, M. Murphey-Corb, and T. M. Folks.** 1994. Infection of a laboratory worker with simian immunodeficiency virus. *N. Engl. J. Med.* **330:**172–177.
26. **Kroneman, A., L. A. Cornelissen, M. C. Horzinek, R. J. de Groot, and H. F. Egberinck.** 1998. Identification and characterisation of a porcine torovirus. *J. Virol.* **72:**3507–3511.
27. **Lanza, R. P., D. K. Cooper, and W. L. Chick.** 1997. Xenotransplantation. *Sci. Am.* **277:**54–59.
28. **Le Tissier, P., J. P. Stoye, Y. Takeuchi, C. Patience, and R. A. Weiss.** 1997. Two sets of human-tropic pig retrovirus. *Nature* **389:**681–682.
29. **Levy, J. A.** 1998. *HIV and the Pathogenesis of AIDS.* ASM Press, Washington, D.C.
30. **Levy, J. A.** 1999. Xenotropism: the elusive viral receptor finally uncovered. *Proc. Natl. Acad. Sci. USA* **96:**802–804.
31. **Lieber, M. M., C. J. Sherr, G. J. Todaro, R. E. Benveniste, R. Callahan, and H. G. Coon.** 1975. Isolation from the asian mouse *Mus caroli* of an endogenous type C virus related to infectious primate type C viruses. *Proc. Natl. Acad. Sci. USA* **72:**2315–2319.
32. **Martin, J., E. Herniou, J. Cook, R. W. O'Neill, and M. Tristem.** 1999. Interclass transmission and phyletic host tracking in murine leukemia virus-related retroviruses. *J. Virol.* **73:**2442–2449.
33. **Martin, U., V. Kiessig, J. H. Blusch, A. Haverich, K. von der Helm, T. Herden, and G. Steinhoff.** 1998. Expression of pig endogenous retrovirus by primary porcine endothelial cells and infection of human cells. *Lancet* **352:**692–694.
34. **McClure, M. O., P. D. Bieniasz, T. F. Schulz, I. L. Chrystie, G. Simpson, A. Aguzzi, J. G. Hoad, A. Cunningham, J. Kirkwood, and R. A. Weiss.** 1994. Isolation of a new foamy retrovirus from orangutans. *J. Virol.* **68:**7124–7130.
35. **Meng, X. J., P. G. Halbur, M. S. Shapiro, S. Govindarajan, J. D. Bruna, I. K. Mushahwar, R. H. Purcell, and S. U. Emerson.** 1998. Genetic and experimental evidence for cross-species infection by swine hepatitis E virus. *J. Virol.* **72:**9714–9721.
36. **Meng, X. J., R. H. Purcell, P. G. Halbur, J. R. Lehman, D. M. Webb, T. S. Tsareva, J. S. Haynes, B. J. Thacker, and S. U. Emerson.** 1997. A novel virus in swine is closely related to the human hepatitis E virus. *Proc. Natl. Acad. Sci. USA* **94:**9860–9865.
37. **Moennig, V., H. Frank, G. Hunsmann, P. Ohms, H. Schwarz, and W. Schafer.** 1974. C-type particles produced by a permanent cell line from a leukemic pig. II. Physical, chemical, and serological characterization of the particles. *Virology* **57:**179–188.
38. **Nichol, S. T., C. F. Spiropoulou, S. Morzunov, P. E. Rollin, T. G. Ksiazek, H. Feldmann, A. Sanchez, J. Childs, S. Zaki, and C. J. Peters.** 1993. Genetic identification of a hantavirus associated with an outbreak of acute respiratory illness. *Science* **262:**914–917.
38a. **Paradis, K., G. Langford, Z. Long, W. Heneine, P. Sandstrom, W. M. Switzer, L. E. Chapman, C. Lockey, D. Onions, and E. Otto.** 1999. Search for cross-species transmission of porcine endogenous retrovirus in patients treated with living pig tissue. *Science* **285:**1236–1241.
39. **Patience, C., G. S. Patton, Y. Takeuchi, R. A. Weiss, M. O. McClure, L. Rydberg, and M. E. Breimer.** 1998. No evidence of pig DNA or retroviral infection in patients with short-term extracorporeal connection to pig kidneys. *Lancet* **352:**699–701.
40. **Patience, C., Y. Takeuchi, W. Switzer, W. Heneine, T. Folks, and R. A. Weiss.** Multiple types of endogenous retroviral genome in the DNA of swine and other species of Suiformes. Submitted for publication.
41. **Patience, C., Y. Takeuchi, and R. A. Weiss.** 1997. Infection of human cells by an endogenous retrovirus of pigs. *Nature Med.* **3:**282–286.
42. **Patience, C., D. A. Wilkinson, and R. A. Weiss.** 1997. Our retroviral heritage. *Trends Genet.* **13:**116–120.

43. **Philbey, A. W., P. D. Kirkland, A. D. Ross, R. J. Davis, A. B. Gleeson, R. J. Love, P. W. Daniels, A. R. Gould, and A. D. Hyatt.** 1998. An apparently new virus (family *Paramyxoviridae*) infectious for pigs, humans, and fruit bats. *Emerg. Infect. Dis.* **4:**269–271.
44. **Rosenblum, L., and M. O. McClure.** 1999. Non-lentiviral primate retroviruses, p. 251–279. *In* A. G. Dalgleish and R. A. Weiss (ed.), *HIV and the New Viruses.* Academic Press, London, United Kingdom.
45. **Simpson, G. R., C. Patience, R. Lower, R. R. Tonjes, H. D. Moore, R. A. Weiss, and M. T. Boyd.** 1996. Endogenous D-type (HERV-K) related sequences are packaged into retroviral particles in the placenta and possess open reading frames for reverse transcriptase. *Virology* **222:**451–456.
46. **Stoye, J. P., and J. M. Coffin.** 1995. The dangers of xenotransplantation. *Nature Med.* **1:**1100.
47. **Sverdlov, E. D.** 2000. Retroviruses and primate evolution. *BioEssays* **22:**161–171.
48. **Takeuchi, Y., C. Patience, S. Magre, R. A. Weiss, P. T. Banerjee, P. Le Tissier, and J. P. Stoye.** 1998. Host range and interference studies of three classes of pig endogenous retrovirus. *J. Virol.* **72:**9986–9991.
49. **Todaro, G. J., R. E. Benveniste, M. M. Lieber, and C. J. Sherr.** 1974. Characterization of a type C virus released from the porcine cell line PK(15). *Virology* **58:**65–74.
50. **Van der Kuyl, A. C., J. T. Dekker, and J. Goudsmit.** 1995. Distribution of baboon endogenous virus among species of African monkeys suggests multiple ancient cross-species transmissions in shared habitats. *J. Virol.* **69:**7877–7887.
51. **Venables, P. J., S. M. Brookes, D. Griffiths, R. A. Weiss, and M. T. Boyd.** 1995. Abundance of an endogenous retroviral envelope protein in placental trophoblasts suggests a biological function. *Virology* **211:**589–592.
52. **Weiss, R. A.** 1993. *Cellular Receptors and Viral Glycoproteins Involved in Retrovirus Entry,* vol. 2. Plenum Press, New York, N.Y.
53. **Weiss, R. A.** 1998. Transgenic pigs and virus adaptation. *Nature* **391:**327–328.
54. **Weiss, R. A., and R. W. Wrangham.** 1999. The origin of HIV-1: from *Pan* to pandemic. *Nature* **397:**385–386.
55. **Wilson, C. A., S. Wong, J. Muller, C. E. Davidson, T. M. Rose, and P. Burd.** 1998. Type C retrovirus released from porcine primary peripheral blood mononuclear cells infects human cells. *J. Virol.* **72:**3082–3087.
56. **Zhu, T., B. T. Korber, A. J. Nahmias, E. Hooper, P. M. Sharp, and D. D. Ho.** 1998. An African HIV-1 sequence from 1959 and implications for the origin of the epidemic. *Nature* **391:**594–597.

Xenotransplantation
Edited by Jeffrey L. Platt

Chapter 14

Potential Medical Impact of Endogenous Retroviruses

Rima Abu-Nader and Carlos V. Paya

Xenotransplantation has established itself as a fundamental part of transplantation research. The concept of transplanting organs from animal species into humans is in part prompted by a shortage of human donor organs. Different types of animal species have been considered for this purpose, but more recently, focus has been directed toward swine as the most favorable candidate. Pigs are found in preponderance and can be derived by caesarean section, deprived of colostrum, and raised in a pathogen-free environment, thereby minimizing the risk of commonly acquired infections. However, unlike grafts obtained from baboons, chimpanzees, and other non-human primates, porcine grafts are far more discordant, when compared to the others, with respect to human organs. Thus, they are easier targets for hyperacute rejection, which is characterized by extensive vascular endothelial injury usually occurring within minutes of tissue or organ implantation (33, 34). In addition to the phylogenetic and immunologic disparity between human and pig organs, the latter may harbor organisms that are otherwise undetectable by available tests and that could be potentially deleterious to the future human recipient. The recent in vitro observation that porcine endogenous retroviruses (PERV) can infect human cells (22, 31, 51) has ignited tremendous fear among investigators in the xenotransplantation field and health officials. Active research projects in the field were put under tight scrutiny, moratoriums on this research were proposed, and most of all, future clinical trials of whole organ xenotransplantation were halted, pending further in vitro and animal model data evaluation. While this situation may be considered as of extreme caution, with recent data indicating the unlikelihood that an organism such as PERV can be transmitted into humans by xenografting (49), it is clear that few data are available about the potential of endogenous retrovirus being transmitted and becoming virulent in the transplanted host. This chapter will review the available experience with other endogenous retroviruses in different animal situations, with the aim of better understanding the potential impact of such organisms in the field of xenotransplantation.

Rima Abu-Nader and Carlos V. Paya • Division of Infectious Diseases, Mayo Clinic, 200 First St., SW, Rochester, MN 55905.

EVOLUTION OF ENDOGENOUS RETROVIRUSES: LESSONS FROM THE PAST

Endogenous retroviruses are widely distributed among vertebrate species (Table 1). All mammals that have been examined so far, including pigs and baboons, have endogenous retrovirus DNA sequences integrated in their genomes (6, 11). Although transmitted in the germ line, they exhibit a very significant sequence homology to exogenous retroviruses. The true source of endogenous retroviruses remains to be elucidated. One hypothesis is that they are viral remnants of remote infections with exogenous forms of the virus. Alternative explanations include that retroviruses may be derived from retrotransposons or that endogenous retroviruses are the precursors of exogenous retroviral agents (42–44). In contrast to the horizontal transmission commonly observed with exogenous retroviruses, endogenous retroviruses exhibit a vertical mode of transmission, whereby the viral genome is carried over to the offspring in a Mendelian fashion. They are classified according to morphology as types A, B, C, and D (11). Type A particles are not strict virions, but rather more like retrotransposons, lacking the envelope genes. They are abundantly found in mice and in certain cell types, including mature B cells (9).

Type B particles are represented by the mature virions of mouse mammary tumor virus (MMTV), which was the first mammalian retrovirus to be discovered (6). Mammalian type C viruses, a group of type C retroviruses, include human endogenous retrovirus (HERV-K), PERV, baboon endogenous virus (BaEV), and RD-114 in domestic cats, among others (6).

Long before the xenotransplantation era, several investigators warned about the potential harmful effects of endogenous retroviruses on laboratory experiments, due to their ability for expression and growth in various cell lines, including human cells (48). For instance, BaEV replicates in human cells, reaching high titers of infectious virions, whereas in its natural host, it is only present at a low copy number (5 to 15 copies per cell) and appears to be rather innocuous (46, 47). However, this in vitro observation has not been reproduced in vivo as of yet, and therefore, the implications on xenotransplantation are poorly understood. The first trials of primate-to-human xenotransplantation suggested that, since BaEV was found transiently and only in association with baboon mitochondria in one patient, this argues against reactivation and infection of the human host (3, 27).

Because non-human primates harbor many strains of retrovirus, both endogenous (e.g., BaEV) and exogenous (e.g., simian immunodeficiency virus and simian foamy virus), they fell out of favor as candidate donors for xenotransplantation. Instead, they have become the animal models of choice for xenotransplantation experiments.

In swine, there are approximately 50 integrated copies of type C endogenous retroviruses in their genomes. Porcine cell lines have been shown to produce C-type particles, including the proviruses PERV-A, B, and C, based on differences in their envelope genes (1, 28, 42).

Table 1. Summary of characteristics of different types of endogenous retroviruses

Source of ERV	Average no. of proviral copies per cell/replication in heterologous cells	Xenotropic infection in vivo	Virulence	Oncogenesis
Murine	1,000/+ + + (6, 20)	+ + + (45)	+ + + (20)	Yes (20)
Baboon	5–15/+ + + (46, 47)	? ± (14, 46, 47)	?	No
Porcine	50/+ (22, 31, 51)	?	?	No

While PERV-A and PERV-B were first characterized in a porcine cell line (42), PERV-C was first isolated from miniature swine lymphocytes and swine lymphoma (1, 2). Furthermore, these retroviruses infect human cells in vitro using different host cell receptors. Two pig kidney-derived cell lines, PK-15 and MPK, are both capable of producing porcine endogenous retroviruses in vitro. Yet, these different types of retrovirus differ in cell tropism since only the supernatant from PK-15 cells (containing PERV-A and PERV-B) infected human embryonal kidney cells (HEK293) whereas MPK supernatant (containing PERV-C) did not (28, 32). Primary porcine lymphocytes are also capable of releasing the virus and infecting human cells with experimental induction (51). Moreover, cocultivation of primary porcine endothelial cells with HEK293 cells released virus and infected human cells (24) in the absence of mitogenic stimulation.

ENDOGENOUS RETROVIRUS AS A POTENTIAL PATHOGEN: THEORETICAL CONSIDERATIONS

Recombination and Replication

The majority of endogenous retroviruses act as colonizers in the germ line of the host and are, therefore, defective or, in other words, noninfectious. Reasons underlying this inactivity include the existence of spontaneous deletions and/or point mutations or host-directed cellular mechanisms such as methylation of CG sequences in the provirus leading to the arrest of transcription (6).

The exact functions of the remaining "competent" or partially defective endogenous retroviruses remain enigmatic. It is speculated that, among a number of possible functions, they may enhance the pathogenicity of exogenous retroviruses by the recombination and production of a hybrid virus with altered receptor specificity and species tropism, now capable of infecting a new range of hosts. Therefore, the possibility that a recombinant virus could arise from ERV and human retroviral or even normal genetic sequences, when those two are present in proximity to each other, cannot be underscored. In vitro, ERV sequences have been shown to provide deletion-defective exogenous retroviruses with functional proviral DNA sequences, facilitating their replication in NIH/3T3 cells (50).

In cats, endogenous feline leukemia virus (FeLV) is unable to replicate by itself, but in the presence of exogenous FeLV-A, recombination occurs and highly pathogenic, tumor-inducing viruses are generated (36). Both FeLV-A and a recombinant product between FeLV-A and endogenous sequences have been frequently detected in these tumors. Other examples of replication-competent endogenous retrovirus are type C murine leukemia virus (MLV) and type B MMTV. From the studies of these two retroviruses, a strong association between endogenous retroviruses and tumorigenesis was demonstrated in mice (20). MMTV has been implicated in the induction of mammary adenocarcinomas and T-lymphomas in mice. Although horizontal transmission via milk from the mother is well established, mice that are nursed on virus-free milk still developed mammary tumors (6). The mechanisms leading to these two different types of tumors were long investigated, and recombination was not found to be a prerequisite, but rather MMTV caused disease, while still in its germ-line form, by vertical transmission. Furthermore, it was noted that rearrangements in the long terminal repeat (LTR) region led to changes in tissue specificity from the mammary gland to the T cell, thus manifesting as T-cell lymphomas. There is also firm evidence that endogenous proviruses are involved in the development of spontaneous leukemia in various strains of mice. This time, recombinant viruses, known as mink cell focus-forming viruses, are formed from several endogenous proviruses following a series of complex events (41).

Although the role of endogenous retroviruses in oncogenesis is clearly evident in rodent models, it should be emphasized that most retroviruses do not cause disease. One should also take into account that the murine species is much richer in endogenous retroviruses than, for example, humans and pigs combined (18), which may partly explain the high incidence of disease observed in mice due to these viruses.

Xenotropism

Many endogenous retroviruses are dormant in their native hosts but do replicate, reaching high titers in a heterologous cell line, a phenomenon known as xenotropism. At present, xenotropism cannot be prospectively studied, short of phase III xenotransplantation trials. However, naturally occurring cross-species transmission of ERV during the course of evolution can be used as valid references. A best example for xenotropism would be the sequence of events leading to the existence of the gibbon ape leukemia virus (GALV), an exogenous type C retrovirus. It appears that it has originated from a cross-species infection of gibbons with an endogenous retrovirus of a mouse species (7, 23). Other interesting naturally occurring xenogeneic infections are those in cats of the endogenous feline oncoretroviruses, endogenous FeLV and RD-114, which are thought to be transmitted from Asian mice and Old World monkey ancestors, respectively (14, 46, 47). Apparently, RD-114 bears strong homology to BaEV, confirming speculations that cross-species transmission and subsequent germ-line fixation occurred many years ago, when simians and felines were clustered together in the same habitat (14, 46, 47). Furthermore, it has long been shown that when human tumor xenografts are grown in immunodeficient mice, they become contaminated with mouse ERV (45). Similarly, reverse transcription activity of RD-114 has been detected in a human tumor (rhabdomyosarcoma cells) xenograft that was passaged into a fetal cat (25). One may extrapolate that a reverse situation, where ERV is released from graft to host, may arise in pig-to-human xenotransplantation. Recently, a striking similarity was demonstrated between the sequences of the exogenous gibbon leukemia virus, the koala retrovirus, and PERV, suggesting a horizontal zoonotic transfer across species lines (24).

Endogenous Retrovirus Reactivation

The mechanisms involved in the regulation of expression of endogenous retroviral sequences are largely unknown. A recent study described a full-length endogenous retrovirus that was recovered from the lymphocytes of miniature swine (PERV-MSL), carrying a strong sequence homology to porcine endogenous retroviruses obtained from cell lines. Tissue expression, i.e., the production of transcribed PERV elements, was evident by Northern blot analysis in various porcine organs, except perhaps for fetal brain cells (1, 49). The amount of constitutive expression of PERV by each organ differs, however; these organ-specific differences cannot be translated into clinical relevance. Perhaps the organ that has the largest number of proviral copies would confer the highest risk of viral transmission to the recipient host. The fact remains that most porcine tissues that are of potential use in xenotransplantation contain the full-size PERV transcript, regardless of the number of copies. Therefore, no one tissue or organ can be, at the present moment, considered a superior choice for xenotransplantation.

Immunosuppression

It is well established that a given state of immunosuppression heightens the risk of opportunistic infections and their complications. From experience with human allotransplantation, endogenous viruses (present in the recipient or within the donor organ) may reactivate from latency and cause significant morbidity and mortality in the transplant recipient. In the case of xenotransplantation, the human recipient of an animal organ will be exposed to new potential pathogens that are present in the xenograft. Sequelae related to the time and closeness of contact between discordant cells from the graft and the recipient are totally unpredictable. Although no cases of human infection with endogenous retroviruses have ever been described in the literature, the mere fact that they have now crossed the physical barrier and that they are not kept in check by the immune system, due to ongoing immunosuppression with drugs, makes it a possibility. The species-specificity boundaries that apply to viruses have been deranged in many instances, whereby healthy animal-care workers acquired persistent infection with either simian immunodeficiency or simian foamy virus (both exogenous retroviruses) following occupational exposure (7, 15, 19, 37). Recently, a prevalence of 1.8% for infection with the simian foamy virus (SFV) among laboratory handlers of non-human primates was found (15). There is also growing evidence to support the hypothesis of cross-species transmission of HIV-1 from chimpanzees to humans (12, 52). Even though these viruses are exogenous in nature and despite the fact that no clinical disease or further transmission to the household resulted from these infections, even after 20 years in some cases, it is impossible to predict the same outcome for endogenous retroviruses in immunosuppressed xenotransplant human recipients.

CLINICAL XENOTRANSPLANTATION TRIALS: A LEARNING EXPERIENCE

Overall, experience with xenotransplantation, mainly with whole organ transplantation, has not been, to date, associated with long-term success. Initially, baboons were the favored contenders for organ donation, by virtue of their phylogenetic proximity to humans. The first attempts were carried out with baboon and chimpanzee kidneys (17, 39) and hearts (4, 5). The death rate was high, shortly after the surgical procedure (hours to days), and was attributed to sepsis. The observation that non-human primates are resistant to infection with human immunodeficiency virus (HIV) and hepatitis B led to the transplantation of a baboon liver into an AIDS patient suffering from hepatitis B–induced liver failure in 1992 (38). A second baboon-liver xenotransplantation was subsequently performed on another patient (40). Survival rate did not exceed 70 days in both instances, with death occurring as a result of infectious complications. In a retrospective analysis of tissue specimens obtained from those two patients after the liver transplantation, BaEV as well as SIV and SFV were detected in different tissue compartments, along with baboon mitochondrial DNA (3). The presence of the latter, which may be indicative of a latency state rather than a true infection, raises a significant concern.

Pancreatic islet cells from pigs were implanted as an attempt to treat 10 patients with diabetes in Sweden, none of whom has developed PERV infection yet (13, 16). Ex vivo pig-liver perfusion has also been used as a bridge to human organ transplantation in a small series of patients with end-stage liver disease (8). Again, survival time was short to allow further evaluation. More recently, clinical studies using porcine cells to treat many diseases, including neurodegenerative diseases (e.g., porcine ventral mesencephalic cells for Parkinson's disease patients) and focal epilepsy, are currently in phase II trials, and the data so far indicate no transmission of PERV to human recipients (49). Reports reflecting the absence of PERV infection in a variety of porcine tissue xenografts in humans are accumulating. Serum samples from 160 patients who had received different types of living pig tissues, some dating back to a decade ago, tested negative for PERV by reverse transcriptase–polymerase chain reaction and immunoblot analysis (29). Furthermore, serial molecular and serological testing of blood samples from two patients with short-term extracorporeal connection to pig kidneys failed to detect PERV DNA and PERV-specific antibodies, respectively (30).

Data presented at the last xenotransplantation subcommittee meeting in June 1999 consistently showed that all specimens tested for PERV were negative by sensitive detection assays. Specimens that were examined came from human hosts of pig islet and neural cells, as well as from non-human primate recipients of different organs. Separate data obtained from hemophiliac patients who regularly receive transfusions of porcine factor 8 had no evidence of PERV infection, even though all preparations of the clotting factor tested positive prior to administration (data communicated at the Xenotransplantation Subcommittee, Bethesda, Md., June 3–4, 1999). In concert with previous observations, these new data illustrate once again the point that what is observed in vitro does not always correlate with events in vivo.

CONCLUSIONS

The initial enthusiasm, triggered by the concept and potential clinical usefulness of xenotransplantation, was somehow deflated by the potential pathogenicity of PERV in in vitro experiments. This concern, while raising a significant number of questions, has been somehow counteracted by the recent studies in humans in whom no evidence of PERV has been noted. However, the possibility of the infectious potential of endogenous retroviruses in xenotransplantation cannot be truly addressed unless properly designed human trials are in place. From the cumulated data on organ xenotransplantation so far, although mostly reassuring, the margin of safety continues to appear thin. Because of the ubiquitous nature of endogenous retroviruses, it is inconceivable to eliminate the reservoir that is present in the animal genome. Further studies of these viruses and attempts to sort out defective from partially defective proviral DNA will help stratify the potential risk of xenotropism and pathogenicity. In addition, caution should be exercised when clinical whole organ xenotransplantation trials are initiated. It would then be imperative to initiate post-xenotransplant surveillance to maximize early recognition of xenogeneic infection, which can be achieved by periodic testing for PERV, specimen archiving, close-contact education, and lifestyle restrictions. Close follow-up and observation should be undertaken for many years after xenotransplantation because of the predictable long latency state of these viruses.

New animal viruses are being discovered on a regular basis, as detection methods are becoming more sophisticated. Several new identifications of porcine viruses have been made that include a porcine torovirus, a swine hepatitis E virus, and two gamma-herpesviruses (10, 21, 26); this probably represents the tip of the iceberg. Similarly, many more animal endogenous retroviruses are yet to be discovered and fully characterized.

On the basis of available evidence so far, a general conclusion about the medical impacts of endogenous retroviruses, on the xenotransplant human recipient and the community at large, cannot be reached at this time.

REFERENCES

1. **Akiyoshi, D. E., M. Denaro, H. Zhu, J. L. Greenstein, P. Banerjee, and J. Fishman.** 1998. Identification of a full-length cDNA for an endogenous retrovirus of miniature swine. *J. Virol.* **72:**4503–4507.
2. **Akiyoshi, D. E., I. Suzuka, N. Shimizu, K. Sekiguchi, H. Hoshino, M. Kodama, and K. Shimotohno.** 1986. Molecular cloning of unintegrated closed circular DNA of porcine retrovirus. *FEBS Lett.* **198:**339–343.
3. **Allan, J. S., S. R. Broussard, M. G. Michaels, T. E. Starzl, K. L. Leighton, E. M. Whitehead, A. G. Comuzzie, R. E. Lanford, M. M. Leland, W. M. Switzer, and W. Heneine.** 1998. Amplification of simian retroviral sequences from human recipients of baboon liver transplants. *AIDS Res. Hum. Retrov.* **14:**82111–82114.
4. **Bailey, L. L., S. L. Nehlsen-Cannarella, W. Concepcion, and W. B. Jolley.** 1985. Baboon-to-human cardiac xenotransplantation in a neonate. *JAMA* **254:**3321–3329.
5. **Barnard, C. N., A. Wolpowitz, and J. G. Losman.** 1977. Heterotopic cardiac transplantation with a xenograft for assistance of the left heart in cardiogenic shock after cardiopulmonary bypass. *S. Afr. Med. J.* **52:**1035–1039.
6. **Boeke, J. D., and J. P. Stoye.** 1997. Retrotransposons, endogenous retroviruses, and the evolution of retroelements, p. 343–435. *In* J. M. Coffin, S. H. Hughes, and H. E. Varmus (ed.), *Retroviruses.* Cold Spring Harbor Press, Cold Spring Harbor, N.Y.
7. **Brown, J., A. L. Matthews, P. A. Sandstrom, and L. E. Chapman.** 1998. Xenotransplantation and the risk of retroviral zoonosis. *Trends Microbiol.* **6:**411–415.
8. **Chari, R. S., B. H. Collins, J. C. Magee, M. DiMaio, A. D. Kirk, R. C. Harland, R. L. McCann, J. L. Platt, and W. C. Meyers.** 1994. Brief report: treatment of hepatic failure with ex-vivo pig-liver perfusion followed by liver transplantation. *N. Engl. J. Med.* **331:**234–237.
9. **Coffin, J. M.** 1992. Structure and classification of retroviruses, p. 19–49. *In* J. A. Levy (ed.), *The Retroviridae,* vol. 1. Plenum Press, New York, N.Y.
10. **Ehlers, B., S. Ulrich, and M. Goltz.** 1999. Detection of two novel porcine herpesviruses with high similarity to gammaherpesviruses. *J. Gen. Virol.* **80**(PT4)**:**971–978.
11. **Friedlander, A., and R. Patarca.** 1999. Endogenous proviruses. *Crit. Rev. Oncol.* **10:**129–159.
12. **Gao, F., E. Bailes, D. L. Robertson, Y. Chen, C. M. Rodenburg, S. F. Michael, L. B. Cummins, L. O. Arthur, M. Peeters, G. M. Shaw, P. M. Sharp, and B. H. Hahn.** 1999. Origin of HIV-1 in the chimpanzee *Pan troglodytes troglodytes. Nature* **397:**436–441.
13. **Groth, C. G., O. Korsgren, A. Tibell, J. Tollemar, E. Moller, J. Bolinder, J. Ostman, F. P. Reinholt, C. Hellerstrom, and A. Andersson.** 1994. Transplantation of porcine fetal pancreas to diabetic patients. *Lancet* **344:**1402–1404.
14. **Hardy, W. D.** 1993. Feline oncoretroviruses, p. 109–180. *In* J. A. Levy (ed.), *The Retroviridae,* vol. 2. Plenum Press, New York, N.Y.
15. **Heneine, W., W. M. Switzer, P. Sandstrom, J. Brown, S. Vedapuri, C. A. Schable, A. S. Khan, N. W. Lerche, M. Schweizer, D. Neumann-Haefelin, L. E. Chapman, and T. M. Folks.** 1998. Identification of a human population infected with simian foamy viruses. *Nature Med.* **4:**403–407.
16. **Heneine, W., A. Tibell, W. M. Switzer, P. Sandstrom, G. V. Rosales, A. Mathews, O. Korsgren, L. E. Chapman, T. M. Folks, and C. G. Groth.** 1998. No evidence of infection with porcine endogenous retrovirus in recipients of porcine islet-cell xenografts. *Lancet* **352:**695–699.
17. **Hitchcock, C. R., J. C. Kiser, R. L. Telander, and E. L. Seljeskog.** 1964. Baboon renal grafts. *JAMA* **189:**158–161.
18. **Isacson, O., and X. O. Breakefield.** 1997. Benefits and risks of hosting animal cells in the human brain. *Nature Med.* **3:**964–969.
19. **Khabbaz, R. F., W. Heneine, J. R. George, B. Parekh, T. Woods, W. M. Switzer, H. M. McClure,**

M. Murphey-Corb, and T. M. Folks. 1994. Brief report: infection of a laboratory worker with simian immunodeficieny virus. *N. Engl. J. Med.* **330:**172–177.

20. **Kozak, C. A., and S. Ruscetti.** 1992. Retroviruses in rodents, p. 405–481. *In* J. A. Levy (ed.), *The Retroviridae*, vol. 1. Plenum Press, New York, N.Y.
21. **Kroneman, A., L. A. H. M. Cornelissen, M. C. Horzinek, R. J. de Groot, and H. F. Egberink.** 1998. Identification and characterization of a porcine torovirus. *J. Virol.* **72:**3507–3511.
22. **Le Tissier, P., J. P. Stoye, Y. Takeuchi, C. Patience, and R. A. Weiss.** 1997. Two sets of human-tropic pig retrovirus. *Nature* **389:**681–682.
23. **Lieber, M. M., C. J. Sherr, G. J. Torado, R. E. Benveniste, R. Callahan, and H. G. Coon.** 1975. Isolation from the Asian mouse *Mus caroli* of an endogenous type C virus related to infectious primate type C viruses. *Proc. Natl. Acad. Sci. USA* **72:**2315–2319.
24. **Martin, J., E. Herniou, J. Cook, R. W. O'Neill, and M. Tristem.** 1999. Interclass transmission and phyletic host tracking in murine leukemia virus-related retroviruses. *J. Virol.* **73:**2442–2449.
25. **McAllister, R. M., M. Nicolson, M. B. Gardner, R. W. Rongey, S. Rasheed, P. S. Sarma, R. J. Huebner, M. Hatanaka, S. Oroszlan, R. V. Gilden, A Kabigting, and L. Vernon.** 1972. C-type virus released from cultured human rhabdomyosarcoma cells. *Nature New Biol.* **235:**3–6.
26. **Meng, X.-J., R. H. Purcell, P. G. Halbur, J. R. Lehman, D. M. Webb, T. S. Tsareva, J. S. Haynes, B. J. Thacker, and S. U. Emerson.** 1997. A novel virus in swine is closely related to the human hepatitis E virus. *Proc. Natl. Acad. Sci. USA* **94:**9860–9865.
27. **Michaels, M. G.** 1997. Infectious concerns of cross-species transplantation: xenozoonoses. *World J. Surg.* **21:**968–974.
28. **Onions, D., D. Hart, C. Mahoney, D. Galbraith, and K. Smith.** 1998. Endogenous retroviruses and the safety of porcine xenotransplantation. *Trends Microbiol.* **6:**430–431.
29. **Paradis, K., G. Langford, Z. Long, W. Heneine, P. Sandstrom, W. M. Switzer, L. E. Chapman, C. Lockey, D. Onions, the XEN 111 Study Group, and E. Otto.** 1999. Search for cross-species transmission of porcine endogenous retrovirus in patients treated with living pig tissue. *Science* **285:**1236–1241.
30. **Patience, C., G. S. Patton, Y. Takeuchi, R. A. Weiss, M. O. McClure, L. Rydberg, and M. E. Breimer.** 1998. No evidence of pig DNA or retroviral infection in patients with short-term extracorporeal connection to pig kidneys. *Lancet* **352:**699–701.
31. **Patience, C., Y. Takeuchi, and R. A. Weiss.** 1997. Infection of human cells by an endogenous retrovirus of pigs. *Nature Med.* **3:**282–286.
32. **Patience, C., Y. Takeuchi, and R. A. Weiss.** 1998. Zoonosis in xenotransplantation. *Curr. Opin. Immunol.* **10:**539–542.
33. **Platt, J. L.** 1994. A perspective on xenograft rejection and accomodation. *Immunol. Rev.* **141:**127–149.
34. **Platt, J. L.** 1998. New directions for organ transplantation. *Nature* **392:**11–17.
35. **Reemtsma, K., B. H. McCracken, J. U. Schlegel, M. A. Pearl, C. W. Pearce, C. W. DeWitt, P. E. Smith, R. L. Hewitt, R. L. Flinner, and O. Creech, Jr.** 1964. Renal heterotransplantation in man. *Ann. Surg.* **160:**384–410.
36. **Rosenberg, N., and P. Jolicoeur.** 1997. Retroviral pathogenesis, p. 475–585. *In* J. M. Coffin, S. H. Hughes, and H. E. Varmus (ed.), *Retroviruses.* Cold Spring Harbor Press, Cold Spring Harbor, N.Y.
37. **Schweizer, M., V. Falcone, J. Gange, R. Turek, and D. Neumann-Haefelin.** 1997. Simian foamy virus isolated from an accidentally infected human individual. *J. Virol.* **71:**4821–4824.
38. **Starzl, T. E., J. Fung, A. Tzakis, S. Todo, A. J. Demetris, I. R. Marino, H. Doyle, A. Zeevi, V. Warty, M. Michaels, S. Kusne, W. A. Rudert, and M. Trucco.** 1993. Baboon-to-human liver transplantation. *Lancet* **341:**65–71.
39. **Starzl, T. E., T. L. Marchioro, G. N. Peters, C. H. Kirkpatrick, W. E. C. Wilson, K. A. Porter, D. Rifkind, D. A. Ogden, C. R. Hitchcock, and W. R. Waddell.** 1964. Renal heterotransplantation from baboon to man: experience with 6 cases. *Transplantation* **2:**752–776.
40. **Starzl, T. E., A. Tzakis, J. J. Fung, S. Todo, A. J. Demetris, R. Manez, I. R. Marino, L. Valdivia, and N. Murase.** 1994. Prospects of clinical xenotransplantation. *Transplant. Proc.* **26:**1082.
41. **Stoye, J. P., C. Moroni, and J. M. Coffin.** 1991. Virological events leading to spontaneous AKR thymomas. *J. Virol.* **65:**1273–1285.
42. **Takeuchi, Y., C. Patience, S. Magre, R. A. Weiss, P. T. Banerjee, P. Le Tissier, and J. P. Stoye.** 1998. Host range and interference studies of three classes of pig endogenous retrovirus. *J. Virol.* **72:**9986–9991.
43. **Temin, H. M.** 1980. Origin of retroviruses from cellular moveable genetic elements. *Cell* **21:**599–600.

44. **Temin, H. M.** 1992. Origin and general nature of retroviruses, p.1–18. *In* J. A. Levy (ed.), *The Retroviridae,* vol. 1. Plenum Press, New York, N.Y.
45. **Tralka, T. S., C. L. Yee, A. B. Rabson, N. A. Wivel, K. J. Stromberg, A. S. Rabson, and J. C. Costa.** 1983. Murine type C retroviruses and intracisternal A-particles in human tumors serially passaged in nude mice. *J. Natl. Cancer Inst.* **71:**591–596.
46. **van der Kuyl, A. C., J. T. Dekker, and J. Goudsmit.** 1996. Baboon endogenous virus evolution and ecology. *Trends Microbiol.* **4:**55–59.
47. **van der Kuyl, A. C., J. T. Dekker, and J. Goudsmit.** 1995. Full-length proviruses of baboon endogenous virus (BaEV) and dispersed reverse transcriptase retroelements in the genome of baboon species. *J. Virol.* **69:**5917–5924.
48. **Weiss, R. A.** 1978. Why cell biologists should be aware of genetically transmitted viruses. *Natl. Cancer Inst. Monogr.* **48:**183–189.
49. **Weiss, R. A.** 1999. Xenografts and retroviruses. *Science* **285:**1221–1222.
50. **Wilkinson, D. A., D. L. Mager, and J. A. C. Leong.** 1994. Endogenous human retroviruses, p. 465–535. *In* J. A. Levy (ed.), *The Retroviridae,* vol. 3. Plenum Press, New York, N.Y.
51. **Wilson, C. A., S. Wong, J. Muller, C. E. Davidson, T. M. Rose, and P. Burd.** 1998. Type C retrovirus released from porcine primary peripheral blood mononuclear cells infects human cells. *J. Virol.* **72:**3082–3087.
52. **Zhu, T., B. T. Korber, A. J. Nahmias, E. Hooper, P. M. Sharp, and D. D. Ho.** 1998. An African HIV-1 sequence from 1959 and implications for the origin of the epidemic. *Nature* **391:**594–597.

Xenotransplantation
Edited by Jeffrey L. Platt

Chapter 15

Prevention of Infection in Xenotransplantation

Jay A. Fishman

Infection and cancer are the major complications of the long-term immune suppression used to prevent the rejection of transplanted organs and tissues (23). Infection develops as a result of exposure to organisms derived from the environment, from the graft, and via the activation of latent infections carried by the graft recipient. The most common malignancies in the transplant recipient, including the post-transplantation lymphoproliferative disorders (largely B-cell lymphomas), squamous cell carcinoma, cervical carcinoma, and hepatoma, also have an association with previous viral infection. As in allotransplantation, the risk of infection in xenotransplantation is a function of the nature and intensity of exposures to potential pathogens, the native virulence of these organisms, and the immune deficits present in the recipient. Because immunosuppressed individuals tolerate established infection poorly, the prevention of infection is critical to the ultimate success of clinical transplantation (22, 23). The aspect of infectious risk that is unique in xenotransplantation is the potential exposure of the recipient and, subsequently, the general population to novel infectious agents derived from non-human species (21, 59, 101).

The central hypothesis for this discussion is that some of the infectious risks associated with xenotransplantation can be assessed before the broad application of this emerging technology. The ability to characterize novel human pathogens in preclinical models or from clinical xenotransplant recipients will facilitate the development of strategies for the prevention of infection, including antimicrobial prophylaxis and exclusion of potential pathogens during animal husbandry. Such microbiological data will serve to enhance the safety of clinical xenotransplantation and may also have implications for studies of infection in allograft recipients.

BACKGROUND: INFECTION IN ALLOTRANSPLANTATION

In contrast with the natural spread of infection between species (zoonosis), transplantation poses a unique epidemiologic hazard due to the efficiency of transmission of pathogens, particularly viruses, with viable cellular grafts. The risk of infection in transplantation is determined by the interaction of two factors: the pathogens to which the individual is exposed

Jay A. Fishman • Infectious Disease Division and Transplantation Unit, Massachusetts General Hospital and Harvard Medical School, Boston, MA 02114.

(epidemiologic exposures) and a measure of the individual's susceptibility to infection (net state of immunosuppression) (1–3, 23). The relationship between these factors is semiquantitative. Thus, any manipulation that allows the use of lesser amounts of exogenous immune suppression (e.g., tolerance induction) may be expected to reduce the risk of infection.

Epidemiologic exposures in the transplant recipient take two forms: those occurring within the hospital or the community, and those exposures carried with the transplanted organ. Within the community, acute exposures include respiratory viruses; foodborne pathogens including *Salmonella* spp., *Listeria monocytogenes*, and *Campylobacter jejuni*; and remote and current exposures to such organisms as the geographically restricted systemic mycoses (*Blastomyces dermatitidis*, *Coccidioides immitis*, and *Histoplasma capsulatum*), *Mycobacterium tuberculosis*, and *Strongyloides stercoralis* (1, 5, 7). Within the hospital, exposures occur on the hospital unit where the patient is housed and during travel to clinical procedures (e.g., surgery, radiology). Nosocomial infections reflect contamination of the air or potable water supply with pathogens such as *Aspergillus* spp., *Legionella* spp., or gram-negative bacilli such as *Pseudomonas aeruginosa*, and by person-to-person spread or via contaminated equipment by vancomycin-resistant *Enterococcus faecium*, methicillin-resistant *Staphylococcus aureus*, and *Clostridium difficile*. By contrast, exposures to organisms in xenotransplantation depend on knowledge of previous exposures of the donor animal or herd to pathogens that are then carried to the recipient. These organisms must then replicate within the xenograft; the likelihood of significant infection is enhanced by the immunosuppressed status of the host.

The net state of immunosuppression is a function of multiple factors, the most important of which are the nature of the immunosuppressive therapy (the dose, duration, and temporal sequence of individual agents); the presence or absence of infection with the immunomodulating viruses, most notably cytomegalovirus (CMV), but also including Epstein-Barr virus (EBV), hepatitis B and C (HBV and HCV), and the human immunodeficiency virus (HIV). The residua of technical complications (e.g., devitalized or injured tissues, undrained fluid collections, and the need for indwelling drains and vascular or urinary catheters) from the transplant operation also contribute to the risk of infection. The sum of these factors constitutes the patient's net state of immunosuppression. In xenotransplantation, the same factors apply, with added consideration of the novel immune modifications that may be made to either the donor or the recipient and of the histocompatibility disparity of donor and host, which may affect immune function and/or the pathogenesis of infection in an unpredictable manner.

Timeline of Infections: Known Pathogens after Xenotransplantation

As immunosuppressive regimens for allotransplantation have become more standardized, it has become apparent that common infections occur in a predictable pattern at different points in the post-transplant course (23). The resultant timeline of expected infections reflects the predictable course of immunosuppression and common epidemiologic exposures of the allograft recipient. The timeline is modified by alterations in maintenance immunosuppression due to treatment of graft rejection or graft-versus-host disease or by periods of prolonged neutropenia (e.g., following bone marrow transplantation or due to drug toxicity). Immune suppression in xenotransplantation will vary with the type of graft (e.g., cells vs. vascularized organ), the use of source animals modified by genetic engineering, modification of the recipient by tolerance induction or antibody depletion, or other treatments in addition to pharmacologic immune suppression, resulting in changes in the relative risk of infection over time.

On the basis of experience with human allograft recipients and with immunosuppressed miniature swine, common infections in the first month after xenotransplantation are likely to be due to bacteria and fungi common to swine and to primates: staphylococci, streptococci, *Candida* spp., *Aspergillus* spp., *Salmonella* spp., and *Actinomyces* spp., which are routinely isolated from swine and from non-human primates (45, 47, 84, 85). These common pathogens are likely to cause clinically recognizable syndromes when they occur. Microbiological assays are available for the detection of these organisms, whether they occur in human or non-human hosts or tissues.

After the first month post-transplant, a broad spectrum of latent pathogens may emerge in the setting of persistent immune suppression or immune reactivity. The specific infections observed will reflect the epidemiology of the host and the graft and the ultimate level of immune suppression needed to maintain xenograft function in the human host. A major factor in the risk of infection is the presence or absence of immunomodulating viral infection. These are particularly troublesome in transplantation because of the frequency of latent carriage by viable tissue grafts. In the transplant recipient, viral infection has been associated with viral syndromes (flu-like or mononucleosis-like illness) or direct tissue injury (retinitis, hepatitis); graft injury (e.g., nephritis, carditis, pneumonitis); development of graft rejection; and systemic immunosuppression, which predisposes to other opportunistic infections (e.g., *Pneumocystis carinii*, *Aspergillus* spp., or *Nocardia asteroides*); or it may contribute to the development of malignancy. In allotransplantation, the major pathogen of this group is human cytomegalovirus (HCMV). Other viruses important to transplantation include herpes simplex and varicella viruses, EBV, human herpes virus 6, hepatitis viruses (notably B and C), adenovirus, respiratory syncytial virus, parvovirus, and influenza and parainfluenza viruses. Human immunodeficiency virus (HIV-1 and -2) and human T-cell lymphotropic virus (HTLV1) have, until recently, been considered relative contraindications to transplantation.

In the xenograft recipient, CMV infections will depend on the presence or absence of latent virus in the human recipient (measured serologically) and the donor species; for example, porcine CMV (PCMV) or primate CMV (e.g., cercopithicine herpesvirus 3 of baboons or SA6). Given the limited host range (species specificity) of the herpesviruses, CMV might be expected to infect only tissues from the native species. A porcine gammaherpesvirus has also been identified. Other herpesviruses, adenovirus, papillomavirus, and the hepatitis viruses are also likely to emerge, with the species specificity of each remaining to be determined (10, 14, 15, 20, 37, 66, 72, 80). In the xenograft recipient, as in allotransplant recipients, the ultimate effects of viral infection will reflect the type of virus and the tissues infected. The ability of a virus derived from non-human species to cause infection in humans outside the xenograft cannot be predicted with assurance.

In addition to viral pathogens, and regardless of whether the source species is swine or primate, emerging opportunistic infections may include mycobacterial species, *Brucella* spp. (*abortus* and *suis*), and *Leptospira* sp., as well as systemic fungal infections caused by *Candida* sp., *Mucor* sp., and *Cryptococcus* sp., and the geographic fungi including *Histoplasma capsulatum*. In addition to these common infections, swine and primates are susceptible to many common human zoonotic parasitic infections, some of which are caused by major pathogens in the immunocompromised human host: *Toxoplasma gondii*, *Strongyloides stercoralis*, coccidial species (*Isospora belli*, *Isospora suis*, and *Cryptosporidium parvum*),

Table 1. Nonrecognition of infection associated with xenograft transplantation

Previously unknown or unrecognized pathogens
New syndromes or altered clinical manifestations in the transplant recipient
Low incidence or scattered or sporadic cases
Masked symptoms due to coinfection with other opportunistic pathogens
Absence of specific diagnostic tests for animal-derived organisms
High background rate of opportunistic infection
Common syndromes (respiratory, liver, gastrointestinal)
Latency or carrier (colonization) state

Babesia sp., and *Trypanosoma* sp. Microbiologic assays exist for these common pathogens. However, serologic tests developed for use in humans are not likely to be useful in screening source animals for latent infection with these pathogens; species-appropriate assays must be developed.

Relative Infectious Risk in Xenotransplantation versus Allotransplantation

A number of factors serve to increase the risk of infection in xenotransplantation beyond that associated with allotransplantation. (i) The xenograft itself serves as a permissive focus from which organisms gain access to and may persist in the human host, avoiding the need for a vector to achieve disease transmission. (ii) There is a deficiency in microbiologic data regarding the behavior of novel pathogens from donor species in humans. In particular, there may be organisms that may infect the human xenograft recipient but may not cause disease in the native host species (i.e., xenotropic organisms). Further, there may be organisms that acquire new characteristics (genetic recombination or mutation) within the xeno-host (40, 41, 44, 68, 87). (iii) Clinical laboratory testing for most organisms derived from non-human species is not generally available (e.g., antibodies, molecular probes, or culture systems for species-specific organisms, or serologic tests for human antibodies against animal pathogens). (iv) Novel clinical syndromes may result from infection by new pathogens in the immunocompromised host; these syndromes may not be recognized by the clinician (see Table 1). (v) Clinical manifestations may be muted by the immune suppression needed to maintain xenograft function. (vi) The high, intrinsic rate of infection in transplant recipients (e.g., pulmonary, gastrointestinal, and urinary tract syndromes; surgical complications; nosocomial infections) may mask the presence of novel infection. (vii) The recipient may lack preexisting immunity to novel pathogens, making the host more susceptible to infection. (viii) Species disparity of histocompatibility antigens may be associated with diminished cellular immune function by the host against organisms within the xenograft (22).

LESSONS OF ZOONOTIC EXPOSURES

Given the prolonged exposure of humans to both swine and primates, some data regarding the transmissibility of infection between species should be available. Few prospective data exist. Studies in non-human primates have focused on investigations of epidemics (AIDS, Ebola virus, Marburg virus) or on laboratory accidents and accidental exposures (splashes, bites) with laboratory animals. Some of these exposures have been considered under the rubric of emerging infections, as discussed by the Institute of Medicine (38). Many primate-borne pathogens are capable of infecting humans (Table 2). Some, such as foamy virus, are apparently without symptomatic sequelae, while B virus encephalitis is fatal unless treated appropriately (30). At present, primates have been excluded as xenograft donors in the United States.

A number of accidental human exposures to animal-derived viruses have been reported. One well-characterized exposure was the contamination of the Salk polio vaccine virus and adenovirus vaccines with simian virus 40 (SV40). SV40 was secreted by the rhesus monkey cells used to grow vaccine strains of virus. SV40 was undetected because the virus causes no cytopathic effect in the monkey cell lines used for vaccine production. SV40, an oncogenic agent in monkeys, was ingested by or injected into over one million individuals without adverse effects on morbidity or mortality, including leukemia or other forms of carcinoma up to 10 years following exposure (25, 78, 91). Careful analysis is complicated by the presence of cross-reacting antigens for serologic testing and by the relatively short follow-up period. More recent data suggest a possibly increased frequency of SV40 DNA sequence in mesothelioma (9). There are no data to support a role for such exposures in the development of HIV and AIDS (as has been suggested in the lay press). However, human infections due to non-human primate viruses have been well documented with regard to Marburg virus from African green monkey kidneys used for vaccine production, herpes B virus, and simian immunodeficiency virus. This topic is discussed further below.

The relative paucity of sequence data on viral organisms of swine makes it difficult to assess the amount or frequency of incorporation of porcine sequences or porcine retroviral sequences into the human genome. The suggestion that the exchange of genetic information is ongoing is supported by homologies between genomic sequences of humans and of non-human primates. One recent example is the similarity of sequences of *Herpesvirus saimiri* and of the EBV BLDF1 gene to unique sequences found in human Kaposi's sarcoma tissues (11). It should be noted that these are large DNA viruses, not retroviruses. The integration of foreign sequences into human genomes would appear to be a long-standing, ongoing event. It seems likely that long-term physical and environmental contacts (e.g., via mosquitoes, retroviruses, respiratory viruses, transfusions, ingestion) have already resulted in the entry of non-human sequences into the human gene pool. Further epidemiologic data are needed in this area.

Many organisms found in swine have also been associated with infection in humans (Table 3). In considering infections likely to cause disease in xenograft recipients, a number of swine–human contacts may be instructive: Swine-derived infections of humans due to occupational exposures (breeders, meat handlers) or ingestion; the impact of exposures to animal-derived products (e.g., heart valves, vascular grafts, skin xenografts, temporary xenografts, insulin) or infection (swine influenza); and unexpected infections in human transplantation recipients.

Infections in Immunocompromised Miniature Swine and Non-Human Primates

Bacteria and Fungi

Miniature swine have been developed for studies of transplantation immunology and are being developed commercially as potential organ donors for humans (57, 73, 90). Infections have been studied in these animals and in non-human primates (baboons and macaque monkeys) following bone marrow and solid organ transplantation. Each animal receives

Table 2. Infectious considerations for non-human primates in xenotransplantation[a]

Herpesviruses[b]
Herpesvirus simiae (B virus, *Herpesvirus cercopithecus* 1)
Herpes simplex 1 and 2
SA8 (African, *Herpesvirus cercopithecus* 2)
Herpesvirus tamarinus (New World)
Herpesvirus saimiri (New World)
Epstein-Barr virus (EBV)
Varicella-zoster (human, simian)
Cytomegalovirus (rhesus, chimpanzee, SA6-African)
Herpesvirus papio 2 (simian EBV)
SA12
Human herpesvirus 8
Retroviruses[b]
Simian viruses (SRV 1–5)
Simian T-cell leukemia virus (STLV-1)
Simian immunodeficiency virus (macaque, green monkey, sooty mangabey)
HIV-1, -2 (human immunodeficiency virus)
Baboon endogenous virus (type C, SRV type D)
Other viruses[b]
Rubeola (measles)
Rubella
Adenovirus
Influenza A, B
Respiratory syncytial virus
SV40 (parvovirus)
SV5 (parainfluenza)
Lymphocytic choriomeningitis (arenavirus)
Monkeypox (also epidermal monkeypox, Yaba, tanapox)
Molluscum, smallpox
Foamy virus (spumavirus)
Rabies (vesicular stomatitis virus)
Parvovirus B19
Arboviruses
Filoviruses (Ebola, Marburg, simian hemorrhagic fever virus)
Hepatitis A, B, C, E
Reovirus
Dengue, yellow fever (Flavivirus)
Picornavirus (coxsackie, poliovirus)
Encephalomyocarditis
Polyoma
Bacteria
Mycobacterium (*tuberculosis*, *leprae*, *intracellulare*, *scrofulaceum*)
Brucella spp.
Salmonella spp.
Leptospira spp.
Pseudomonas pseudomallei
Yersinia spp.
Treponema spp. (syphilis, yaws, pinta)
Antibiotic-resistant organisms
Clostridium tetani
Neisseria (*gonorrhoeae*, *meningiditis*)

Table 2. *Continued*

Parasites
Toxoplasma sp.
Strongyloides sp.
Filariasis
Isospora belli
Schistosoma sp.
Trypanosoma sp.
Leishmania sp.
Cryptosporidium sp.
Babesia sp.
Plasmodium sp. (malaria)
Fungi
Histoplasma spp.
Aspergillus spp.
Nocardia spp.
Coccidioides spp.
Cryptococcus spp.
Mucor spp.
Pneumocystis spp.
Other
Rickettsiae
Mycoplasma spp.
Prions

[a] Appropriate to species.
[b] Not all organisms are known to be associated with human infection or disease.

intensive clinical care through periods of neutropenia, graft rejection, graft-versus-host disease, immune suppression with cyclosporine A, corticosteroids and other immunosuppressive therapies, and following the induction of tolerance to the donor using bone marrow xenografts (in collaboration with Dr. David H. Sachs, Transplantation Biology Research Center, Massachusetts General Hospital, Boston). All graft recipients receive prophylaxis with first-generation cephalosporin in the perioperative period and daily fluoroquinolone antimicrobial agent (ofloxacin, orally or via gastrostomy tube) and oral Nystatin (bid) during immune suppression and/or total white blood cell counts (WBC) of less than 1,000/mm^3. In addition, bone marrow transplant recipients receive trimethoprim-sulfamethoxazole for 7 days before transplantation. Screening cultures of mouth, nares, and rectum are obtained quarterly from all animals in the colony. In addition, in any animals demonstrating evidence of infection (fever, elevated WBC, wound infection), blood and urine cultures are obtained, and cultures are obtained from potentially infected sites (e.g., surgical incisions, intravenous catheters, gastrostomy tubes).

During a period before the initiation of the described regimen, animals received antimicrobial prophylaxis with broad-spectrum antibiotics including piperacillin and gentamicin. Multiple infections related to surgical sites and intravenous catheters developed due to gram-negative bacteria resistant to multiple antimicrobial agents including *Klebsiella pneumoniae* and *P. aeruginosa.* In addition, bacteremic infections were demonstrated to be due to *Enterococcus faecalis*, *S. aureus*, *Streptococcus suis*, *Actinomyces pyogenes*, *Pasteurella multocida*, and *Candida albicans*—all common cutaneous colonizing flora of

Table 3. Microbial agents of swine known to cause infection in humans

Bacteria
Actinobacillus spp.
Actinomyces pyogenes
Bacillus anthracis
Brucella suis
Campylobacter coli
Campylobacter jejuni
Chlamydia psittaci
Clostridium perfringens
Clostridium septicum
Clostridium tetani
Erysipelothrix rhusiopathiae
Haemophilus spp.
Listeria monocytogenes
Mycobacterium avium complex
Mycobacterium bovis
Mycobacterium tuberculosis
Pasteurella multocida
Pseudomonas aeruginosa
Pseudomonas pseudomallei
Salmonella enterica serovar Choleraesuis
Salmonella enterica serovar Enteritidis
Salmonella enterica serovar Typhimurium
Shigella spp.
Staphylococcus aureus
Streptococcus group E
Streptococcus pneumoniae
Streptococcus suis
Yersinia enterocolitica
Yersinia pseudotuberculosis
Viruses
Encephalomyocarditis virus
Foot-and-mouth disease virus
Parainfluenza virus-1
Rabies virus
Swine influenza virus (H_1N_1, H_3N_2)
Fungi
Aspergillus spp.
Candida albicans
Coccidioides immitis
Cryptococcus neoformans
Histoplasma capsulatum
Microsporum nanum (ringworm)
Nocardia asteroides
Petriellidium boydii
Pneumocystis carinii (possibly species specific)
Prototheca spp. (algae)
Zygomycetes (*Mucor, Rhizopus, Absida*)
Parasites (protozoa/helminths)
Ascaris suum
Cryptosporidium sp.
Gnathostoma spinigerum
Isospora sp.
Paragonimus westermani
Sarcocystis suihominis
Spirometra sp.
Schistosoma japonicum
Toxoplasma gondii
Trichinella spiralis

swine and in each case related to wound or catheter-site infections. Screening cultures from asymptomatic, normal swine also revealed all of these organisms (in addition to antibiotic-resistant *Escherichia coli* and anaerobic bacteria) by 5 to 7 days following entry into the colony.

Following restriction of the routine use of broad-spectrum antimicrobial agents (including antifungals), routine isolation of antibiotic-resistant bacteria from mouth, nares, and rectum has been eliminated. Gram-negative aerobic bacteria are no longer isolated in oral and nasal cultures. *E. coli, Candida* sp., *Actinomyces* sp., and *Pasteurella* sp. are routinely isolated from the skin, rectum, and nares of normal and prophylaxed swine.

A variety of cultured organisms isolated from immunosuppressed swine could not be completely speciated by the Clinical Microbiology Laboratory of the Massachusetts General Hospital. These swine-specific organisms included aerobic *Streptococcus* sp., *Haemophilus* sp., *Campylobacter* sp., and *Pasteurella* sp. and many anaerobic streptococci. Human serologic testing to porcine-specific organisms and porcine serologies to human-specific pathogens are not available. Thus,

- Antibiotic use has had adverse effects on the microbial ecology of an inbred population of swine.
- Spread of antimicrobial resistance within a closed breeding colony is rapid.
- New microbial pathogens will require the development of new diagnostic techniques for clinical use. These tests must include culture and molecular techniques, as serologic testing for animal-derived organisms in humans is generally unavailable or unreliable. Serologic tests are often falsely negative in the immunocompromised host.
- Xenotransplantation from swine to non-human primates and rodents (in my laboratory) has not been associated with evidence of unusual infections. However, while survival of non-human primates receiving swine kidneys has reached multiple months, this represents a relatively limited period of observation for the emergence of latent infection.

Cytomegalovirus

As was noted, viral pathogens are of great importance in organ transplantation recipients. PCMV infection, which is common in swine (the laboratory marker being seropositivity), is propagated by the respiratory route and produces fever, respiratory distress, and death in young pigs but causes relatively benign disease in older animals. As in humans, the pathology of PCMV infection is systemic, with infected cells in blood vessel endothelia, spleen, kidney, liver, and lungs. Latent virus is observed in porcine alveolar macrophages and alveolar epithelial cells (17, 18). The recrudescence of PCMV excretion has occurred after the administration of corticosteroids to latently infected animals. In this setting, virus can be recovered from the macrophages of asymptomatic, seropositive pigs. Both an indirect immunofluorescence test and an ELISA have been described for PCMV (2, 43).

In miniature swine receiving mismatched allogeneic bone marrow transplants, a syndrome of interstitial pneumonitis has been observed following marrow engraftment, generally 20 to 90 days after transplantation. Alveolar macrophages collected by bronchoalveolar lavage from such animals demonstrate productive infection due to PCMV. PCMV was cultured from porcine alveolar macrophages on porcine fallopian tube (PFT) cells and detected using polyclonal antisera to PCMV (2, 6, 18, 43, 62). Stocks of PCMV sufficient to lyse 100% of PFT or swine testis (ST) cells in vitro cause no apparent cytopathic effect or productive infection (by immunofluorescence) in human-derived cell lines including HEL or WI-38 (lung fibroblastoid) cells. Similarly, HCMV stocks of Towne strain and from a recent clinical isolate of CMV do not appear to infect PFT, ST, or IB-RS-2D10 (porcine kidney cells) cell lines. These observations support the species specificity of PCMV in vitro. The behavior of PCMV in immunocompromised human hosts may be altered, but data suggest that infection by some pathogens is likely to be restricted to the xenograft.

Zoonotic Infections from Swine

Zoonotic infections of humans due to swine-derived pathogens have been observed in meat handlers, farmers, and individuals ingesting undercooked pork. Ingestion has resulted in many bacterial and parasitic infections, including those due to *Salmonella enterica* serovar Choleraesuis, *Brucella* spp., and *Trichinella spiralis*. Significant infections in butchers and farmers have included rabies, anthrax, brucellosis, *Salmonella* spp., *Campylobacter* and *Cryptosporidium* gastroenteritis, toxoplasmosis, leptospirosis, listeriosis, erysipeloid, salmonellosis, and yersiniosis (13, 56, 70, 92, 94). Infections due to *S. suis* are considered an occupational hazard for European meat handlers (45, 47). An excess mortality has been associated in Europe with the occupation of pork butchers over other meat handlers and the general population (28). This increase was notable for lung cancer and a variety of other tumors. However, butchers in general appeared to have excess mortality due to dietary habits (drinking alcohol, eating red meat, cigarette smoking) as well. No excess mortality due to infection has been described in pork butchers.

Swine influenza (generally H1N1 or H3N2 subtypes) is a group influenza A virus infection of humans and pigs. Influenza in swine was observed in the human influenza pandemic of 1918–1919 and, more recently, in military recruits at Fort Dix (33, 61, 67, 79). Animals develop conjunctivitis, pharyngitis, pneumonitis, and fever with low mortality (67, 99). Up to 20% of slaughterhouse workers and 25% of swine have serologic evidence of exposure to these agents (67, 76). Recombinant strains of influenza (H1N2) have been observed in swine populations in which H1N1 strains are endemic and coinfection from humans with other strains (H3N2) occurs (33, 88). There is no evidence of increased virulence of these "new" strains. However, such populations of swine may serve as a reservoir for human infection. In a recent outbreak (1997) in Hong Kong, avian "flu" was transmitted to humans directly from chickens without intervening pig infection and resulted in at least eight deaths. The rapidity of the spread of such infections would rapidly outpace the development of relevant vaccine programs.

Infection in Discordant Xenotransplantation

Few data are available regarding the activation of infection following xenotransplantation. Infections including *Aspergillus* fungemia and bacterial peritonitis following biliary anastamotic leaks have complicated the recoveries of immunosuppressed recipients of livers from non-human primates (84, 85). Patients have not developed serologic evidence of infection due to B virus or other unsuspected pathogens, but further studies of the recipients (nucleic acid hybridization or polymerase chain reaction amplification) for such pathogens are needed.

Screening of caesarean-derived porcine fetal tissues intended for human xenotransplantation has been reported for pancreatic islet cells implanted into the kidney capsule or portal vein (5, 19, 27, 32, 52, 60). These investigators have focused on the reduction or elimination of common pathogens of swine in tissue preparation. Bjoersdorff and coworkers used a serologic and microbiologic screening program for preparations of islet-like cell clusters (5). In donor swine, antibodies were found to *Leptospira interrogans* and *Aspergillus fumigatus*. Bacterial cultures from the endometrium or amniotic fluid were rarely (4%) positive, and negative from the transplanted cell preparations. Viral, fungal, and parasitic evaluations were also negative. When cells were transplanted into humans, no infections were reported. One patient experienced mild abdominal pain following intraportal injection, with transient transaminase elevation and depression of the platelet count. Transplantation of porcine fetal brain cells for the treatment of refractory Parkinson's disease has been achieved and reported in the news media. The screening protocol for these tissues includes stringent testing for neurotropic viruses and, in the recipients, episodic screening for new viral pathogens. Transplantation into the central nervous system may be less subject to immune rejection or cellular inflammation than other tissues. The impact of this location on the activation of infection cannot be predicted.

The "archiving" of tissue and serum samples from donor animals and recipients will assist in the tracking of any unsuspected pathogen.

Experience with Animal-Derived Products

Immunologic barriers to human transplantation from miniature swine are most evident in regard to immunologic hyperacute rejection expected in the setting of transplantation between discordant species. This reaction reflects the presence of preformed antibodies to the antigens of swine. Further antibodies to antigens of swine are likely to be observed in recipients of porcine heart valves, insulin and enzymatic replacements, skin xenografts for treatment of burn injuries, and food products. The intensive exposure to products derived from pigs and other non-human species has had no demonstrable adverse effects on individuals or the general population. However, other than foods, and unlike xenograft tissues, each of these products represents killed tissues or processed drug products that can be reliably tested for the absence of microbiologic contaminants.

XENOSIS—NOVEL PATHOGENS IN XENOTRANSPLANTATION

Immunocompromised hosts have served as sentinels for the recognition of many new pathogens and clinical syndromes in infectious disease. Thus, AIDS patients have developed infections due to newly described protozoa (microsporidia, *Cryptosporidium* sp.), viruses (JK, human herpesvirus 8, cytomegalovirus), bacteria (*Bartonella* sp., *Rhodococcus* sp.), and fungi (*Penicillium* sp.) and infections of enhanced severity compared with normal hosts. Similarly, the ability of unknown pathogens to replicate in the immunocompromised human host following xenotransplantation might be expected, and the biological behavior of organisms introduced with xenografts is not predictable. Recombination or *trans*-regulation between viruses, selective pressures favoring mutant strains, and xenotropic viruses, for example, cannot be confidently excluded.

The term xenosis (also direct zoonosis or xenozoonosis) was coined to reflect the unique epidemiology of infection from organisms carried by xenogeneic tissues (21, 59, 100). Given the goal of prevention of infection in these highly susceptible hosts, strategic decisions must be made regarding the exclusion of potential pathogens in source animal breeding and/or the development of prophylactic regimens in the post-xenograft setting. The likely human

Table 4. Categories of potential pathogens resulting from xenotransplantation

Traditional zoonosis	Well-characterized clinical syndromes of humans (e.g., *Toxoplasma gondii*) Specific diagnostic tests generally available
Species-specific	Incapable of causing infection outside the xenograft (e.g., porcine cytomegalovirus) Some tests available, few standardized tests available for human use
Potential pathogens	Organisms of broad "host range" that may spread beyond the xenograft e.g., adenovirus Few specific tests available
Unknown pathogens	New virulence characteristics within the host, e.g., xenotropic viruses Not known to be present or pathogenic (e.g., protozoa or retroviruses) Viral recombinants Resulting from intentional genetic modification of donor Diseases resulting from multiple simultaneous infections (e.g., lymphosis of cattle due to *Babesia* sp. and viral coinfection)

pathogens derived from animals can be categorized according to the predicted behavior or importance of each pathogen in the transplant recipient (Table 4). Without confirmation in animal models or in humans, such predictions are merely educated guesses based on experience with human allotransplantation. Specifically, the ability of each pathogen to cause productive infection and to cause disease in the human recipient must be assessed. The virulence of specific organisms may tend to increase with passage in a new host (evolutionary adaptation) while diminishing over time in the native host (16). Thus, there are likely to be a number of novel organisms derived from animals that are unknown at present and/or that have not been recognized to cause disease in humans, and that may cause disease in the immunocompromised transplant recipient.

Based on the issues discussed above, a group of "exclusion criteria" (Table 5) can be generated for organisms likely to cause disease in xenograft recipients and lists of organisms created to guide the breeding of source animals for xenotransplantation. Such lists, while inexact in the absence of clinical experience, serve a variety of purposes in the progress of xenotransplantation. (i) Organisms thought to pose an unacceptable risk to the recipient can be bred out of a donor herd prospectively (designated pathogen-free or DPF). (ii) Microbiologic assays for these organisms can be developed. (iii) Studies of these organisms in xenograft models may clarify the biologic behavior of these organisms and uncover new potential pathogens. (iv) Knowledge gained may be applicable to the care of allograft recipients. The exclusion list will vary with the donor species and the use intended for the xenograft. Thus, encapsulated cells placed in the brain may provide a risk different from that posed by a xenografted liver or heart. Such lists of designated pathogens (e.g., for swine and non-human primates) (Tables 2 and 6) provide a basis for microbiologic screening of source animals and/or of cells and tissues intended for xenotransplantation. Such

Table 5. Screening xenograft source animals: microbiologic exclusion criteria

Known pathogens of humans (e.g., rabies, *Mycobacterium tuberculosis*)
Known pathogens of immunocompromised human hosts (e.g., *Toxoplasma gondii*, *Strongyloides* sp.)
Similar to pathogens of transplant recipients (e.g., porcine cytomegalovirus, adenovirus)
Antibiotic-resistant organisms
Viruses at high risk for recombination (e.g., parvovirus, rotavirus)
Organ-specific exclusion list (e.g., *Mycoplasma* spp. in lung donors)

Table 6. Designated-pathogen-free miniature swine for xenotransplantation

Exclude the presence of:
Brucella suis
Leptospira spp.
Listeria monocytogenes
Mycobacterium bovis
Mycobacterium tuberculosis
Mycobacterium avium-intracellulare complex
Mycoplasma hyopneumoniae (lung transplant)
Salmonella enterica serovars Typhi, Typhimurium, and Choleraesuis
Shigella spp.
Aspergillus[a] spp.
Candida[a] spp.
Histoplasma capsulatum
Ascaris suum
Cryptosporidium parvum
Neospora spp.
Strongyloides ransomi
Toxoplasma gondii
Trichinella spiralis
Adenovirus (porcine)
Cytomegalovirus (porcine)
Encephalomyocarditis virus
Influenza virus (porcine and human)
Porcine parvovirus
Porcine reproductive and respiratory syndrome virus
Pseudorabies virus
Rabies virus
Rotavirus

[a]Exclude animals with lesions.

microbiological standards must be dynamic—rigorously tested and subject to revision based on experimental and clinical data and reflecting the evolution of testing strategies and adjusted for differences in the use of specific tissues and the geographic region in which tissues are procured.

SOURCE ANIMAL SELECTION AND EXCLUSION OF LIKELY PATHOGENS

The choice of the optimal donor species for xenotransplantation has not been resolved. The recent cloning of farm animals suggests that animals developed through genetic engineering or traditional breeding methods may radically alter concepts of animal selection. Issues of availability, cost, infectious risk, and ethical concerns require careful consideration. The selection of the appropriate source species for xenotransplantation is central to the design of microbiological testing regimens and to the nature of the immune suppression selected to maintain graft function.

Thus far, non-human primates and swine have received the greatest attention as potential source animals. The use of concordant (primate) source animals carries the advantage of decreased immunologic barriers and the possibility of improved metabolic compatibility with human recipients. By contrast with the non-human primates, the use of discordant species poses a greater immunologic barrier in exchange for fewer ethical concerns and ease of breeding. Transplantation from swine is complicated by the existence in humans of preformed or "natural" antibodies to the α-1,3-Gal sugar that is present on the endothelial surfaces of all vascularized tissues of swine. This barrier, though approachable via the removal of the antibodies or via genetic engineering of the donor animals, has been a major hurdle to transplantation from swine to primates.

Primates

Primates have the disadvantages of relatively slow reproduction with long gestation periods, single births, and the requirement for extensive socialization and exercise areas—all of which make the development of large numbers of such animals difficult and costly. Thus, the task of breeding large numbers of primates (generally baboons) of appropriate size and that are free of known human pathogens is daunting. The theoretical argument has also been made that pathogens adapted to primates will infect humans more readily than organisms derived from more phylogenetically distant species. Several endogenous and exogenous retroviruses of primates have been identified (see Table 2) that are infectious for humans and for which high seroprevalence has been documented, including simian foamy viruses, simian T-cell lymphotropic viruses, baboon endogenous virus, and simian endogenous retrovirus. Current breeding programs are not capable of providing animals free of these potential pathogens. Further, the presence of herpesviruses pathogenic for humans and of a newly identified baboon reovirus merit further consideration in the use of non-human primates as xenograft donors.

Of note regarding this source species, the single baboon-to-human bone marrow transplant for AIDS has not been associated, as of yet, with infection by any of these pathogens. However, the duration of survival of the baboon cells in the recipient was brief, the conditioning mild, and many transplant and AIDS patients fail to establish serologic evidence following infectious exposure. A key question remains as to whether infection in the absence of clinical disease (e.g., simian foamy virus) is sufficiently worrisome so as to block the use of most non-human primates as xenograft donors (30).

Swine

Large numbers of swine can be bred in microbiological isolation at relatively modest cost; genetic modification systems are available for swine, and microbiologic testing is generally available for many common pathogens. Animal husbandry for swine is advanced. The immunologic barriers to xenotransplantation from swine have formed the basis of extensive research to overcome hyperacute rejection, delayed vascular rejection, and chronic rejection, using a combination of genetic engineering of donor tissues and host manipulations including immune suppression, tolerance induction, and removal of preformed antibodies to pig antigens. Each of these strategies carries a potential risk in terms of infection that is discussed below.

Given the number and variety of potential pathogens that may be carried by xenograft tissues as described above, the design of schemes for the breeding of pathogen-free source animals for xenotransplantation is complex. Tests are available in veterinary clinical laboratories for many organisms, which, therefore, can be excluded prospectively from donor herds. By contrast, wild-caught animals or those maintained in open herds (e.g., corrals) may be infected by organisms that are pathogenic in xenograft recipients. Thus, swine or primates maintained outdoors have unregulated contact with insects, rodents, amphibians, farm animals, and humans. The spread of organisms between closely quartered animals is rapid and may occur over great distances (12, 26). The risk of introducing antibiotic-resistant organisms can be reduced by limiting the use of such agents in herd maintenance. The benefits of vaccination of source animals must be balanced against the need to use serologic testing to detect entry of specific pathogens into a colony. The risk of acquiring human pathogens from animals can also be reduced by the prospective screening and contact precautions by animal handlers. Meat by-products must be excluded from animal diets to avoid the potential for the spread of prions.

These observations suggest a need for herd isolation and continuous surveillance of animals intended for organ derivation and place a significant burden on the developers of animals for human organ donation, particularly in the use of primates. Meticulous record-keeping of all breeding conditions and archived specimens of animal tissues and sera must be maintained to allow prospective and retrospective evaluation of infectious hazards from each animal and/or herd. While barrier facilities for isolated herds of animals appear essential, it seems likely that the manner in which the level of safety created by the exclusion criteria or lists of organisms is achieved need not be uniform as long as the transplanted tissues do not pose a microbiologic hazard to the recipient. For example, the need to develop pathogen-free herds of animals may be reduced if the absence of potential pathogens can be demonstrated, or such organisms removed, during processing. Thus, cellular transplants (e.g., bone marrow, microencapsulated tissues) pose a different set of opportunities and challenges than do vascularized organ grafts. The goal is, therefore, not to establish the use of a single technology for animal husbandry but to achieve the microbiologic endpoint of optimal safety. Achievement of microbiological standards must be monitored through the routine screening of sentinel animals from the donor herds. In addition, food sources must be carefully selected to avoid the introduction of organisms and prions. The development of breeding technology includes a variety of facilities for the isolation of herds from other animals (including rodents) and arthropod vectors. The development and use of such facilities must be documented so as to comply with regulatory authorities and to ensure optimal animal welfare standards. Health screening must not be limited to infectious disease risks. In-breeding may increase the incidence of congenital malformations or of inborn errors of metabolism that must be identified and excluded from source animals.

The goal of animal husbandry for xenotransplantation is to exclude potential pathogens for the human recipient and to prevent the contamination of such herds and of other animals by human-derived pathogens. A scheme for such testing is presented in Table 7.

XENOSIS AND THE RETROVIRUSES

With prolonged xenograft survival, the susceptibility of the xenograft recipient to infection reflects the individual's epidemiologic exposures and the immune suppression and manipulations of donor and host needed to prevent graft rejection. While breeding strategies, discussed above, may enhance the safety of xenotransplantation, the greatest potential risk to the recipient and to the general community by xenograft-derived organisms may be due to infection by unknown pathogens that cause minimal or novel clinical syndromes and for which clinical laboratory testing is not available. Further, the possibility exists for

Table 7. Microbiologic screening of animal handlers

Serologies
Hepatitis viruses (A, B, C)
Measles
Mumps
Rubella
Epstein-Barr virus
Herpes simplex
Histoplasma capsulatum
Varicella-zoster virus
Cytomegalovirus
Toxoplasma gondii
HIV-1, -2 (voluntary, anonymous)
Parvovirus B19
Syphilis
Other
Mycobacterium tuberculosis (skin testing)
Possible swine pathogens (selected examples)
Porcine cytomegalovirus
Swine influenza
Porcine rotavirus
Transmissible gastroenteritis
Possible primate pathogens (selected examples)
B virus
SA8
Herpesvirus papio
Simian immunodeficiency virus
Foamy virus
Simian retrovirus/baboon endogenous virus

the emergence of new strains of organisms with altered virulence characteristics (e.g., due to recombination or mutation) as has been observed, for example, for the development of antiviral resistance by CMV in transplant patients, or mutations by EBV in the pathogenesis of oral hairy leukoplakia in AIDS.

While pathogens of a variety of types may be capable of developing in the xenograft recipient, concern has focused on the potential for the spread of retroviruses to the recipient and to the general population as the result of xenotransplantation. Recent viral epidemics and outbreaks (i.e., AIDS, Ebola) may have contributed to this concern. The activation and behavior of the retroviruses in transplantation have not been well studied in vivo. However, conditions present in transplantation may increase the likelihood of retroviral activation if any intact and infectious proviruses are present (81). These conditions include immune suppression, graft-versus-host disease, graft rejection, viral coinfection, and cytotoxic therapy (34–36, 63). However, the course of accidentally transmitted infection due to HIV-1 has been accelerated in transplant recipients, manifesting disease within 6 months (8, 77). The activation of latent virus and the development of clinical manifestations, if any, may be delayed for over a decade and may not occur during the life span of the recipient. Further, the manifestations of retroviral infection, commonly including immune suppression, altered gene regulation, oncogenesis, or recombination with other viruses, may be clinically inapparent.

Retroviral infections by human endogenous retroviruses (HERV) have not been a major concern in human allotransplantation given the absence of known full-length replicating HERVs (with the exception of the expression of open reading frames for the HERV-K in placental tissues). By contrast, endogenous retroviruses that are infectious for human cells in vitro have been described in other mammalian species including swine (PERV), baboons (BaEV), cats (RD114), and mice (murine ERV). The activation of latent retroviruses and the development of clinical manifestations of infection, if any, may be delayed for over a decade, and transmission may be "silent" in that the manifestations of retroviral infection may be clinically inapparent. Pathogenic endogenous retroviruses would be expected to be selected against (i.e., those that are detrimental) in the native host species, but interspecies transmission of such retroviruses (i.e., xenotropic virus) has been identified in a number of models, including seroconversion of humans to simian immunodeficiency virus (46); human foamy virus genes inducing encephalopathy in mice; pseudotyping of Rous sarcoma virus (95) with avian and murine tumor viruses (49); pseudotyping of HIV with murine amphotropic retrovirus (51, 83); simian agent 8 in baboons (48); and infection of cells of baboons, apes, and New and Old World monkeys by HIV-1 and -2 (4, 54). Recent data have demonstrated asymptomatic spread of simian foamy viruses to 1.8% of tested, immunologically normal animal handlers with significant occupational exposures (30). These foamy virus infections were detected serologically and by the isolation of proviral DNA and viral RNA many years after initial exposure and did not result in detectable spread to sexual contacts.

Strategies developed to reduce the level of rejection occurring after xenotransplantation may alter the risk of viral activation. Transgenic animals developed to minimize acute rejection of xenografts may alter the expression of latent virus as a result of insertion or deletion of genes (55). These transgenes may also encode receptors for new pathogens; for example, decay-accelerating factor (DAF) is the receptor for human measles virus (69), while CD46 binds morbillivirus. In humans, natural antibodies to Galα1-3Galβ1-4G1cNAc-R epitopes (called anti-α-galactosyl antibody) may be a part of an intrinsic defense mechanism against exogenous retroviral (and bacterial) infections (3, 25, 29, 71, 75, 82, 96, 97). These antibodies determine the ability of human sera to lyse retrovirally infected cells and to neutralize free virus (65). These same antibodies provide a major transplantation barrier to the use of vascularized organ grafts from swine that express the endothelial Galα1-4Gal sugars in humans. Techniques that remove these sugars or antibodies may alter the risk of retroviral activation (74).

Retroviruses of primates have been more thoroughly characterized than those of swine. In part due to studies related to AIDS, up to 30 strains of lentiviruses have been described in primates. A number of the common primate retroviruses are infectious for human cells in vitro, including SIV (in human T cells) and baboon foamy virus (human fibroblasts). The ubiquitous nature and genetic homologies of the primate immunodeficiency viruses (SIV, simian T-cell leukemia virus, endogenous viruses) and the ability of these pathogens to infect other species suggest a potential risk for human infection. However, none of the recipients of tissues from non-human primates have had such infections detected thus far.

The potential retroviral risks associated with the use of tissues from swine in humans are beginning to be explored. A virus from the PK15 cell line and another derived from a malignant lymphoma-derived cell line (Shimozuma cells) have been described (7, 50, 89, 93).

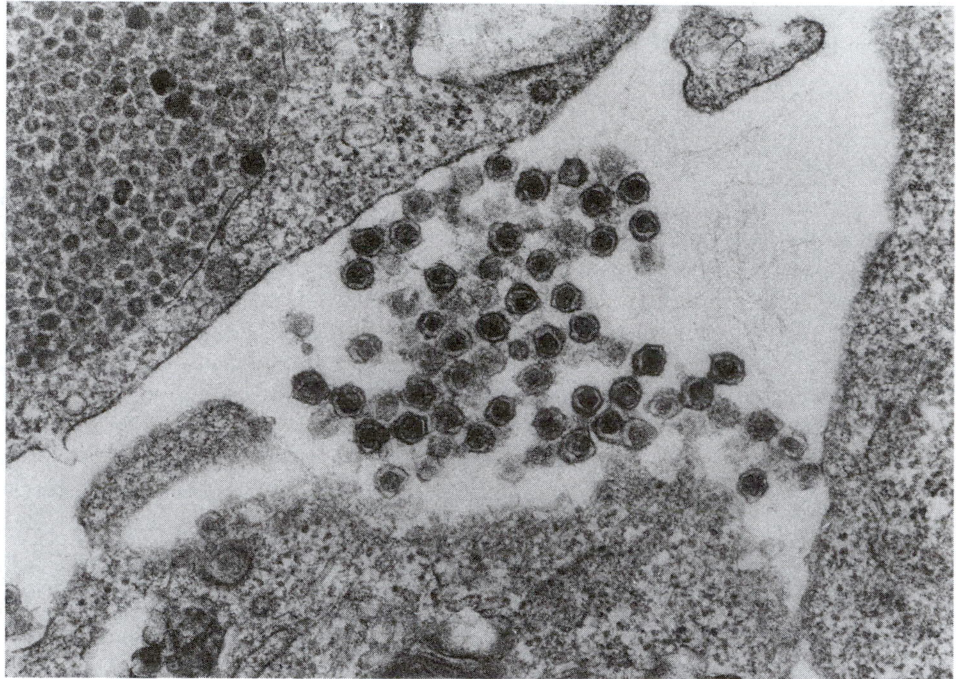

Figure 1. Porcine endogenous retrovirus replicating in human 293 kidney cells (×60,000). Provided by Drs. K. Boller, R. R. Tonjes, J. Denner, Paul-Ehrlich Institute, Langen, Germany.

The latter isolate, Tsukuba-1, has caused B- and T-cell lymphomas in wild boars (42). A family of C-type porcine endogenous retroviruses has been identified, some of which induce productive infection of human cells in vitro (see Fig. 1) (1, 65, 98). The full-length cDNA porcine endogenous retroviral sequence from miniature swine lymphocytes (PERV-MSL) is 8,132 base pairs. The nucleotide sequences of PERV-MSL, PK15-ERV, and Tsukuba-1 (Genbank: AF038600, AF038601, AF038599) have structural features identical to those of related C-type retroviruses (1). The sequences (both nucleotide and deduced amino acid) with the greatest similarity to PERV-MSL are from the gibbon ape leukemia virus (GALV), followed by several murine leukemia viruses, including the Moloney murine leukemia virus. Important to infectivity is variation in the envelope region (*env* gene), which encodes two polypeptides, the SU (gp70) polypeptide and transmembrane protein (TM; p15E). Typically, the SU polypeptide, which contains the receptor-binding domain, is heavily glycosylated. Eight of the nine potential glycosylation sites (Asn-x-Thr/Ser) in PERV-MSL *env* are located in the gp70 protein.

Expression of PERV is found both in porcine kidney-derived cell lines (PK15) and in the cells and tissues of normal swine (Fig. 2). PERV has been detected in all strains of swine tested, with some variability in the copy number of possible full-length proviral sequences (range 8 to 20). Infection of human cells in vitro is associated with altered viral antigenicity after a single passage. It is not known whether these viruses can cause disease in humans. A number of characteristics of this family have been identified.

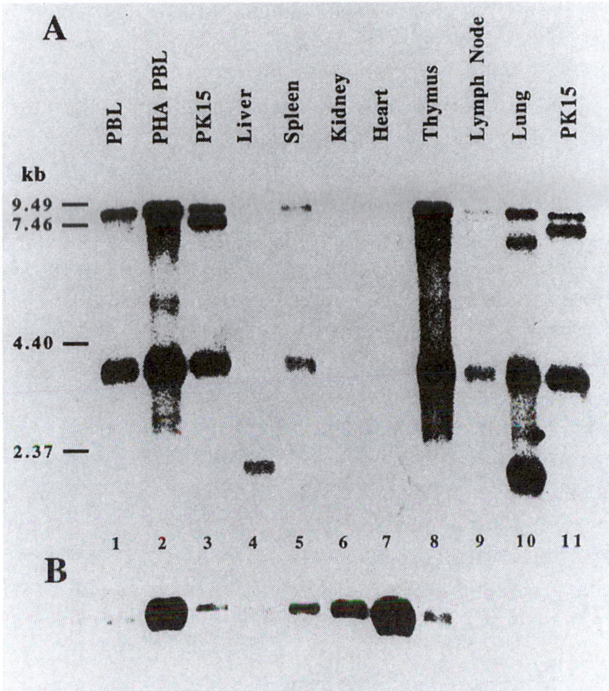

Figure 2. Northern analysis of the expression of PERV-MSL (PERV C) in various tissues. A probe for the *env* region of PERV was hybridized to poly-A+ RNA (0.5 μg) from each tissue indicated and from normal peripheral blood lymphocytes (PBL, lane 1) and PHA-activated lymphocytes (PHA PBL, lane 2), PK15 cells (0.04 μg, lanes 3 and 11). Expression of PERV was detected in all porcine cells and tissues analyzed (including kidney and heart with longer exposures). The expression of PERV is increased by stimulation with the mitogen PHA (reprinted from reference 1, with permission).

- Three closely related, functional PERV sequences (PERV A, B, C) have been identified based largely on variation in the envelope glycoprotein open reading frame in the gp70/SU region of PERV, which is responsible for receptor binding by the virus to target cells and variation in antigenicity (J. Stoye and R. Weiss, personal communication).
- All three viruses are capable of infecting porcine cells; PERV A and B also infect human cells with decreased infectivity (65) but, in a limited series of experiments, have not infected a limited number of established (non-primary) cell lines from non-human primates, including 26CB1 (baboon), cynomK1 (cynomolgus monkey), cos-7 and Vero (African green monkey), and FRhK (rhesus monkey) (R. Weiss, personal communication). By contrast, murine cells (NIH3T3, *M. dunni*), mink cells (Mv-1-lu), rat cells (HSN, NKK), and a variety of porcine cells (ST) have been infected to varying degrees. Preliminary data suggest that primary cell lines from baboons may be infectable by PERV.
- PERV mRNA is expressed spontaneously in all pig tissues under consideration for xenotransplantation in all types of swine tested to date (1). This includes liver, kidney,

heart, lung, thymus, bone marrow and hematopoietic cells, pancreas, and endothelial cells (1, 53).

- The number and distribution of partial and full-length copies of sequences homologous with PERV-MSL vary between swine leukocyte antigen (SLA, the major histocompatibility loci of swine) types and between swine within a given haplotype. The presence of such variation between siblings (i.e., over a short time period) suggests that ongoing horizontal infection due to PERV is occurring in addition to germ-line inheritance and gradual mutation of germ-line copies of proviral sequences (86, 87).
- In addition to full-length transcripts, variably sized shorter transcripts were found in a consistent pattern in some tissues that might represent alternatively spliced transcripts: 3 kb (approximately) transcripts from lymphocytes, 2 and 7 kb from lung, and 2 kb from liver. These transcripts suggest some degree of tissue-specific determination of PERV expression.
- Viral expression is amplified by stimulation of swine peripheral blood lymphocytes by phytohemagglutinin (1).
- Normal porcine endothelial cells are actively infected with PERV and can infect human (HEK293) cells when cocultured in vitro (53). However, no evidence of human infection in vivo has been established by PCR (polymerase chain reaction) analysis or other techniques, and no disease due to this family of viruses has been described in swine or humans to date (31, 64). Studies of individuals exposed to extracorporeal porcine splenic perfusion for a variety of illnesses and to porcine skin grafting for burns have demonstrated remarkable persistence (years) of porcine cells in some patients. No evidence of PERV infection has been found based on DNA and mRNA assays of peripheral blood leukocytes.
- Infection is best detected by cocultivation of cells expressing PERV with permissive swine cells; infection of cells from other species is more difficult to detect, and infection using sera or supernatants of cultured porcine cells is unreliable.

These observations suggest that PERV infection is either difficult to detect with presently available assays or is not transferred to humans by limited exposures to porcine cells or tissues, or that such infection is delayed for years in terms of detectable expression. However, the limited number of patients, the limited duration of exposure to pig tissues, the absence of immune suppression comparable to that required for whole organ transplantation, and the limited numbers of tissue sampled may bias against the detection of PERV in clinical samples. Thus, the final word on human infection by PERV remains unresolved.

SAFETY IN CLINICAL TRIALS OF XENOTRANSPLANTATION

Clinical trials of cellular xenografts are ongoing, while bone marrow and whole organ transplantation protocols, artificial liver devices that incorporate porcine cells, and other applications of this technology are under development. Three of a number of problems merit discussion as xenotransplantation moves toward broader clinical trials. (i) The differentiation of infection of host cells from expression of virus by cells derived from the donor, i.e., chimerism (the coexistence of donor and recipient cells and tissues in the xenograft recipient), remains difficult. (ii) It is uncertain as to the nature of routine investigations which should be conducted in xenograft recipients. (iii) The development of contingency plans is essential for the optimal management of xenograft recipients who develop signs or symptoms of infection (e.g., viremia, fever, pneumonia, hepatitis, gastroenteritis).

Chimerism and False Positive Assays for Infection of the Host

Concern regarding xenosis has centered on the demonstration of active replication of animal-derived organisms in human cells, i.e., will donor-derived agents attach to, and replicate in or on human recipient cells? Because some organisms are expressed constitutively (PERV) or under conditions of immune suppression (porcine CMV), infection of human cells may be difficult to detect, especially if this is an infrequent event or expression is at low levels. The sensitivity of molecular assays has been of great benefit in the clinical diagnosis of infections, particularly by organisms that grow poorly in vitro. The sensitivity of such assays for single-copy genes or for low levels of mRNA expression allows the detection of a single cell from the xenograft donor in 10^5 to 10^6 host cells in this laboratory. Given the presence of 100 to 200 copies of PERV fragments per porcine cell (up to 20 potentially full-length copies) and high-level expression of mRNA for PERV in each cell tested, the detection of single, integrated copies of PERV in human DNA or expression of PERV mRNA in a human cell may be difficult to detect against the high background. The presence of free virus in the circulation, if any, may further confound viral assays. Thus, assays performed on blood samples taken in the presence of persistent lymphohematopoietic chimerism—the simultaneous presence of blood elements from donor and recipient—may provide false positive or uninterpretable results. The induction of chimerism may be used as a mechanism by which to induce donor-specific tolerance in allo- and xenotransplantation, increasing the need for highly specific assays. Techniques including in situ PCR and hybridization or fluorescence-activated cell sorting may be needed to provide the necessary level of resolution for this problem.

A number of assays have been developed to determine whether PERV infection of baboon xenograft recipient's cells occurs after xenotransplantation. Such assays must detect PERV expression against a background of baboon and swine cells. In this system, *gag* and *env* PCR primers specifically amplify fragments of the expected size from reaction tubes spiked with porcine cells. By Southern analysis, the detection limit of PERV is 1 porcine cell in 40,000 baboon cells. Samples containing no DNA or only baboon genomic DNA are negative. As the PERV proviral copy number (all size fragments) in miniature swine haplotype d/d is estimated to be approximately 200 copies, 1 porcine cell equivalent corresponds to about 200 proviral elements (viral fragments) with up to 20 (approximately) potentially full-length sequences. Using either the *gag* or *env* primers, the detection limit of the PERV-MSL plasmid is about 2 copies, which is comparable to the detection of porcine cytochrome b-specific PCR primers used to monitor the presence of porcine cells. The porcine mitochondrial cytochrome b gene is a housekeeping gene and present at 100 to 200 copies per cell (39).

Routine Monitoring for Xenogeneic Infection

In xenograft recipients as for allograft recipients, the risks of infection, graft dysfunction, and rejection are lifelong and necessitate lifelong monitoring for infection and cancer. In addition to the recipients, some individuals are potentially at heightened risk for infection derived from either the donor animals or the recipient. This includes first-degree relatives or sexual contacts of recipients and xenograft donor animal handlers, and these individuals need to be considered for inclusion in any monitoring scheme. Individuals should be monitored at fixed intervals and for periods of increased risk of infection: during symptomatic infections and during periods of increased immune suppression as in the treatment of graft rejection.

The tests to be performed will be of four types: (i) cultures to identify and isolate organisms for further study; (ii) nucleic acid amplification; (iii) antigen detection tests, which are particularly useful for the detection of organisms not easily isolated by available culture techniques; and (iv) serologic testing for epidemiologic evaluation of exposures to novel organisms. The frequency of routine testing for the recipient might be weekly for 3 months, alternate weeks for 3 months, monthly for 6 months, and quarterly thereafter, consistent with a common schedule for post-transplantation clinical care. Following periods of fever or of clinical infection (see below), monitoring would be increased to weekly for 1 to 2 months and then revert to the previous level of surveillance. Samples could be stored from relatives, intimate contacts, and animal handlers every 6 months, with more frequent monitoring (monthly) if the animals or recipients developed signs of infection or were determined to be infected with a xenograft-derived pathogen.

Testing should include archiving of specimens for future study, routine bacterial, fungal, and viral cultures on cells of human and donor origin, PCR for PERV using both sera and leukocytes, and cocultivation of peripheral blood leukocytes with human and donor cell lines. The spectrum of organisms of non-human primates that may infect humans will necessitate a larger panel of PCR screens. In the United States, the Centers for Disease Control and Prevention is intimately involved in the procurement, storage, and testing of samples for retroviral infection resulting from exposure to pig-derived tissues.

Optimal assays for PERV have not been defined; reverse transcribed PCR may be more informative regarding viral infection and standard (DNA) PCR subject to more artifact from donor cellular contamination. Each assay must be standardized and certified as to reliability. Each positive assay for PERV must be confirmed in independent assays before informing the physicians and the patient and acting on the possibility of xenogeneic infection.

Paradigm for the Management of Patients with Signs of Infection

Recipients of solid organ and hematopoietic transplants frequently manifest signs of infection in the form of fever (often without clear source); neutropenia; thrombocytopenia; unexplained leukocytosis; pulmonary, gastrointestinal, and urinary tract infections; sepsis; or hepatitis. Graft rejection, post-transplantation lymphoproliferative disorder, and other etiologies of organ dysfunction may be indistinguishable on clinical grounds. These may also present as myocarditis, pneumonitis, brochiolitis, or nephritis and are separable histologically by tissue biopsy. In xenograft recipients, these signs may be manifestations of common, community-acquired infections or of latent infections reactivated from the recipient. However, the risk that these signs represent infections due to novel organisms will require an organized management strategy similar to that diagrammed in Fig. 3. The key features of this scheme are not dissimilar to the approach taken for allograft recipients:

- Full microbiologic evaluation prior to the initiation of antimicrobial therapy
- Radiologic studies, often accompanied by invasive diagnostic testing (needle or surgical biopsies)

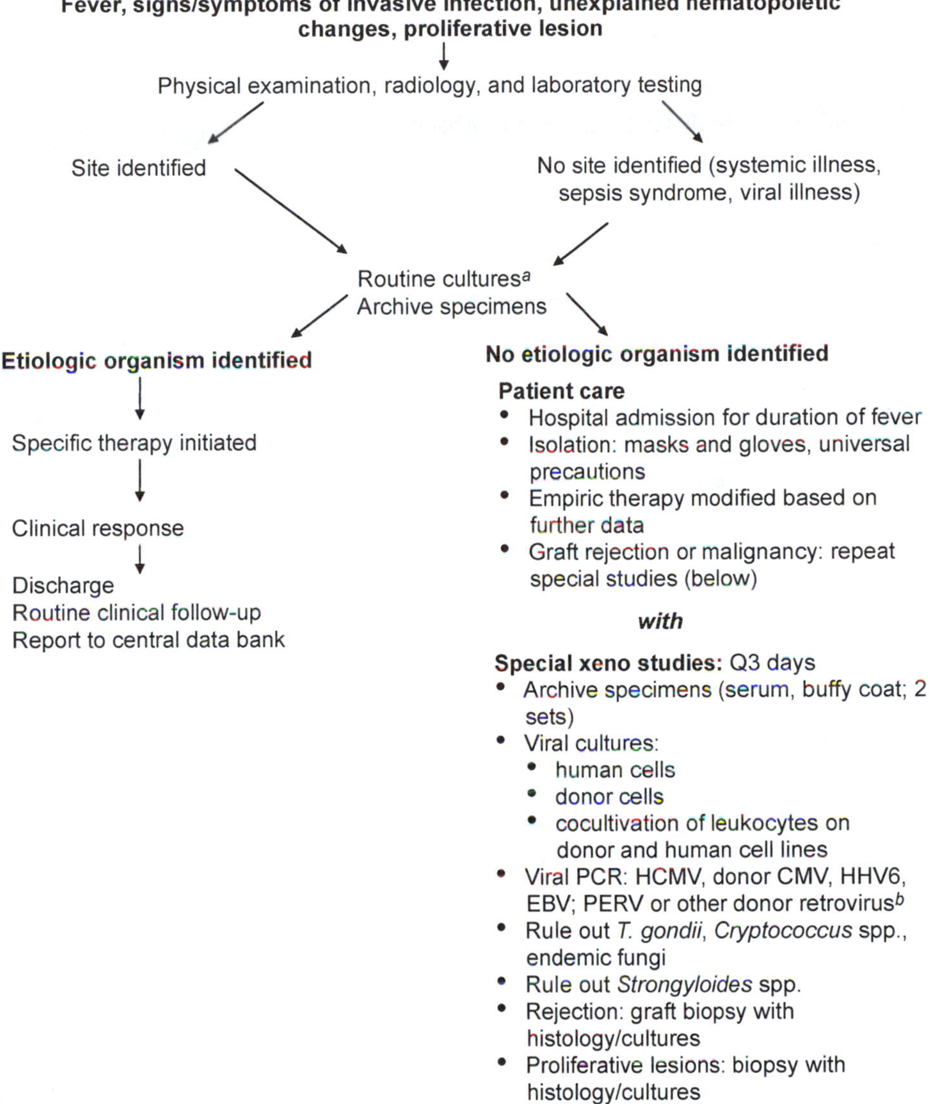

[a] Routine evaluation: Bacterial cultures of blood, urine, sputum, stool; cerebrospinal fluid if indicated clinically; viral cultures of blood/buffy coat on permissive cells of human origin; HCMV assay—antigenemia or PCR; consider PCR for HHV6, HHV7, other human pathogens.

[b] PCR, polymerase chain reaction; HCMV, human cytomegalovirus; HHV, human herpesvirus; PERV, porcine endogenous retrovirus.

Figure 3. Strategy for the evaluation of xenograft recipients with signs or symptoms of infection.

- Early empiric antimicrobial therapy directed at the most likely pathogens
- Hospital admission and isolation from other patients until the nature of the process is further defined; special precautions (e.g., respiratory, secretions, neutropenia) dictated by the patients' clinical presentation
- Universal precautions for all patients

Special testing will be dictated by the donor species and available data from the breeding colony and physical and laboratory examinations. In the event of the recognition of a novel recombinant organism or severe infectious illness without explanation, strict isolation with HEPA filtration will be required.

RECIPIENT SELECTION

Infectious risk to the xenograft recipient and possibly to the community may be increased by preexisting immunodeficiency states or chronic infections (e.g., hepatitis, diabetes, *Pseudomonas* sp. in cystic fibrosis) in these candidates. These are likely to be the same underlying conditions that caused the organ dysfunction necessitating transplantation. Such factors must be considered in developing criteria used for recipient selection. For example, the use of xenografts in older recipients may be advocated given that individuals with limited projected life spans might not survive beyond the period of retroviral latency. As candidates for xenografting, the increased infectious risks of common opportunistic infections in persons with HIV (1 or 2) or with hepatitis B or C, or more common infections with EBV or herpes simplex viruses, may render these individuals poor choices for initial studies (72). However, it is equally apparent that the urgency for transplantation may be greatest in these virally infected hosts. The greatest benefits of xenotransplantation may be the potential resistance to reinfection by the xenograft tissues from disparate species. Persons with cancers other than of hematopoietic origin are generally excluded as recipients of allografts because of enhanced tumor growth in the immunosuppressed host. The resolution of these ethical dilemmas will be important to the success of early clinical trials.

Because lifelong surveillance may be needed to assess the incidence of opportunistic infections or of other complications of xenotransplantation, the recipient must be willing to participate in such an enduring experiment.

THE ADVANTAGES OF XENOTRANSPLANTATION

Despite the potential risks, clinical xenotransplantation may provide some tangible benefits in the clinical care of patients with progressive organ failure. Many patients die while awaiting cadaver donor organs. In addition to an unlimited supply of properly sized organs, xenogeneic organs may be resistant to infection with viral pathogens of humans, including HIV (1 and 2), HTLV, hepatitis viruses, and herpesviruses including HCMV (discussed above). For example, human hepatitis B virus does not appear to infect baboons in vivo (58). This species specificity may reflect the absence of receptors or of cellular machinery necessary for viral replication in a novel host.

At present, cadaver donor organs are derived from hospitalized patients potentially infected with nosocomial pathogens. Similarly, transplant recipients often have prolonged in-hospital waiting times for allografts. During this time they become colonized with nosocomial organisms and may develop infection related to intravenous and urinary catheters or respiratory and cardiac-assist devices. Patients receiving xenografts can receive their transplants at the time of greatest clinical need; surgery can be timed to avoid infections, to receive vaccination against potential pathogens, to store blood products, and to optimize the patient physically. The source animal can be derived free of known infectious hazards.

STRATEGIES FOR THE FUTURE: MINIMIZING THE RISKS TO PATIENTS AND THE COMMUNITY

Can the degree of risk for each potential organism derived from a donor species be stratified in a useful manner? Routine opportunistic infections of allograft recipients are often difficult to treat in the transplant patient but generally pose little threat to the immunologically normal general public. Thus, common bacteria, fungi, viruses, and parasites in the xenograft recipient will require prompt and aggressive treatment but pose no unique hazard for the general population. Unique risks exist only because of the possibility that novel organisms may infect xenograft recipients and spread to the community. These organisms pose a greater risk if infection occurs in the absence of clinical symptoms. Only prospective monitoring will detect the novel organisms (viruses, bacterial, fungi, protozoa, algae, cyanobacteria, others) of the types that have been detected in other immunosuppressed hosts. Thus, the screening of donor animals for known organisms may only marginally reduce the risk to the community.

The assessment of the risks associated with xenotransplantation is essential to public acceptance of this therapy. In the absence of data, it is difficult to develop a meaningful dialogue regarding the risks to the recipient or to the community at large. Research is essential regarding the behavior of organisms known to be present in prospective donor species in xenograft recipients and on the detection of novel potential pathogens. Some of the potential areas for study include the following.

- Studies of infection should be conducted in the "appropriate" preclinical models. Thus, viral activation and susceptibility to infection can be realistically assessed only in xenograft models although in vitro studies may be very informative (e.g., mixed lymphocyte or stimulated cultures). Models including swine-to-primate, primate-to-primate, and scid mice reconstituted with human, swine, and/or primate cells will be informative.
- The presence of unknown pathogens must be considered and strategies to identify such organisms developed.
- Diagnostic assays, preferably molecular or antigen-based, as well as serologic, must be developed for the assessment of both source animals and humans.
- The activity of available antimicrobial agents against pathogens (e.g., PERV) derived from the donor species should be assessed.
- Stringent peer review and oversight of clinical protocols are needed to ensure the protection of the patient and appropriate attention to public health concerns.
- Clinical trials must include careful archiving of source animal and recipient sera and tissues to aid in microbiologic and epidemiologic studies of emerging infections in xenograft recipients. Similar samples may be needed from medical personnel and the recipient's family, sexual, and social contacts.

- Efforts to minimize the immune suppression needed to maintain graft function must be emphasized.
- The effects of genetic manipulation on susceptibility to infection must be assessed.
- Source animals must be protected from human pathogens.

Significant dangers of infection exist for all transplant recipients given the available immunosuppressive regimens. Careful source animal selection and studies in preclinical models may allow the risks to the recipient and to the community to be reduced, and may confer substantial benefits when the potential of xenotransplantation is recognized. The development of clinical xenotransplantation from the infectious disease perspective is viewed as an example of the potential risks of new technologies in the emergence of novel infection. However, in the absence of further data, the risks remain theoretical. Thus, fundamental research using innovative preclinical models and careful examination of clinical research subjects will provide a rational basis for decision making in this field as for allotransplantation over the past 20 years.

REFERENCES

1. **Akiyoshi, D. E., M. Denaro, H. Zhu, J. L. Greenstein, P. Banerjee, and J. A. Fishman.** 1998. Identification of a full-length cDNA for an endogenous retrovirus of miniature swine. *J. Virol.* **72:**4503–4507.
2. **Assaf, R., A. M. P. Bouillant, and E. DiFranco.** 1982. Enzyme linked immunosorbent assay (ELISA) for the detection of antibodies to porcine cytomegalovirus. *Can. J. Comp. Med.* **46:**183–185.
3. **Barbacid, M., D. Bolognesi, and S. A. Aaronson.** 1980. Humans have antibodies capable of recognizing oncoviral glycoproteins: demonstration that these antibodies are formed in reponse to cellular modification of glycoproteins rather than as consequence of exposure to virus. *Proc. Natl. Acad. Sci. USA* **77:**1617–1621.
4. **Barnett, S. W., K. K. Murthy, B. G. Herndier, and J. A. Levy.** 1994. An AIDS-like condition induced in baboons by HIV-2. *Science* **266:**642–646.
5. **Bjoersdorff, A., O. Korsgren, R. Feinstein, A. Andersson, J. Tollemar, A.-S. Malmborg, A. Ehrnst, and C. G. Groth.** 1995. Microbiological characterization of porcine fetal islet-like cell clusters for intended clinical xenografting. *Xenotransplantation* **2:**26–31.
6. **Bouillant, A. M. P., A. S. Greig, and P. Genest.** 1973. Biological characterization of cell line derived from the pig oviduct. *In Vitro* **9:**92–102.
7. **Bouilant, A. M. P., A. S. Grieg, M. M. Lieber, and G. J. Todaro.** 1975. Type-C virus production by a continuous line of pig oviduct cells (PFT). *J. Gen. Virol.* **27:**173–180.
8. **Bowden, R. A., R. W. Coombs, B. H. Nikora, C. Bigelow, G. E. Sale, D. Thomas, J. D. Meyers, and L. Corey.** 1990. Progression of human immunodeficiency virus type-1 infection after allogeneic marrow transplantation. *Am. J. Med.* **88:**5-49N–5-52N.
9. **Carbone, M., H. I. Pass, P. Rizzo, M. Marinetti, M. DiMuzio, D. J. Mew, A. S. Levine, and A. Procopio.** 1994. Simian virus-40-like DNA sequences in human pleural mesothelioma. *Oncogene* **9:**1781–1790.
10. **Cen, H., M. C. Breinig, R. W. Atchinson, M. Ho, and J. L. C. McKnight.** 1991. Epstein-Barr virus transmission via the donor organs in solid organ transplantation polymerase chain reaction and restriction fragment length polymorphism analysis of IR2, IR3 and IR4. *J. Virol.* **65:**976–980.
11. **Chang, Y., E. Cesarman, M. S. Pessin, F. Lee, J. Culpepper, D. M. Knowles, and P. S. Moore.** 1994. Identification of herpesvirus-like DNA sequences in AIDS- associated Kaposi's sarcoma. *Science* **266:**1865–1869.
12. **Christensen, L. S., K. J. Sorensen, B. S. Strandby-Gaard, C. A. Henrikson, and J. B. Anderson.** 1990. Evidence of long distance airborne transmission of Aujeszky's disease virus-1, identification of emerging strains, p. 206. *Proc. 11th Int. Congr. Pig Vet. Soc.* University of Iowa, Ames.
13. **Christensen, S. G.** 1987. Co-ordination of a nationwide survey on the presence of *Yersinia enterocolitica* 0:3 in the environment of butcher shops. *Contrib. Microbiol. Immunol.* **9:**26–29.
14. **Dummer, J. S., J. Armstrong, J. Somers, S. Kusne, B. J. Carpenter, J. T. Rosenthal, and M. Ho.** 1987. Transmission of infection with herpes simplex by renal transplantation. *J. Infect. Dis.* **155:**202–206.

15. **Dummer, J. S., S. Erb, M. K. Breinig, M. Ho, C. R. Rinaldo, Jr., P. Gupta, M. V. Ragni, A. Tzakis, L. Makowka, D. Van Thiel, et al.** 1989. Infection with human immunodeficiency virus in the Pittsburgh transplant population. *Transplantation* **47:**134–139.
16. **Ebert, D.** 1998. Experimental evolution of parasites. *Science* **282:**1432–1435.
17. **Edington, N., S. Broad, A. E. Wrathall, and J. T. Done.** 1988. Superinfection with porcine cytomegalovirus-initiation by transplacental infection. *Vet. Microbiol.* **16:**189–193.
18. **Edington, N., A. E. Wrathall, and J. T. Done.** 1988. Porcine cytomegalovirus (PCMV) in early gestation. *Vet. Microbiol.* **17:**117–128.
19. **Emery, D. W., M. Sykes, D. H. Sachs, and C. LeGuern.** 1994. Mixed swine/human long-term bone marrow cultures. *Transplant. Proc.* **26:**1313–1314.
20. **Erice, A., F. S. Rhame, R. C. Heussner, D. L. Dunn, and H. H. Balfour.** 1991. Human immunodeficiency virus infection in patients with solid-organ transplants: report of five cases and review. *Rev. Infect. Dis.* **13:**7–47.
21. **Fishman, J. A.** 1994. Miniature swine as organ donors for man: strategies for prevention of xenotransplant-associated infections. *Xenotransplantation* **1:**47–57.
22. **Fishman, J. A.** 1997. Xenosis and xenotransplantation: addressing the infectious risks posed by an emerging technology. *Kidney Int.* **51**(Supp 58):41–45.
23. **Fishman, J. A., and R. H. Rubin.** 1998. Infection in organ transplant recipients. *N. Engl. J. Med.* **338:**1741–1751.
24. **Fraumeni, J. F., Jr., F. Ederer, and R. W. Miller.** 1963. An evaluation of the carcinogenicity of simian virus 40 in man. *JAMA* **185:**713–718.
25. **Galili, U., M. R. Clark, S. B. Shohet, J. Buehler, and B. A. Macher.** 1987. Evolutionary relationship between the natural anti-Gal antibody and the GalαGal epitope in primates. *Proc. Natl. Acad. Sci. USA* **84:**1369–1373.
26. **Gloster, J., R. F. Sellers, and A. I. Donaldson.** 1982. Long distance transport of foot-and-mouth disease virus over sea. *Vet. Rec.* **100:**47–52.
27. **Groth, C. G., O. Korsgren, A. Tibell, J. Tollemar, E. Moller, J. Bolinder, J. Ostman, F. P. Reinholt, C. Hellerstrom, and A. Andersson.** 1994. Transplantation of porcine fetal pancreas to diabetic patients. *Lancet* **344:**1402–1404.
28. **Guberan, E., M. Usel, L. Raymond, and G. Fioretta.** 1993. Mortality and incidence of cancer among a cohort of self employed butchers from Geneva and their wives. *Br. J. Ind. Med.* **50:**1008–1016.
29. **Hamadeh, R. M., G. A. Jarvis, U. Galili, R. E. Mandrell, P. Zhou, and J. M. Griffiss.** 1992. Human natural anti-Gal IgG regulates alternative complement pathway activation on bacterial surfaces. *J. Clin. Invest.* **89:**1223–1235.
30. **Heneine, W., W. M. Switzer, P. Sandstrom, J. Brown, S. Vedapuri, C. A. Schable, A. S. Khan, N. W. Lerche, M. Schweizer, D. Neumann-Haefelin, L. E. Chapman, and T. M. Folks.** 1998. Identification of a human population infected with simian foamy viruses [see comments]. *Nature Med.* **4:**403–407.
31. **Heneine, W., A. Tibell, W. M. Switzer, P. Sandstrom, G. Vazquez Rosales, A. Mathews, O. Korsgren, L. E. Chapman, T. M. Folks, and C. G. Groth.** 1998. No evidence of infection with porcine endogenous retrovirus in recipients of porcine islet-cell xenografts. *Lancet* **352:**695–699.
32. **Henretta, J., T. McFadden, K. Pittman, J. Thomas, and F. Thomas.** 1994. Six- to eight-month survival of discordant pig islet xenografts documented by differential species, insulin, and C-peptide in animals given short-term immunosuppression. *Transplant. Proc.* **26:**1138–1139.
33. **Hinshaw, V. S., W. J. Bean, Jr., R. G. Webster, and B. C. Easterday.** 1978. The prevalence of influenza viruses in swine and the antigenic and genetic relatedness of influenza viruses from man and swine. *Virology* **84:**51–62.
34. **Hirsch, M. S.** 1976. Immunologic activation of endogenous oncogenic viruses. *Ann. N.Y. Acad. Sci.* **276:**529–535.
35. **Hirsch, M. S., D. A. Ellis, P. A. Black, A. P. Monaco, and M. L. Wood.** 1973. Leukemia virus activation during homograft rejection. *Science* **180:**500–502.
36. **Hirsch, M. S., S. M. Phillips, C. Solnik, P. H. Black, R. S. Schwartz, and C. B. Carpenter.** 1972. Activation of leukemia viruses by graft-versus-host and mixed lymphocyte reactions in vitro. *Proc. Natl. Acad. Sci. USA* **69:**1069–1072.
37. **Ho, M., G. Miller, R. W. Atchison, M. K. Breinig, J. S. Dummer, W. Andiman, T. E. Starzl, R. Eastman, B. P. Griffith, R. L. Hardesty, et al.** 1985. Epstein-Barr virus infections and DNA hybridization studies in

post transplantation lymphoma and lymphoproliferative lesions the role of primary infection. *J. Infect. Dis.* **152:**876–886.

38. **Institute of Medicine.** 1992. *Emerging Infections: Microbial Threats to Health in the United States.* National Academy Press, Washington, D.C.
39. **Irwin, D. M., T. D. Kocher, and A. C. Wilson.** 1991. Evolution of the cytochrome B gene of mammals. *J. Mol. Evol.* **32:**128–144.
40. **Isfort, R., D. Jones, R. Kost, R. Witter, and H. Kung.** 1992. Retrovirus insertion into herpesvirus in vitro and in vivo. *Proc. Natl. Acad. Sci. USA* **89:**991–995.
41. **Javier, R. T., F. Sedarati, and J. G. Stevens.** 1986. Two avirulent herpes simplex viruses generate lethal recombinants in vivo. *Science* **234:**746–748.
42. **Kaeffer, B., E. Bottreau, L. P. Thanh, M. Olivier, and H. Salmon.** 1990. Histocompatible miniature boar model: selection of transformed cell lines of B and T lineages producing retrovirus. *Int. J. Cancer* **46:**481–488.
43. **Kanitz, C. L., and M. E. Woodruff.** 1976. Cell culture indirect fluorescence antibody studies of porcine cytomegalovirus, p. 9. *In Proc. 4th Int. Pig Vet. Soc. Congress.* University of Iowa, Ames.
44. **Katz, R. A. and A. M. Skalka.** 1990. Generation of diversity in retroviruses. *Annu. Rev. Genet.* **24:**409–405.
45. **Kaufhold, A., R. Lutticken, and S. Litterscheid.** 1988. Systemic infection caused by *Streptococcus suis. Deutsche Med. Wochenschrift* **113:**1642–1643.
46. **Khabbaz, R. F., W. Heneine, J. R. George, B. Parekh, T. Rowe, T. Woods, W. M. Switzer, H. M. McClure, M. Murphey-Corb, and T. M. Folks.** 1994. Infection of a laboratory worker with simian immunodeficiency virus. *N. Engl. J. Med.* **330:**172–177.
47. **Kohler, W., H. Queisser, E. Kunter, R. Sawitzki, and G. Frach.** 1989. Type 2 *Streptococcus suis* (R-streptococci) as pathogens of occupational diseases. Report of a case and a review of the literature. *Zeitschrift Gesamte Inn. Med. Grenzgebiete* **44:**144–148.
48. **Levin, J. L., J. K. Hilliard, S. L. Lipper, T. M. Butler, and W. J. Goodwin.** 1988. A naturally occurring epizootic of simian agent 8 in the baboon. *Lab. Animal. Sci.* **38:**394–397.
49. **Levy, J. A.** 1977. Murine xenotropic type C viruses. III. Phenotypic mixing with avian leukosis and sarcoma viruses. *Virology* **77:**811–825.
50. **Lieber, M. M., C. H. Sherr, R. E. Benveniste, and C. J. Todaro.** 1975. Biologic and immunologic properties of porcine type C virus. *Virology* **66:**616.
51. **Lusso, P., F. Di Marzo Veronese, B. Ensoli, G. Franchini, C. Jemma, S. E. DeRocco, V. S. Kalyanaraman, and R. C. Gallo.** 1990. Expanded HIV-1 cellular tropism by phenotypic mixing with murine endogenous retroviruses. *Science* **247:**848–852.
52. **Marchetti, P., D. W. Scharp, J. Longwith, C. Swanson, B. Olack, A. Gerasimidi-Vazeou, E. H. Finke, and P. E. Lacy.** 1992. Prevention of contamination of isolated porcine islets of Langerhans. *Transplantation* **53:**1364–1366.
53. **Martin, U., V. Kiessig, J. H. Blusch, A. Haverich, K. von der Helm, T. Herden, and G. Steinhoff.** 1998. Expression of pig endogenous retrovirus by primary porcine endothelial cells and infection of human cells. *Lancet* **352:**692–694.
54. **McClure, M. O., Q. J. Sattentau, P. C. Beverley, J. P. Hearn, A. K. Fitzgerald, A. J. Zuckerman, and R. A. Weiss.** 1987. HIV infection of primate lymphocytes and conservation of the CD4 receptor. *Nature* **330:**487–489.
55. **McCurry, K. R., D. L. Kooyman, C. G. Alvarado, A. H. Cotterell, M. J. Martin, J. S. Logan, and J. L. Platt.** 1995. Human complement regulatory proteins protect swine-to-primate cardiac xenografts from humoral injury. *Nature Med.* **1:**423–427.
56. **Merilahti-Palo, R., R. Lahesmaa, K. Granfors, C. Gripenberg-Lerche, and P. Toivanen.** 1991. Risk of *Yersinia* infection among butchers. *Scand. J. Infect. Dis.* **23:**55–61.
57. **Metzger, J. J., G. L. Gilliland, J. K. Lunney, B. A. Osborne, S. Rudikoff, and D. H. Sachs.** 1981. Transplantation in miniature swine. IX. Swine histocompatibility antigens isolation and purification of papain-solubilized SLA antigens. *J. Immunol.* **127:**769–775.
58. **Michaels, M. G., R. Lanford, A. J. Demetris, D. Chavez, K. Brasky, J. Fung, and T. E. Starzl.** 1996. Lack of susceptibility of baboons to infection with hepatitis B virus. *Transplantation* **61:**350–351.
59. **Michaels, M. G., and R. L. Simmons.** 1994. Xenotransplant-associated zoonoses: strategies for prevention. *Transplantation* **57:**1–7.

60. **Morsiani, E., L. Cappellari, L. Fogli, D. Ricci, C. Puviani, and G. Azzena.** 1992. Xenograft of piscine insular tissue in nude streptozotocin-diabetic mice: a transplantation model. *Transplant. Proc.* **24:**672–673.
61. **Murphy, B. R., and R. G. Webster.** 1990. Orthomyxoviruses, p. 1091–1152. *In* B. N. Fields and D. M. Knipe (ed.), *Virology.* Raven Press, Ltd., New York, N.Y.
62. **Narita, M., M. Shimizu, H. Kawamura, M. Haritani, and M. Moriawaki.** 1987. Pathologic changes in pigs with prednisolone-induced recrudescence of herpesvirus infection. *Am. J. Vet. Res.* **48:**1398–1402.
63. **Olding, L. B., F. C. Jensen, and M. B. Oldstone.** 1975. Pathogenesis of cytomegalovirus infection. I. Activation of virus from bone-derived lymphocytes by in vitro allogeneic reaction. *J. Exp. Med.* **141:**561–566.
64. **Patience, C., G. S. Patton, S. Takeuchi, R. A. Weiss, M. O. McClure, L. Rydberg, and M. E. Breimer.** 1998. No evidence of pig DNA or retroviral infection in patients with short-term extracorporeal connection to pig kidneys. *Lancet* **352:**699–701.
65. **Patience, C., Y. Takeuchi, and R. A. Weiss.** 1997. Infection of human cells by an endogenous retrovirus of pigs. *Nature Med.* **3:**276–282.
66. **Pereira, B. J. G., E. L. Milford, R. L. Kirkman, and A. S. Levey.** 1991. Transmission of hepatitis C virus by organ transplantation. *N. Engl. J. Med.* **325:**454–460.
67. **Pirtle, E. C.** 1973. Incidence of antibody to swine influenza virus in Iowa breeder and butcher pigs correlated with signs of influenza-like illness. *Am. J. Vet. Res.* **34:**83–85.
68. **Rando, R. F., A. Srinivasan, J. Feingold, E. Gonczol, and S. Plotkin.** 1990. Characterization of multiple molecular interactions between human cytomegalovirus (HCMV) and human immunodeficiency virus type 1 (HIV-1). *Virology* **176:**87–97.
69. **Rosengard, A. M., N. R. B. Cary, G. A. Langford, A. W. Tucker, J. Wallwork, and D. J. G. White.** 1995. Tissue expression of human complement inhibitor, decay-accelerating factor, in transgenic pigs. A potential approach for preventing xenograft rejection. *Transplantation* **59:**1325–1333.
70. **Rothe, J., P. J. McDonald, and A. M. Johnson.** 1985. Detection of *Toxoplasma* cysts and oocysts in an urban environment in a developed country. *Pathology* **17:**497–499.
71. **Rother, R. P., W. L. Fodor, J. P. Springhorn, C. W. Birks, E. Setter, M. S. Sandrin, S. P. Squinto, and S. A. Rollins.** 1995. A novel mechanism of retrovirus inactivation in human serum mediated by anti-α-galactosyl natural antibody. *J. Exp. Med.* **182:**1345–1355.
72. **Rubin, R. H., and N. E. Tolkoff-Rubin.** 1988. The problem of human immunodeficiency virus (HIV) infection and transplantation. *Transplant. Immunol.* **1:**36–38.
73. **Sachs, D. H., G. Leight, J. Cone, S. Schwarz, L. Stuart, and S. Rosenberg.** 1976. Transplantation in miniature swine: I. Fixation of the major histocompatibility complex. *Transplantation* **22:**559–567.
74. **Sandrin, M. S., W. L. Fodor, E. Mouhtouris, N. Osman, S. Cohney, S. A. Rollins, E. R. Guilmette, E. Setter, S. P. Squinto, and I. F. C. McKenzie.** 1995. Enzymatic remodelling of the carbohydrate surface of a senogenic cell substantially reduces human antibody binding and complement-mediated cytolysis. *Nature Med.* **1:**1261–1267.
75. **Sandrin, M. S., H. A. Vaughan, and I. F. C. McKenzie.** 1994. Identification of Gal(α1,3)Gal as the major epitope for pig-to-human vascularised xenografts. *Transplant. Rev.* **8:**134–149.
76. **Schnurrenberger, P. R., G. T. Woods, and R. J. Martin.** 1970. Serologic evidence of human infection with swine influenza virus. *Am. Rev. Respir. Dis.* **102:**356–361.
77. **Schwarz, A., G. Offermann, F. Keller, I. Bennhold, J. L'Age-Stehr, P. H. Krause, and M. J. Mihatsch.** 1993. The effect of cyclosporine on the progression of human immunodeficiency virus type 1 infection transmitted by transplantation—data on four cases and review of the literature. *Transplantation* **55:**95–103.
78. **Shah, K. V., H. L. Ozer, H. S. Pond, L. D. Palma, and G. P. Murphy.** 1971. SV40 neutralizing antibodies in sera of US residents without history of polio immunization. *Nature* **231:**448–449.
79. **Shope, R. E.** 1931. Swine influenza. III. Filtration experiments and etiology. *J. Exp. Med.* **54:**373–380.
80. **Simonds, R. J., S. D. Holmberg, R. L. Hurwitz, T. R. Coleman, S. Bottenfield, L. J. Conley, S. H. Kohlenberg, K. G. Castro, B. A. Dahan, C. A. Schable, et al.** 1992. Transmission of human immunodeficiency virus type I from a seronegative organ and tissue donor. *N. Engl. J. Med.* **326:**726–732.
81. **Smith, D. M.** 1993. Endogenous retroviruses in xenografts. *N. Engl. J. Med.* **328:**141–142.
82. **Snyder, H. W., Jr., and E. Fleissner.** 1980. Specificity of human antibodies to oncovirus glycoproteins: recognition of antigen by natural antibodies directed against carbohydrate structures. *Proc. Natl. Acad. Sci. USA* **77:**1622–1626.

83. **Spector, D. H., E. Wade, D. A. Wright, V. Koval, C. Clark, D. Jaquish, and S. A. Spector.** 1990. Human immunodeficiency virus pseudotypes with expanded cellular and species tropism. *J. Virol.* **64:**2298–2308.
84. **Starzl, T. E., J. Fung, A. Tzakis, S. Todo, A. J. Demetris, I. R. Marino, H. Doyle, A. Zeevi, V. Warty, M. Michaels, et al.** 1993. Baboon to human liver transplantation. *Lancet* **341:**65–71.
85. **Starzl, T. E., A. Tzakis, J. J. Fung, S. Todo, A. J. Demetris, R. Manez, I. R. Marino, L. Valdivia, and N. Muase.** 1994. Prospects of clinical xenotransplantation. *Transplant. Proc.* **26:**1082–1088.
86. **Stoye J. P., and J. M. Coffin.** 1988. Polymorphism of murine endogenous proviruses revealed by using virus class-specific oligonucleotide probes. *J. Virol.* **62:**168–175.
87. **Stoye, J. P., and J. M. Coffin.** 1985. Endogenous viruses, p. 357. *In* R. Weiss, N. Teich, H. Varmus, and J. Coffin (ed.), *RNA Tumor Viruses.* Cold Spring Harbor Laboratory, Cold Spring Harbor, N.Y.
88. **Sugimura, T., H. Yonemochi, T. Ogawa, Y. Tanaka, and T. Kumagai.** 1980. Isolation of a recombinant influenza virus (Hsw1N2) from swine in Japan. *Arch. Virol.* **66:**271–274.
89. **Suzuka, I., K. Sekiguchi, and M. Kodama.** 1985. Some characteristics of a porcine retrovirus from a cell line derived from swine malignant lymphomas. *FEBS* **183:**124–128.
90. **Suzuki, T., T. M. Sundt, E. O. Kortz, A. Mixon, M. A. Eckhaus, R. E. Gress, T. R. Spitzer, and D. H. Sachs.** 1989. Bone marrow transplantation across an MHC barrier in miniature swine. *Transplant. Proc.* **21:**3076–3078.
91. **Sweet, B. H., and M. R. Hilleman.** 1960. The vacuolating virus: SV40 (26128). *Proc. Soc. Exp. Biol. Med.* **105:**420–427.
92. **Tacal, J. V., Jr., M. Sobieh, and A. el-Ahraf.** 1987. Cryptosporidium in market pigs in southern California, USA. *Vet. Rec.* **120:**615–616.
93. **Todaro, G. J., R. E. Benveniste, M. M. Lieber, and C. J. Sherr.** 1974. Characteristics of a type C virus released from the porcine cell line PK(15). *Virology* **58:**65–74.
94. **Todd, K. H., and P. D. Lyde.** 1989. Brucellosis and thrombocytopenic purpura: case report and review. *Texas Med.* **85:**37–38.
95. **Weiss, R. A., and A. L. Wong.** 1977. Phenotypic mixing between avian and mammalian RNA tumor viruses: 1. Envelope pseudotypes of Rous sarcoma virus. *Virology* **76:**826–834.
96. **Welsh, R. M., N. R. Cooper, F. C. Jensen, and M. B. A. Oldstone.** 1975. Human serum lyses RNA tumour viruses. *Nature* **257:**612–614.
97. **Welsh, R. M., F. C. Jensen, N. R. Cooper, and M. B. A. Oldstone.** 1976. Inactivation and lysis of oncornaviruses by human serum. *Virology* **74:**432–440.
98. **Wilson, C. A., S. Wong, J. Muller, C. E. Davidson, T. M. Rose, and P. Burd.** 1998. Type C retrovirus released from porcine primary peripheral blood mononuclear cells infects human cells. *J. Virol.* **72:**3082–3087.
99. **Winkler, G. C., and N. F. Cheville.** 1986. Ultrastructural morphometric investigation of early lesions in the pulmonary alveolar region of pigs during experimental swine influenza infection. *Am. J. Pathol.* **122:**541–552.
100. **Ye, Y., M. Niekrasz, S. Kosanke, R. Welsh, H. E. Jordan, J. C. Fox, W. C. Edwards, C. Maxwell, and D. K. C. Cooper.** 1994. The pig as a potential organ donor for man. A study of potentially transferable disease from donor pig to recipient man. *Transplantation* **57:**694–703.
101. **Ye, Y., M. Niekrasz, R. Welsh, S. Kosanke, C. Maxwell, N. Zuhdi, and D. K. C. Cooper.** 1994. A practical study of zoonoses that could complicate pig-to-man organ transplantation. *Transplant. Proc.* **26:**1312.

INDEX

D

E